**Napier University
Learning Information Services**

ST/ 〉LOAN

D1325442

CONTINGENCY MANAGEMENT IN SUBSTANCE ABUSE TREATMENT

CONTINGENCY MANAGEMENT IN SUBSTANCE ABUSE TREATMENT

EDITED BY

Stephen T. Higgins
Kenneth Silverman
Sarah H. Heil

Foreword by Joseph V. Brady

THE GUILFORD PRESS
New York   London

©2008 The Guilford Press
A Division of Guilford Publications, Inc.
72 Spring Street, New York, NY 10012
www.guilford.com

Printed in the United States of America

This book is printed on acid-free paper.

Last digit is print number: 9 8 7 6 5 4 3 2 1

The authors have checked with sources believed to be reliable in their efforts to provide
information that is complete and generally in accord with the standards of practice that
are accepted at the time of publication. However, in view of the possibility of human
error or changes in medical sciences, neither the authors, nor the editor and publisher,
nor any other party who has been involved in the preparation or publication of this
work warrants that the information contained herein is in every respect accurate or
complete, and they are not responsible for any errors or omissions or the results obtained from the use of such information. Readers are encouraged to confirm the information contained in this book with other sources.

Library of Congress Cataloging-in-Publication Data

Contingency management in substance abuse treatment / edited by Stephen T. Higgins,
Kenneth Silverman, Sarah H. Heil.
    p. cm.
  Includes bibliographical references and index.
  ISBN-13: 978-1-59385-571-0 (hardcover : alk. paper)
  ISBN-10: 1-59385-571-0 (hardcover : alk. paper)
    1. Substance abuse—Treatment. 2. Behavior modification. I. Higgins, Stephen T.
II. Silverman, Kenneth, 1953–   III. Heil, Sarah H.
  RC564.C666 2007
  616.86′06—dc22
                                                            2007021361

ABOUT THE EDITORS

Stephen T. Higgins, PhD, joined the faculty of the University of Vermont in 1986, where he is now a Professor of Psychiatry and Psychology. Dr. Higgins has received numerous national awards for research excellence, including the Joseph Cochin Award from the College on Problems of Drug Dependence, the Dan Anderson Award from the Hazelden Foundation, the Don Hake Award from the Division of the Experimental Analysis of Behavior of the American Psychological Association, and a MERIT Award from the National Institutes of Health. He is currently President of the College on Problems of Drug Dependence and principal and coinvestigator on numerous grants from the National Institute on Drug Abuse (NIDA). He has published extensively on furthering scientific understanding of the behavioral and pharmacological processes involved in substance use disorders.

Kenneth Silverman, PhD, served as a staff fellow in the Clinical Trials Section of NIDA's Intramural Research Program in Baltimore from 1991 to 1993. He is currently Professor of Psychiatry and Behavioral Sciences at Johns Hopkins University School of Medicine, where he has maintained a faculty appointment since 1991. Dr. Silverman's research at Johns Hopkins has been funded primarily by grants from NIDA, and focuses on developing operant treatments to address the interrelated problems of poverty and drug addiction. His primary research has focused on the development and evaluation of abstinence reinforcement interventions for heroin and cocaine addiction in poor, inner-city adults, and the integration of those abstinence reinforcement contingencies into model employment settings.

Sarah H. Heil, PhD, is a Research Assistant Professor of Psychiatry and Psychology at the University of Vermont. Dr. Heil completed an NIDA postdoctoral fellowship in behavioral pharmacology at the University of Vermont and joined the faculty there in 2002. Funded by NIDA, her research interests include the behavioral and pharmacological processes involved in substance use disorders, with a special focus on pregnant and recently postpartum women. She is a regular contributor to the scientific literature on drug abuse and has received several honors and awards for research excellence, including the NIDA Women and Gender Junior Investigator Award.

CONTRIBUTORS

Sheila M. Alessi, PhD, Department of Psychiatry, University of Connecticut Health Center, Storrs, Connecticut

Leslie Amass, PhD, Schering Plough Global Medical Affairs, Kenilworth, New Jersey

George E. Bigelow, PhD, Department of Psychiatry and Behavioral Sciences, Johns Hopkins University School of Medicine, Baltimore, Maryland

Alan J. Budney, PhD, Center for Addiction Research, Department of Psychiatry, College of Medicine, University of Arkansas for Medical Sciences, Little Rock, Arkansas

Kathleen M. Carroll, PhD, Department of Psychiatry, Yale University School of Medicine, New Haven, Connecticut

Dana Cavallo, PhD, Substance Abuse Center, Yale Universtiy School of Medicine, New Haven, Connecticut

Laura Chivers, MA, Department of Psychology, Harvard University, Cambridge, Massachusetts

Jesse Dallery, PhD, Department of Psychology, University of Florida, Gainesville, Florida

Wendy D. Donlin, PhD, Center for Learning and Health, Johns Hopkins University School of Medicine, Baltimore, Maryland

Charles Drebing, PhD, New England Mental Illness Research Education and Clinical Center, Bedford VA Medical Center, Bedford, Massachusetts

Amy M. Duhig, PhD, Department of Psychiatry, Yale University School of Medicine, New Haven, Connecticut

David H. Epstein, PhD, Clinical Pharmacology and Therapeutics Research Branch, National Institute on Drug Abuse Intramural Research Program, Baltimore, Maryland

Sarah H. Heil, PhD, Departments of Psychiatry and Psychology, University of Vermont, Burlington, Vermont

Stephen T. Higgins, PhD, Departments of Psychiatry and Psychology, University of Vermont, Burlington, Vermont

Jonathan B. Kamien, PhD, BioPsych Consulting, Califon, New Jersey

Scott Kellogg, PhD, Department of Psychology, New York University, New York, New York

Todd W. Knealing, PhD, Department of Psychology, Briarcliff University, Sioux City, Iowa

Suchitra Krishnan-Sarin, PhD, Department of Psychiatry, Yale University School of Medicine, New Haven, Connecticut

Richard J. Lamb, PhD, Departments of Psychiatry and Pharmacology, University of Texas Health Science Center at San Antonio, San Antonio, Texas

Douglas B. Marlowe, JD, PhD, Treatment Research Institute, University of Pennsylvania, Philadelphia, Pennsylvania

Jesse B. Milby, PhD, Department of Psychology, University of Alabama at Birmingham, Birmingham, Alabama

Thomas Newton, MD, Department of Psychiatry and Biobehavioral Sciences, David Geffen School of Medicine, University of California at Los Angeles, Los Angeles, California

Nancy M. Petry, PhD, Department of Psychiatry, University of Connecticut Health Center, Farmington, Connecticut

Kenzie L. Preston, PhD, Clinical Pharmacology and Therapeutics Research Branch, National Institute on Drug Abuse Intramural Research Program, Baltimore, Maryland

Richard K. Ries, MD, Department of Psychiatry and Behavioral Sciences, University of Washington, and Harborview Medical Center, Seattle, Washington

Randall E. Rogers, PhD, Department of Psychiatry, University of Vermont, Burlington, Vermont

John M. Roll, PhD, Washington Institute for Mental Illness Research and Training, Washington State University, Spokane, Washington

Marc Rosen, MD, Department of Psychiatry, VA Connecticut Healthcare System, West Haven, Connecticut

Robert Rosenheck, MD, Department of Psychiatry, Yale University School of Medicine, New Haven, Connecticut

Bruce J. Rounsaville, MD, Department of Psychiatry, Yale University School of Medicine, New Haven, Connecticut

Joseph Schumacher, PhD, Division of Preventive Medicine, University of Alabama at Birmingham, Birmingham, Alabama

Stacey C. Sigmon, PhD, Departments of Psychiatry and Psychology, University of Vermont, Burlington, Vermont

Kenneth Silverman, PhD, Center for Learning and Health, Johns Hopkins University School of Medicine, Baltimore, Maryland

Catherine Stanger, PhD, Center for Addiction Research, Department of Psychiatry, College of Medicine, University of Arkansas for Medical Sciences, Little Rock, Arkansas

Maxine L. Stitzer, PhD, Department of Psychiatry and Behavioral Sciences, Behavioral Pharmacology Research Unit, Johns Hopkins Bayview Medical Center, Baltimore, Maryland

Jennifer W. Tidey, PhD, Center for Alcohol and Addiction Studies, and Department of Psychiatry and Human Behavior, Brown University, Providence, Rhode Island

Conrad J. Wong, PhD, Department of Behavioral Science, University of Kentucky College of Medicine, Lexington, Kentucky

Jin H. Yoon, PhD, Department of Psychiatry, University of Vermont, Burlington, Vermont

FOREWORD

Almost a half-century has passed since a pioneering group of young investigators, Charles R. Schuster and Travis Thompson among them, sought to explore the role of basic behavior analysis principles in laboratory models of drug dependence and abuse. Among the early experimental subjects addressed were the reinforcing functions of pharmacological agents in laboratory animals and the exploration of drug self-infusion through an indwelling vascular catheter. The publication in *Science* some 50 years ago that reported the results of these seminal studies has since been followed by a vast literature detailing the reinforcing functions of pharmacological agents in experimental and applied settings. The results of these studies have shown clearly that research participants, both animal and human, will self-administer a wide range of commonly abused substances and that such drug seeking and drug taking are sensitive to environmental consequences. Extensive research has confirmed that drug self-administration can be increased or decreased by the same range of environmental outcomes that influence other behavioral interactions.

This extensive experimental evidence base has provided the scientific foundation for development of clinical interventions with drug-dependent individuals by arranging differential reinforcing consequences contingent upon drug abstinence or drug use. The state of our knowledge regarding such contingency management (CM) interventions for the treatment of drug abuse and dependence was last updated and summarized in an edited volume by Stephen Higgins and Kenneth Silverman in 1999. At that time, senior investigators in the field documented the broad effectiveness and potential usefulness of this approach to the treatment of substance abuse disorders. Over the past decade, however, not only has research on the application of CM interventions expanded rapidly, but also the maturation and sophistication of the studies undertaken reflect a significant enhancement in the quality, diversity, and scope of the methodologies employed. The current timely volume, under the editorship of the experienced contributing authors Stephen Higgins, Kenneth Silverman, and Sarah Heil, provides a remarkably comprehensive, insightful, and updated summary of the progress that has been made in the application of CM procedures in the treatment of substance abuse since the turn of the century.

The preeminent research contributors to this volume not only have carefully reviewed the relevant literature but also have provided a range of perspectives informed by years of investigative experience in the field. The chapters in Part I of this three-part volume emphasize the use of CM interventions to promote abstinence from commonly abused drugs such as cocaine, marijuana, methamphetamine, alcohol, the opioids, and smoked nicotine. This section of the book also provides important coverage of the use of CM procedures to promote highly effective but grossly underutilized substance abuse treatment medications, notably disulfiram and naltrexone.

Part II documents the broad utility and diversity of CM interventions across a range of special populations. The studies described with adolescents, pregnant women, homeless individuals, and people with mental illness demonstrate the effectiveness of these interventions with groups in desperate need of treatment that have been extremely difficult to treat effectively with conventional therapeutic approaches.

Part III provides a discursive review and discussion of the encouraging, rapidly expanding, and widespread dissemination of CM approaches to substance abuse treatment. Practical innovations to reduce costs associated with CM interventions are introduced at the very beginning of this third section of the volume to facilitate integration into community drug abuse treatment programs. Reducing the costs of CM interventions for community clinics with limited resources increases the likelihood that they will avail themselves of the treatment-enhancing benefits of these interventions. The cost-reducing measures described include deposit contracting or fee rebate procedures through which the patient, as the primary beneficiary of the treatment intervention, bears some of the costs involved. In addition to seeking community support through donated gifts, programs can also allay financial burdens by reducing the magnitude of the contingent reinforcement used. An important and impressive milestone in the application of lower-cost CM interventions has recently been demonstrated in a multisite randomized control study conducted as part of the National Institute on Drug Abuse Clinical Trial Network. The resourceful approaches to financing and disseminating the benefits of CM interventions described in the remaining chapters capitalize on high-magnitude, reinforcing consequences available in settings beyond community drug abuse treatment programs. Examples are detailed in the book chapters describing CM integration with the U.S. Department of Veterans Affairs' Compensated

Work Therapy program, as well as with drug courts and community workplace projects.

The overall content of this volume provides convincing evidence of the broad utility and remarkable effectiveness of CM interventions in the treatment of substance abuse disorders. Few behavioral or psychosocial treatment approaches to health problems are as extensively grounded in such diverse and rigorous empirical support as CM interventions. There is, of course, work still to be done in developing procedures to ensure long-term success in achieving abstinence and enhancing practical applications to community-based programs. The substantial scientific foundation provided by the progress reported in this volume will contribute importantly to this continuing development. The scholarly and expert reviews by the authors and editors of this timely reference book also make available to clinicians, scientists, and students an invaluable contemporary resource catalogue of effective CM treatment strategies for application to a range of substance abuse problems, populations, and settings.

JOSEPH V. BRADY, PHD
Johns Hopkins University
School of Medicine

PREFACE

Substance use disorders have devastating consequences on public health in the United States. Annual economic costs of drug abuse are in the billions of dollars, and in terms of unrealized individual potential, ruined families, and other outcomes, the costs are incalculable. Contingency management (CM) is a treatment approach derived from basic principles of learning that has proven in controlled studies to be efficacious with a wide variety of substances and populations. CM is effective, for example, in reducing abuse of alcohol, cocaine, cannabis, methamphetamine, opioids, and tobacco. Special subpopulations of substance abusers, such as adolescent, pregnant, homeless, and mentally ill individuals, offer unique treatment challenges, and CM is proving to be efficacious with them as well. This volume characterizes recent advances in research and clinical efforts on the use of CM with each of these substances and clinical populations.

Proper motivation to change is essential to effective treatment for substance use disorders. CM is a powerful, science-based method for increasing motivation to change. CM procedures arrange for the systematic application of reinforcing or punishing consequences that are ethical, human, and effective for promoting drug abstinence and other therapeutic behavior change. Interest in the approach is growing exponentially among substance abuse researchers, clinicians, and policymakers. This interest is a product of the excellent controlled studies that have been conducted demonstrating the efficacy of CM for producing therapeutic changes among even the most recalcitrant forms of substance abuse and subpopulations of abusers. CM has as much or more empirical support for its efficacy as any approach to treatment of substance use disorders. This volume provides detailed overviews of the most efficacious and innovative of these interventions from projects being conducted throughout the United States. Each of the chapters is sufficiently detailed, in depth, and current to be of value to researchers, clinicians, and policymakers alike, including those who might be interested in adopting the intervention. Contributors to this volume were selected because of their respective areas of scientific and clinical expertise.

Of course, a volume of this nature comes to fruition only through the hard work and support of many. We extend our sincere gratitude to the contributors for taking time from their demanding schedules to prepare their respective chapters. We thank the National Institute on Drug Abuse, especially Cece McNamara Spitznas, PhD, for supporting most of the research projects described in this volume and for assisting us in sponsoring a meeting on this topic in Burlington, Vermont, on October 7 and 8, 2004. The planning and discussions that eventually led to this volume began during that meeting. We also thank the many behavior analysts and behavioral pharmacologists who conducted the basic research that provided the scientific foundation for CM. We thank everyone at The Guilford Press for their patience and guidance, especially Jim Nageotte, our editor. Finally, but by no means least, I (S. T. H.) thank Tamra, Tara, and Lucy; I (K. S.) thank Anne, Jake, and Danny; and I (S. H. H.) thank Andy, Emma, and Katie for their loving support and patience.

CONTENTS

PART II. SPECIAL POPULATIONS

PART III. DISSEMINATION

CONTINGENCY MANAGEMENT IN SUBSTANCE ABUSE TREATMENT

CHAPTER 1

INTRODUCTION

Stephen T. Higgins *and* Kenneth Silverman

Substance use disorders (SUDs) represent a highly prevalent and costly public health problem in almost all modern societies. In the United States, for example, approximately 18% of the population experiences an SUD at some point in their lifetime (e.g., Anthony & Chen, 2004), with the economic costs due to lost productivity and increased morbidity and mortality estimated to be approximately $500 billion annually (Office of National Drug Control Policy, 2004).

There has been excellent progress in overcoming the social stigma associated with SUDs and recognizing them as chronic medical disorders and also in developing effective, scientifically based treatments. Nevertheless, much work remains to be done. Many who have an SUD still fail to seek formal treatment. Among those who do seek treatment, premature treatment termination, ongoing drug use, and relapse back to drug use following treatment termination remain common problems. While such recalcitrance is not unique to SUDs and is also seen with other chronic medical disorders such as diabetes and hypertension, the serious adverse consequences associated with SUDs demand an ongoing and concerted effort to develop more effective interventions to prevent and treat them (McLellan, Lewis, O'Brien, & Kleber, 2000).

1

CONTINGENCY MANAGEMENT FOR SUDs

One strong need in the area of treatment development for SUDs is for interventions that motivate individuals to change their behavior. Indeed, a waxing and waning commitment to and ambivalence about change are common characteristics of SUDs. Contingency management (CM) is one effective approach to addressing this need. CM interventions are based on operant conditioning and involve the systematic application of behavioral consequences to promote changes in drug use or other therapeutic goals such as attendance at therapy sessions and medication compliance, among others. This volume provides detailed reviews on the most creative and efficacious approaches to using CM to treat SUDs. Nationally and internationally recognized experts authored each of the chapters, and they cover a strikingly wide range of different types of SUDs, patient populations, and treatment settings. Indeed, this breadth of CM is an impressive feature of this treatment approach that we fully anticipate will be underscored further in the future as still others among the myriad individual and societal problems associated with SUDs are tackled using CM.

Scientific Rationale

The scientific rationale for CM is rooted in an extensive scientific literature demonstrating a robust role for operant conditioning in the genesis and maintenance of drug use, including repeated use, abuse, and dependence. Among the most fundamental scientific observations regarding the role of operant conditioning in SUDs was the revelation that most commonly abused drugs serve as unconditioned positive reinforcers in laboratory animals (Deneau, Yanagita, & Seevers, 1969). For example, normal laboratory animals will learn arbitrary operant responses like pressing a lever or pulling a chain when the only consequence for doing so is the receipt of an injection of a prototypical drug of abuse such as an amphetamine, barbiturate, cocaine, or morphine. When we substitute a drug that humans rarely abuse (e.g., antipsychotic medication), the animals discontinue lever pressing. The animals need not be made physically dependent on abused drugs for them to function as reinforcers. Indeed, relatively little training of any sort is necessary. The animals appear to be biologically prepared for the neuropharmacological effects of most commonly abused drugs to function as positive reinforcers in much the same way as they are prepared for food, water, and sex to do so. Physical dependence, tolerance, and withdrawal influence patterns of drug consumption in these arrangements, but the evidence shows that those states are best understood as consequences of drug use rather than necessary conditions for voluntary drug use to emerge. Perhaps even more striking than the fact that these otherwise normal animals will voluntarily ingest drugs is that they will engage in repeated use that results in serious adverse consequences (Aigner & Balster, 1978). When given unconstrained access to drugs like cocaine and opiates, for example, laboratory animals will consume sufficiently large doses to overdose and will also consume them to the exclusion of basic sustenance and eventual death in the absence of experimenter intervention.

Respondent conditioning, another basic behavioral process, comes into play when an environmental stimulus (person, place, or thing) reliably predicts drug availability and administration. Previously neutral environmental events that predict drug availability and use eventually acquire discriminative stimulus functions (i.e., they become occasion setters) for urges to use drugs as well as drug seeking and use. They also acquire conditioned reinforcing effects that work in concert with the unconditioned reinforcing effects of abused drugs to sustain the often extraordinary efforts of dependent individuals to obtain and consume drugs (e.g., Schindler, Panlilio, & Goldberg, 2002).

Such studies provide compelling evidence for a primary role of operant conditioning in the nonprescription use of drugs that is amply supported by parallel laboratory studies conducted with humans with SUDs. For example, a series of studies was conducted in the 1970s examining the sensitivity of alcohol consumption to environmental consequences among severe alcoholics (e.g., Bigelow, Griffiths, & Liebson, 1975). In these studies, the alcoholics resided on a residential hospital unit where they were permitted to consume alcohol under monitored conditions. Abstinence from voluntary drinking increased when access to an alternative reinforcer (i.e., an enriched environment) was available for doing so, by increasing the amount of work required to obtain alcohol, by providing monetary reinforcement contingent on abstinence, and by imposing brief periods of social isolation contingent upon drinking. Each of these outcomes conformed to predictions based on drug use being a form of operant responding. Results in subsequent studies with cigarette smokers, marijuana abusers, and cocaine and opioid abusers have similarly conformed to predictions based on operant conditioning. In studies in which cocaine users were permitted to make exclusive choices between drug use and money, for example, drug use decreased as an orderly function of increases in the amount of monetary reinforcement offered as an alternative (e.g., Higgins, Heil, & Lussier, 2004; Silverman, Kaminski, Higgins, & Brady, in press).

Overall, these studies confirmed that operant conditioning plays an important role in the genesis and maintenance of drug use, abuse, and dependence. Importantly, though, the research also showed that like other forms of operant responding, drug use even among highly dependent individuals is malleable and sensitive to environmental consequences. The many successful applications of CM to the wide range of different types of SUDs, populations, and settings outlined in this volume are consistent with those conclusions.

A Brief History of the Use of CM to Treat SUDs

The history of using CM to treat SUDs can be traced back to uncontrolled studies in the 1960s where, for example, smokers earned back portions of a monetary deposit contingent upon remaining abstinent from smoking (Elliott & Tighe, 1968). A more programmatic series of controlled studies conducted in the 1970s and 1980s by Stitzer, Bigelow, and colleagues firmly established the efficacy of using contingent access to clinic privileges, medication adjustments, and cash payments among other consequences for increasing abstinence from drug use among opioid-dependent patients enrolled in methadone treatment (see Stitzer & Higgins, 1995, for a review) and also the efficacy of cash payments to increase abstinence from cigarette smoking (e.g., Stitzer & Bigelow, 1982). Recognition of CM as a formal treatment for SUDs was substantially bolstered in the 1990s when a variation that has come to be known as voucher-based reinforcement therapy (VBRT) was demonstrated in randomized controlled trials to be one of few interventions that can reliably increase abstinence from cocaine use among dependent outpatients (e.g., Higgins et al., 1991). Interest and research activity on VBRT as a treatment for SUDs over the 15 years since the first publication on that topic have led to two scientific conferences, with the first conference held on September 14 and 15, 1995, in Bethesda, Maryland, and the second on October 7 and 8, 2004, in Burlington, Vermont. The first conference spurred the publication of an edited volume on the use of CM to treat SUDs (Higgins & Silverman, 1999) and the second conference set the occasion for this volume. A recently published quantitative review of VBRT identified more than 60 reports of controlled studies published in peer-reviewed journals examining VBRT as a treatment for SUDs, with robust evidence supporting its efficacy (Lussier, Heil, Mongeon, Badger, & Higgins, 2006).

Basic Elements of CM

The basic elements that comprise all CM interventions for SUDs have been outlined elsewhere and need not be repeated in detail here (e.g., Higgins, 1999; Petry, 2000). Briefly, CM interventions promote behavior change through the use of one of the following generic types of contingencies administered alone or in combination: positive reinforcement, which involves the delivery of a reinforcing consequence (e.g., monetary-based voucher) contingent upon meeting a therapeutic goal (e.g., abstinence from recent drug use); negative reinforcement, which involves the removal, or a reduction in the intensity, of an aversive event (e.g., job suspension) contingent upon meeting a therapeutic goal (successful completion of treatment); positive punishment, which involves the delivery of an aversive event (e.g., social reprimand) contingent upon evidence of the occurrence of a therapeutically undesirable response (failure to attend therapy sessions); and negative punishment, which involves the removal of a positive condition (forfeiture of clinic privileges) contingent upon the occurrence of an undesirable response (e.g., resumption of drug use).

Reinforcement and punishment interventions are effective, but, by definition, the latter are disliked by patients and often staff and can inadvertently increase treatment dropout. As is amply illustrated in the interventions described in this volume, CM interventions that are comprised of high rates of positive reinforcement and judicious use of negative punishment can be very effective at retaining patients in treatment, reducing drug use, and improving other therapeutic outcomes. To be maximally effective, contingencies need to involve objective verification that the therapeutic target response has occurred, relatively minimal delay in delivering the designated consequence once the response has been verified, and a consequence of sufficient magnitude or intensity to function as a reinforcer or punisher. In a recent meta-analysis of the use of VBRT with SUDs, moderators of treatment effects size were examined (Lussier et al., 2006). Two significant moderators were identified: more immediate delivery of the incentive and greater monetary value of the incentive predicted larger treatment effects. Objective monitoring of the target response in applications with SUDs typically involves some form of testing of biological markers of recent drug use. Delivering the consequence on the same day that testing occurs results in larger effect sizes than waiting until the next day or later. The magnitude of reinforcement or punishment necessary to change behavior will depend on the nature of the behavior change involved, patient population, and so on. The interventions outlined in the different chapters in this volume provide direction in choosing appropriate magnitudes for the various populations and types of therapeutic targets with which one may be working.

THE PRESENT VOLUME

This volume is structured first to address the application of CM to the treatment of SUDs in formal substance abuse treatment clinics and with the major types of SUDs, then to outline the immensely important application of CM with special populations of individuals with SUDs who are especially vulnerable and for whom effective treatments are sorely needed, and wrapping up with a section reviewing a range of creative projects relevant to the dissemination of CM beyond research settings. Each of the chapters characterizes the scope of the specific problem being addressed; provides a detailed review of relevant research findings; discusses ethical or other issues of interest to clinicians, policymakers, and others interested in using CM; and comments on the promise of CM in that particular application.

Applications in Outpatient Substance Abuse Treatment Clinics

Chapter 2 (Higgins, Heil, Rogers, & Chivers) focuses on treating cocaine dependence with VBRT. VBRT was initially developed as one element in a multielement intervention for outpatient treatment of cocaine dependence (Higgins et al., 1991). The chapter traces the development of the use of VBRT to treat cocaine-dependent outpatients enrolled in drug-free and methadone-maintenance clinics starting from the seminal studies up to the more recent multisite trials conducted as part of the National Institute on Drug Abuse's (NIDA) Clinical Trials Network (CTN) (Peirce et al., 2006; Petry et al., 2005; see Stitzer & Kellogg, Chapter 13, this volume). Although there are many remaining issues to be addressed in the successful development and dissemination of VBRT for the treatment of cocaine dependence, the chapter outlines a great deal of success. The positive outcomes obtained in the multisite trials mentioned earlier can be expected to have a positive influence on the dissemination of CM interventions into community treatment clinics. Because of the budgetary constraints under which most community substance abuse treatment clinics must operate, there is strong interest in the type of lower-cost interventions that were used in those multisite trials. The multisite trials demonstrated that lower-cost CM can be efficacious, although as might be expected based on the meta-analysis mentioned previously (Lussier et al., 2006), the size of the treatment effects appeared to be proportionately lower as well (Peirce et al., 2006; Petry et al., 2005).

Methadone and other opioid-replacement therapies are highly effective in treating opioid dependence, but outcomes are enhanced further when pharmacological treatments are combined with behavioral interventions (McLellan, Arndt, Metzger, Woody, & O'Brien, 1993). CM is one behavioral intervention that has extensive empirical support for its efficacy among opioid-dependent patients (Silverman et al., in press). Indeed, many of the seminal studies demonstrating the efficacy of CM in the treatment of illicit drug abuse were conducted with patients enrolled in methadone clinics. Chapter 3 (Epstein & Preston) provides a detailed and insightful overview of this important area of application, covering the use of medication take-home privileges, VBRT, and other efficacious CM interventions.

Recognition of the need for effective treatments for marijuana abuse and dependence is growing (e.g., Budney, Hughes, Moore, & Vandrey, 2004). Chapter 4 (Budney & Stanger) reviews the empirical support for and future promise of CM interventions for addressing that need. The use of VBRT in the treatment of marijuana abuse and dependence among adults, adolescents, and individuals with co-occurring serious mental illness are carefully reviewed. The chapter also discusses important practical issues in the use of CM with marijuana, including the challenge of objectively monitoring recent use given the relatively long metabolic half-life of delta-9-tetrahydrocannabinol and other cannabinoids.

Effective treatments are sorely needed for the growing problem in the United States and elsewhere of methamphetamine use disorders (e.g., Romanelli & Smith, 2006). Chapter 5 (Roll & Newton) provides evidence indicating that, consistent with the positive results obtained with cocaine and other psychomotor stimulants, VBRT is efficacious in treating methamphetamine abuse and dependence. Particularly impressive is that a subset of patients in NIDA's CTN studies mentioned earlier abused methamphetamine. When results from those patients were analyzed they also supported the efficacy of CM (Roll et al., 2006). Based on those findings, CM can be expected to have a substantive role in future efforts to curtail the growing and disturbing problem of methamphetamine use disorders. This is welcome news for a problem that is spreading within the United States and elsewhere and is the focus of much concern among law enforcement and public health officials.

The high rates of morbidity and mortality attributable to tobacco use and dependence are well known. Tremendous headway has been made in the development and dissemination of effective pharmacological and behavioral interventions to promote smoking cessation. That said, the vast majority of patients who attempt to quit smoking fail within the initial days and weeks of the cessation effort. Clearly, improvements in treatment outcome are needed, with a clear role for the use of behavioral interventions (e.g., Stitzer, 1999). Chapter 6 (Sigmon & Lamb) provides a detailed review of the potential of CM to improve smoking-cessation outcomes in the general population of smokers as well as special populations of smokers, including adolescents, pregnant women, individuals with serious mental illness, and opioid- and other drug-dependent individuals. The chapter also provides an informed discussion of the contributions of CM to an experimental analysis of smoking by allowing for effective experimental control over smoking. Also discussed is the potentially useful role that CM may play in promoting sustained abstinence during the initial weeks of a cessation effort. There is extensive evidence among the general population of smokers (Kenford et al., 1994) as well as special populations of smokers (Higgins et al., 2006) that any smoking during the initial 2 weeks of a cessation effort is associated with poor longer-term outcomes.

Efforts to use CM in the treatment of alcohol abuse and dependence began in the early 1970s but did not develop thereafter as well as one might have expected considering the promising initial results (Higgins & Petry, 1999; Silverman et al., in press). Difficulties identifying a reliable method to bioverify abstinence is one obstacle that continues to hamper development in this important area. Chapter 7 (Wong, Silverman, & Bigelow) provides an insightful overview of the use of CM with problem drinking, including results from recent efforts to extend the VBRT-based

Therapeutic Workplace to severely dependent drinkers (Silverman et al., 2005).

In many respects, naltrexone represents one of the most, if not the most, elegant drugs available for treatment of substance use disorders. Naltrexone is well tolerated, largely without agonist effects, and blocks the effects of opioid agonists with once-daily administration. Yet naltrexone's promise as a treatment for opioid dependence has largely gone unrealized save for use with highly motivated subpopulations of abusers such as health care workers. The overarching problem is medication compliance. Naltrexone lacks the reinforcing effects that methadone and comparable agonists have and patients will not reliably comply with the recommended medication regimen in the absence of naturalistic contingencies such as those operating with the health care workers mentioned above. Chapter 8 provides an intriguing and creative overview of efforts to use VBRT to address this problem of compliance with naltrexone, but also with other medications important to the drug-dependent population, including aversive agents (disulfiram), antiretroviral medications, psychotropics, and antibiotics. The strengths and potential weaknesses of CM in addressing the challenges of medication compliance among individuals with SUDs are thoroughly and insightfully discussed.

Applications with Special Populations

There is no question that identifying effective treatments for special populations is an important priority in efforts to develop efficacious interventions for SUDs. This is an area in which CM is showing a striking degree of success and in which the potential for future growth and successful dissemination is particularly promising. Chapter 9 (Milby & Schumacher) reviews efforts to employ CM in developing effective treatments for homeless substance abusers. Of particular interest in this chapter is the description of a programmatic effort to effectively treat homeless cocaine-dependent individuals through contingent access to housing and employment (e.g., Milby, Schumacher, Wallace, Freedman, & Vuchinich, 2005). Homelessness and drug dependence are each daunting problems and when they co-occur the clinical challenges are enormous. Chapter 9 does an excellent job of characterizing those problems and outlining methods for surmounting them.

Pregnant substance abusers represent an especially important and in many ways unique subgroup of substance abusers due to the direct involvement of an innocent and highly vulnerable third party, the fetus. As Chapter 10 (Heil, Yoon, & Higgins) ably illustrates, VBRT has tremendous potential for improving treatment outcomes among pregnant and recently postpartum women with SUDs. One notable program is the Therapeutic Workplace mentioned earlier, which uses VBRT to increase abstinence from cocaine and opioid use while also improving basic academic and vocational skills among pregnant and recently postpartum drug-dependent, inner-city women (Silverman et al., 2005). Also promising are programs using VBRT to increase smoking cessation among pregnant and recently postpartum cigarette smokers (Donatelle, Prows, Champeau, & Hudson, 2000; Higgins, Heil, Solomon, et al., 2004). Cigarette smoking is one of the leading preventable causes of poor pregnancy outcomes in the United States (Cnattingius, 2004). This is a population with whom CM interventions have tremendous potential for providing cost-effective improvements in treatment outcome.

Treating patients with co-occurring serious mental illness and SUDs is as daunting a clinical challenge as any of the others already mentioned. Chapter 11 (Tidey & Ries) provides an excellent overview of the magnitude and complexities of this public health problem (also see Budney & Stangel, Chapters 4; Sigmon, Lamb, & Dallery, Chapter 6; and Drebing, Rounsaville, & Rosenheck, Chapter 16). Among several very promising interventions discussed, Chapter 11 reviews an important effort to develop a self-sustaining CM intervention involving patient disability payments. In this program, the treatment clinic serves as the designated payee for patients with SUDs and serious mental illness who are receiving disability payments (Ries et al., 2004). Disability payments cannot be legally withheld, but in this program constraints are placed on their use while patients are using drugs and those constraints are systematically relaxed contingent on objective evidence of abstinence from recent drug use. The intervention is creative and holds great promise as a model for how to more effectively treat SUDs among those with co-occurring serious mental illness.

Chapter 12 (Krishnan-Sarin, Duhig, & Cavallo) addresses the challenge of treating SUDs among adolescents, a population also addressed to a more limited extent in Chapters 4 and 6. CM interventions have great promise with this population who are often especially ambivalent or indifferent to the need for formal substance abuse treatment but are likely to be motivated by the opportunity to earn material incentives contingent upon behavior change. An important point of focus in Chapter 12 is a creative and groundbreaking program wherein VBRT is being used to promote smoking cessation in a public school setting (Krishnan-Sarin et al., 2006). Here, too, the potential for CM to make a substantive contribution to improving treatment outcomes is clear.

Disseminating CM Interventions Beyond Formal Research Settings

Obviously, a fundamental purpose in developing treatments is to move them into settings in which they can eventually become mainstream treatments, and CM is no exception. The typical sequence is first to conduct efficacy tests, often in well-controlled research settings, then onto effectiveness tests in settings in which the treatment will ultimately be used, and finally onto dissemination in everyday clinical use. Chapter 13 (Stitzer & Kellogg) reviews two major developments in effectiveness testing and dissemination of VBRT into community substance abuse treatment clinics. The effectiveness testing related to the two CTN multisite trials mentioned previously (Peirce et al., 2006; Petry et al., 2005). The chapter provides important new behind-the-scenes insights into the rationales for different aspects of those trials and how researchers and community clinicians worked together in preparing for them. Regarding dissemination, Chapter 13 discusses an important collaborative effort between CM researchers and officials at the New York City Health and Hospitals Corporation, one of the largest municipal providers of substance abuse treatment services in New York City, to establish CM interventions in a number of their community substance abuse treatment clinics. Much has been learned from these two large-scale efforts that should be quite helpful to future efforts to disseminate CM and other interventions.

As was noted earlier, the issue of costs is an obvious and substantive barrier to disseminating VBRT into community substance-abuse treatment clinics. Community substance abuse treatment clinics generally operate on tight budgets that have little room for additional costs in the form of monetary-based incentives or the regular urine toxicology testing needed to implement CM. Chapters 14 (Petry & Alessi) and 15 (Amass & Kamien) describe efforts to reduce costs associated with CM. Chapter 14 reviews several different strategies related to this overarching goal of reducing the costs of CM, but mostly focuses on the creative and programmatic work that went into the development of prize-based CM. Prize-based CM uses a lower-magnitude and less frequent delivery of reinforcement than conventional VBRT interventions. This practice reduces the cost of the intervention while retaining efficacy. That is, the intervention produces discernible improvements in treatment outcome relative to a control condition. As expected, though, the size of the treatment effects obtained with these lower-cost interventions are discernibly smaller than those obtained in comparable populations using more conventional VBRT interventions (see Lussier et al., 2006). Chapter 14 summarizes a compelling body of evidence supporting the efficacy and effectiveness of CM interventions in community substance abuse treatment clinics.

Chapter 15 revisits a practice used in some of the earliest efforts to use CM in the treatment of SUDs, namely, deposit contracting and fee rebates along with obtaining donations from the local community to support VBRT. In the deposit arrangements, patients make a monetary deposit at the start of treatment that is earned back over time contingent upon meeting predetermined therapeutic goals. Similarly, with fee rebates, patients earn partial return of clinic fees that they have already paid contingent upon meeting therapeutic goals. Finally, Chapter 15 details the success of several different projects where donations from community businesses were used to fund VBRT interventions. Programs to treat pregnant women appear to be especially successful in garnering such community support.

Another approach to financing CM interventions has been to identify reinforcers and punishers that are available in community settings outside the drug abuse treatment clinic and to harness those reinforcers and punishers for use in CM interventions. Chapters 16 (Drebing et al.), 17 (Donlin, Knealing, & Silverman), and 18 (Marlowe & Wong) review research designed to integrate CM interventions into three settings that routinely provide relatively high magnitude reinforcers and/or punishers: the U.S. Department of Veterans Affairs' Compensated Work Therapy (CWT) program (Chapter 16), workplace settings (Chapter 17), and the drug court system (Chapter 18).

The U.S. Department of Veterans Affairs' CWT program offers paid supported employment opportunities to chronically unemployed veterans, many of whom have SUDs. The availability of pay in this program provides a unique opportunity to use that pay, or some portion of it, for therapeutic purposes in CM interventions. Chapter 16 describes an effort to situate VBRT within a CWT. Specifically, the chapter focuses on a VBRT intervention designed to increase drug abstinence and vocational goals among veterans with co-occurring SUDs and mental illness enrolled in the Veterans Affairs (VA) CWT program. Evidence from two controlled studies is presented showing that VBRT increases abstinence from drug use and also the rate of obtaining competitive employment. This project offers hope for integrating VBRT into the VA hospital system's vocational rehabilitation program, one of the largest in the United States, which could eventually represent a huge dissemination success. The VA hospital system's drug abuse treatment programs also represent an important future home for contingency management. There is excellent financial support in the VA hospital system relative to other community clinics such that the added costs associated with CM should represent less of an obstacle. There also is excellent infrastructure in the VA settings in the form, for example, of Veteran's canteen services that offer food, beverages, and other retail items at reduced costs and that have the potential to be integrated into incentive programs.

For a variety of reasons, workplaces might be ideal contexts for the application of CM interventions for the treatment of SUDs. Most important, workplaces control high-magnitude reinforcers, most notably wages for work, which could be used to reinforce therapeutic behavior change (e.g., drug abstinence). To arrange employment-based reinforcement, a contingency can be implemented in which an employee is required to emit a desired target behavior (e.g., provide a drug-free urine sample or take a treatment medication) to gain access to work and to earn wages. Chapter 17 reviews the available uncontrolled and controlled research on employment-based reinforcement to promote drug abstinence and medication compliance and then describes features of community workplaces that might facilitate or limit the application of employment-based reinforcement contingencies for the treatment of SUDs in society. Controlled research on employment-based reinforcement has only begun recently, but the data and information reviewed in this chapter illustrate how workplaces offer extremely promising contexts for dissemination of CM interventions.

Last, but certainly not least, the emergence of the U.S. drug court system holds tremendous promise for the successful dissemination of CM into mainstream rehabilitation for SUDs. As detailed in Chapter 18, drug courts are themselves an explicit CM program wherein reinforcers and punishers, termed *incentives* and *sanctions* within the drug court literature, are to be systematically used to leverage nonviolent criminals with SUDs to obtain the treatment that they need. Chapter 18 provides an excellent overview of this relatively new system and insights into how the information gleaned from CM research can inform and improve the efficacy of the drug court system. It is difficult to imagine a better setting for successfully disseminating CM practices.

CONCLUDING COMMENTS

Each of the chapters in this volume has been prepared to stand alone and needs no further introduction by us. As members of the community of researchers examining CM treatments for SUDs, we are heartened and amazed by the tremendous advances that have occurred in this area over the past several decades and proud to be associated with the excellent series of reviews that comprise this volume.

Taken together, the chapters in this volume demonstrate the relevance of basic principles of behavioral science to the treatment of SUDs; the remarkable effectiveness and versatility of CM interventions; and the feasibility of disseminating these interventions in society, both through community treatment clinics and through other settings like workplaces, the VA hospital system, and drug courts. Despite the promise of CM interventions suggested in this extensive body of research, the research reviewed in this volume also shows that more work is needed to find ways to increase the effectiveness of the interventions so that they will succeed with even more patients, to develops methods that will ensure longer-term maintenance of beneficial effects over time, and to continue to develop and refine practical applications that will be used widely in society. Thus, this volume is important because it outlines the great effectiveness and promise of CM interventions as well as the areas in which additional research and more development are needed. As is amply shown in the research in this volume, CM interventions are not a bag of arbitrary tricks but an orderly set of procedures based on fundamental principles of behavioral science. As such, the further improvement and development of these procedures can be guided by the basic scientific principles on which the interventions are based. The broad success the field has achieved to date in applying these basic principles to treat SUDs across populations, drugs, and settings should give great confidence that we can continue to develop and improve these interventions to address the costly and devastating consequences of SUDs that affect virtually all modern societies.

REFERENCES

Aigner, T. G., & Balster, R. L. (1978). Choice behavior in rhesus monkeys: Cocaine vs. food. *Science, 201*, 534–535.

Anthony, J. C., & Chen, C. Y. (2004). Epidemiology of drug dependence. In M. Galanter & H. D. Kleber (Eds.), *Textbook of substance abuse treatment* (3rd ed., pp 55–72). Arlington, VA: American Psychiatric Publishing.

Bigelow, G., Griffiths, R., & Liebson, I. (1975). Experimental models for the modification of human drug self-administration: Methodological developments in the study of ethanol self-administration by alcoholics. *Federation Proceedings, 34*, 1785–1792.

Budney, A. J., Hughes, J. R., Moore, B. A., & Vandrey, R. G. (2004). A review of the validity and significance of the cannabis withdrawal syndrome. *American Journal of Psychiatry, 161*, 1967–1977.

Cnattingius, S. (2004). The epidemiology of smoking during pregnancy: Smoking prevalence, maternal characteristics, and pregnancy outcomes. *Nicotine and Tobacco Research*, 6(Suppl. 2), S125–S140.

Deneau, J., Yanagita, T., & Seevers, M. H. (1969). Self-administration of psychoactive substances by the monkey. *Psychopharmacology, 16*, 30–48.

Donatelle, R. J., Prows, S. L., Champeau, D., & Hudson, D. (2000). Randomised controlled trial using social support and financial incentives for high risk pregnant smokers: Significant other supporter (SOS) program. *Tobacco Control, 9*(Suppl. 3), III67–III69.

Elliott, R., & Tighe, T. (1968). Breaking the cigarette habit: Effects of a technique involving threatened loss of money. *The Psychological Record, 18*, 503–513.

Higgins, S. T. (1999). Introduction. In S. T. Higgins & K. Silverman (Eds.), *Motivating behavior change among illicit-drug abusers: Research on contingency management interventions* (pp. 3–13). Washington, DC: American Psychological Association.

Higgins, S. T., Delaney, D. D., Budney, A. J., Bickel, W. K., Hughes, J. R., Foerg, F., et al. (1991). A behavioral approach to achieving initial cocaine abstinence. *The American Journal of Psychiatry, 148*, 1218–1224.

Higgins, S. T., Heil, S. H., Dumeer, A. M., Thomas, C. S., Solomon, L. J., & Burnstein, I. M. (2006). Smoking status in the initial weeks of quitting as a predictor of smoking cessation outcomes in pregnant women. *Drug and Alcohol Dependence, 85*, 138–141.

Higgins, S. T., Heil, S. H., & Lussier, J. P. (2004). Clinical implications of reinforcement as a determinant of substance use disorders. *Annual Review of Psychology, 55*, 431–461.

Higgins, S. T., Heil, S. H., Solomon, L. J., Bernstein, I. M., Lussier, J. P., Abel, R. L., et al. (2004). A pilot study on voucher-based incentives to promote abstinence from cigarette smoking during pregnancy and postpartum. *Nicotine and Tobacco Research, 6*, 1015–1020.

Higgins, S. T., & Petry, N. M. (1999). Contingency management: Incentives for sobriety. *Alcohol Research and Health, 23*, 122–127.

Higgins, S. T., & Silverman, K. (Eds.). (1999). *Motivating behavior change among illicit-drug abusers: Research on contingency management interventions.* Washington, DC: American Psychological Association.

Kenford, S. C., Fiore, M. C., Jorenby, D. E., Stevens, S. S., Wetter, D., & Baker, T. B. (1994). Predictin smoking-cessation: Who will quit with and without the nicotine patch. *Journal of the American Medical Association, 271,* 589–594.

Krishnan-Sarin, S., Duhig, A., McKee, S., McMahon, T. J., Liss, T., McFetridge, A., et al. (2006). Contingency management for smoking cessation in adolescent smokers. *Experimental and Clinical Psychopharmacology, 14*(1), 306–310.

Lussier, J. P., Heil, S. H., Mongeon, J. A., Badger, G. J., & Higgins, S. T. (2006). A meta-analysis of voucher-based reinforcement therapy for substance use disorders. *Addiction, 101,* 192–203.

McLellan, A. T., Arndt, I. O., Metzger, D. S., Woody, G. E., & O'Brien, C. P. (1993). The effects of psychosocial services in substance abuse treatment. *Journal of the American Medical Association, 269,* 1953–1959.

McLellan, A. T., Lewis, D. C., O'Brien, C. P., & Kleber, H. D. (2000). Drug dependence, a chronic medical illness: Implications for treatment, insurance, and outcomes evaluation. *Journal of the American Medical Association, 284,* 1689–1695.

Milby, J. B., Schumacher, J. E., Wallace, D., Freedman, M. J., & Vuchinich, R. E. (2005). To house or not to house: The effects of providing housing to homeless substance abusers in treatment. *American Journal of Public Health, 95,* 1259–1265.

Office of National Drug Control Policy. (2004). *The economic costs of drug abuse in the United States, 1992–2002* (No. 207303). Washington, DC: Executive Office of the President.

Peirce, J. M., Petry, N. M., Stitzer, M. L., Blaine, J., Kellogg, S., Satterfield, F., et al. (2006). Effects of lower-cost incentives on stimulant abstinence in methadone maintenance treatment: A national drug abuse treatment Clinical Trials Network study. *Archives of General Psychiatry, 63,* 201–208.

Petry, N. M. (2000). A comprehensive guide to the application of contingency management procedures to clinical settings. *Drug and Alcohol Dependence, 58,* 9–25.

Petry, N. M., Peirce, J. M., Stitzer, M. L., Blaine, J., Roll, J. M., Cohen, A., et al. (2005). Prize-based incentives improve outcomes of stimulant abusers in outpatient psychosocial treatment programs: A national drug abuse treatment Clinical Trials Network study. *Archives of General Psychiatry, 62,* 1148–1156.

Ries, R. K., Dyck, D. G., Short, R., Srebnik, D., Fisher, A., & Comtois, K. A. (2004). Outcomes of managing disability benefits among patients with substance dependence and severe mental illness. *Psychiatric Services, 55,* 445–447.

Roll, J. M., Petry, N. M., Stitzer, M. L., Brecht, M. L., Peirce, J. M., McCann, M. J., et al. (2006). Contingency management for the treatment of methamphetamine use disorders. *American Journal of Psychiatry, 163,* 1993–1999.

Romanelli, F., & Smith, K. M. (2006). Clinical effects and management of methamphetamine abuse. *Pharmacotherapy, 8,* 1148–1156.

Schindler, C. W., Panlilio, L. V., & Goldberg, S. R. (2002). Second-order schedules of drug self-administration in animals. *Psychopharmacology, 163,* 327–344.

Silverman, K., Kaminski, B. J., Higgins, S. T., & Brady, J. V. (in press). Behavior analysis of drug addiction. In W. W. Fisher, C. C. Piazza, & H. S. Roane (Eds.), *Handbook of applied behavior analysis.* New York: Guilford Press.

Silverman, K., Wong, C. J., Grabinski, M. J., Hampton, J., Sylvest, C. E., Dillon, E. M., et al. (2005). A web-based therapeutic workplace for the treatment of drug addiction and chronic unemployment. *Behavior Modification, 29,* 417–463.

Stitzer, M. L. (1999). Combined behavioral and pharmacological treatments for smoking cessation. *Nicotine and Tobacco Research, 1,* S181–S187.

Stitzer, M. L., & Bigelow, G. E. (1982). Contingent reinforcement for reduced carbon monoxide levels in cigarette smokers. *Addictive Behaviors, 7,* 403–412.

Stitzer, M. L., & Higgins, S. T. (1995). Behavioral treatment of drug and alcohol abuse. In F. E. Bloom & D. J. Kupfer (Eds.), *Psychopharmacology: The fourth generation of progress* (pp. 1807–1819). New York: Raven Press.

PART I

CONTINGENCY MANAGEMENT ACROSS SUBSTANCES

CHAPTER 2

COCAINE

Stephen T. Higgins, Sarah H. Heil, Randall E. Rogers, *and* Laura Chivers

Cocaine dependence is an entrenched public health problem in the United States (Substance Abuse and Mental Health Services Administration [SAMHSA], 2005) and a more recent problem in many European and other industrialized countries (Haasen et al., 2004; Prinzleve et al., 2004). Cocaine dependence is associated with a wide range of disturbing individual and societal problems, including overdose and premature death, crime, incarceration, violence, homelessness, drug-exposed neonates, and infectious disease (e.g., Karch, 2005; Kruszon-Moran & McQuillan, 2005; Lucas, 2005; Nnadi, Mimiko, McCurtis, & Cadet, 2005; Schiller & Allen, 2005).

The problems related to cocaine dependence that have received so much publicity over the past couple of decades have been largely centered in the United States. After having been confined to small pockets of the subculture for more than half a century, cocaine use began gaining wider popularity in the United States during the end of the 1960s as part of a general increase in the use of illicit drugs (Byck, 1987). Initially touted as a benign, fun drug, with few untoward effects, cocaine's popularity grew rapidly. By the mid-1980s, some 25 million individuals in the United States (12% of residents 12 years and older) reported lifetime cocaine use, and 5.3 million (3%) reported use within the past 30 days (SAMHSA, 1999). However, cocaine's capacity to cause serious adverse health effects and dependence was soon realized. Large numbers of users began presenting in emergency rooms due to cocaine overdose or other medical complications and in substance abuse treatment clinics seeking help with cessation of cocaine use. Fortunately, recognition of these problems was associated with a precipitous decline in the number of current cocaine users from its peak of 5.7 million in 1985 to 1.8 million (0.8%) by 1998 (SAMHSA, 1999). Unfortunately, the prevalence of current use has remained stable since that time. The most recent estimates come from the 2004 National Survey on Drug Use and Health, in which prevalence of current use was 2.0 million (0.8%). Demand for treatment for cocaine dependence appears to have stabilized as well. In 2000, for example, 0.49 million (0.2%) household residents ages 12 years or older received substance abuse treatment for problems related to cocaine use. In 2004, the most recent year for which data are available, the number remained at 0.47 million (0.2%).

CONTINGENCY MANAGEMENT IN THE TREATMENT OF COCAINE DEPENDENCE: HISTORICAL CONTEXT AND CURRENT ISSUES

The focus of the present chapter is on the use of contingency management (CM) to treat cocaine dependence. CM is a treatment approach that arranges for the systematic application of reinforcing or punishing consequences to achieve therapeutic behavior change (Higgins & Silverman, 1999). Specifically, this chapter focuses on what has come to be known as voucher-based reinforcement therapy (VBRT), a form of CM wherein patients earn vouchers redeemable for retail items, or a comparable monetary-based consequence, contingent upon meeting a therapeutic goal—typically abstinence from drug use but also attendance at therapy sessions, medication compliance, and other therapeutic goals (Higgins, Alessi, & Dantona, 2002). VBRT is the most extensively researched and empirically supported CM intervention for treatment of cocaine dependence, but others have been investigated, including, for example, contingent housing with homeless individuals (see Milby & Schumacher, Chapter 9, this volume) and medication take-home privileges with methadone maintenance patients (Stitzer, Iguchi, & Felch, 1992).

Rationale for Using CM to Treat Cocaine Dependence

As demand for treatment for cocaine dependence grew precipitously in the late 1980s and early 1990s, various treatment approaches were explored in residential and outpatient settings. Investigations into the relative merits of residential compared to outpatient care failed to find differences and thus made it difficult to justify the use of the more expensive residential option as a first-line intervention (e.g., Alterman et al., 1994). Instead, outpatient treatment quickly became the recommended first-line approach to managing cocaine dependence and remains so today. However, outpatient treatment of cocaine dependence was hampered by two overarching problems: high rates of early dropout and ongoing cocaine use. The vast majority of interventions tested in efforts to surmount these problems failed miserably (e.g., Mendelson & Mello, 1996; Van Horn & Frank, 1998). This was the context in which clinical investigators first considered using CM as an outpatient approach to treating cocaine dependence.

The scientific rationale for using CM to treat cocaine dependence was bolstered by an extensive literature showing that cocaine and other types of drug use were sensitive to environmental consequences. For example, in well-controlled laboratory studies in which cocaine abusers were permitted to make exclusive choices between using cocaine or earning money, choice of the cocaine option decreased as an orderly, inverse function of the amount of money offered as the alternative (for a review, see Higgins, Heil, & Lussier, 2004). Consistent with results from these laboratory studies, results from several early case studies with health care workers and other professionals also underscored the potential sensitivity of cocaine use to CM interventions (e.g., Anker & Crowley, 1982). In these early investigations, patients did well with a treatment protocol wherein they contracted to undergo random urine toxicology testing and to temporarily forfeit their professional licenses if they tested positive for recent cocaine use. While this intervention included consequences not applicable to the general cocaine-dependent population, the results were encouraging in that conceptually they underscored CM as a potentially fruitful treatment path to explore.

Initial Clinical Trials

Results from the initial controlled trial examining the efficacy of VBRT for cocaine dependence appeared in 1991 (Higgins et al., 1991). That trial involved 25 consecutive admissions to a university-based research clinic specializing in outpatient treatment of cocaine dependence. Thirteen patients received 12 weeks of VBRT + counseling based on the community reinforcement approach (CRA). Their results were compared to those from 15 admissions who received drug abuse counseling. We describe in detail the VBRT program used in that study because it is the model on which most contemporary VBRT interventions are based. The intervention was 12 weeks in duration and explicitly integrated with routine urinalysis testing. Urine specimens were analyzed onsite to minimize delay between obtaining the specimen and delivering appropriate consequences. Cocaine-negative test results earned points that were recorded on vouchers and provided to patients. Points were worth $0.25 each, with the first negative test results earning 10 points or $2.50 in purchasing power. To promote sustained abstinence in the outpatient setting where opportunities to resume use are ubiquitous, the number of points earned increased by 5 with each consecutive cocaine-negative test result and each three consecutive negative test results earned a $10 bonus voucher. Moreover, a cocaine-positive test result or failure to provide a scheduled specimen reset the value of the vouchers back to the initial low level from which it could escalate again according to the same schedule. Five consecutive test results following a reset restored voucher value back to where it was prior to the reset. Money was never given to patients because for many cocaine-dependent individuals cash is a well-established cue for cocaine use. Instead, points were used to purchase retail items in the community, with clinic staff making all purchases. Staff counseled patients to use vouchers to support involvement in healthy activities that could serve as attractive alternatives to cocaine use. If a patient earned all of the points available across 12 weeks, he or she could earn a total of $997.50 in purchasing power, although average earnings were approximately half of the total possible, which we now know is typical in these interventions.

While the number of patients involved was relatively small, the results were striking. Eleven of the 13 (85%) admissions who received VBRT + CRA were retained for the recommended 12 weeks of treatment compared to only 5 of the 15 (33%) who received drug abuse counseling. Moreover, 6 of the 13 (46%) admissions assigned to VBRT + CRA therapy achieved 8 or more weeks of continuous cocaine abstinence verified by urinalysis testing compared to none of those assigned to drug abuse counseling. Interest in this approach was bolstered greatly when a subsequent, fully randomized trial comparing the same two treatment approaches closely replicated the initial results (Higgins et al., 1993).

The research design used in those two initial trials did not permit inferences about the relative contributions to outcome of VBRT versus the intensive behavioral counseling (CRA therapy) that these patients also received. Based on the information from the laboratory studies and clinical case studies mentioned earlier, however, there was a strong likelihood that the VBRT component was an active contributor to the outcomes obtained.

Expanding on the Promise of the Initial Trials

There has been a great deal of research on VBRT during the approximately 15 years since the publication of the seminal studies. Indeed, there has been sufficient interest and research activity to warrant holding two scientific conferences on the use of VBRT to treat substance use disorders, with the first being held on September 14 and 15, 1995, in Bethesda, Maryland, and the second on October 7 and 8, 2004, in Burlington, Vermont. The first conference spurred the publication of an edited volume on the use of CM to treat substance use disorders (Higgins & Silverman, 1999) and the second conference started the ball rolling for the present volume. For completeness we briefly review the material on VBRT treatment of cocaine dependence covered in the first volume, with the remainder of the chapter devoted to an overview of subsequent developments.

The Earlier Volume

The material related to the use of VBRT to treat cocaine dependence covered in the prior volume falls into three general categories. First, the use of VBRT in the treatment of cocaine-dependent outpatients in drug-free clinics that rely primarily on psychosocial interventions was reviewed (Higgins, Roll, Wong, Tidey, & Dantona, 1999). In brief, the trials from the drug-free clinics demonstrated that VBRT delivered in combination with intensive behavioral counseling increased retention in treatment and cocaine abstinence compared to standard drug abuse counseling (Higgins et al., 1991; Higgins et al., 1993), that the VBRT intervention was an active contributor to those positive outcomes (Higgins et al., 1994), and that treatment effects were sustained for at least 6 months after termination of the voucher program (Higgins et al., 1995). This matter of sustaining effects of VBRT continues to be of great interest and more recent developments are reviewed below.

Second, the use of VBRT to treat cocaine dependence in methadone-maintenance clinics was reviewed (Silverman, Preston, Stitzer, & Schuster, 1999). The evidence confirmed that VBRT was efficacious with methadone-maintenance patients and an urban, largely African American population (Silverman et al., 1996; Silverman et al., 1998). Such generality could not be assumed considering that VBRT was originally developed in a drug-free clinic treating a largely rural, white population. There was additional evidence that the target of the VBRT contingency could be expanded to include other drugs of abuse in addition to cocaine without eliminating efficacy (Piotrowski & Hall, 1999), although more recent evidence indicates that doing so reduces the effect size of the VBRT intervention (Lussier, Heil, Mongeon, Badger, & Higgins, 2006).

Third, in addition to the use of VBRT in formal substance abuse clinics, investigators began examining the potential efficacy of VBRT in the treatment of special populations, including those with schizophrenia and other mental illness (Shaner, Tucker, Roberts, & Eckman, 1999), pregnant women and tuberculosis-exposed drug abusers (Elk, 1999), and the homeless (Schumacher et al., 1999). Results with these populations at the time were inconclusive but promising. Considering the tremendous need for effective treatments for special populations, the use of VBRT with them remains an important area of inquiry.

More Recent Developments in the Use of VBRT to Treat Cocaine Dependence

To examine developments since the publication of the prior volume in the use of VBRT to treat cocaine dependence, we conducted a literature search from January 1999 through July 2006 using PubMed as the search engine and *vouchers*, *contingency management*, and *cocaine abuse and dependence* as search terms. We also reviewed the reference sections of all reports located and queried colleagues in the field. Only reports on controlled studies published in peer-reviewed journals since the publication of the last volume were included. As is shown in Table 2.1, we identified 38 reports that met the aforementioned criteria. All the studies identified in our review targeted the intervention on cocaine or cocaine and other drug use, while a subset also targeted participation in therapeutic activities (7/38, 18%) and clinic attendance (3/38, 8%). Thirteen of the 38 studies (34%) involved cocaine-dependent outpatients in drug-free clinics while the remaining studies involved opioid-dependent patients enrolled in agonist-maintenance clinics (63%) or vocational training (5%). Twenty-nine of the 38 studies (76 %) used a schedule of voucher earnings that escalated in value as a function of consecutively negative urine-toxicology tests while 9 of 38 (24%) exclusively used a fixed-value schedule of voucher earnings. Conventional vouchers were used in 32 of the 38 studies (84%) of studies while prize-based VBRT was used in the remaining 6 studies (16%). The most important characteristic of the reports is that 35 of 38 (92%) noted statistically significant improvements in the targeted outcome. Those reliably positive results are consistent with the findings from a recent meta-analysis showing robust support for the efficacy of VBRT in increasing abstinence from the use of cocaine, cocaine and opiates, as well as other substances (Figure 2.1; Lussier et al., 2006).

The 38 reports identified in the literature review addressed at least one of the six different topic areas reviewed here.

Efficacy of VBRT as a Stand-Alone Treatment

As mentioned previously, VBRT was originally introduced as one element of a multielement outpatient treatment for cocaine dependence (Budney & Higgins, 1998). Subsequent studies conducted mostly in methadone-maintenance clinics demonstrated that adding abstinence-contingent vouchers to protocols involving minimal counseling nevertheless resulted in substantial reductions in cocaine use (Silverman et al., 1996; Silverman et al., 1998). The reliable efficacy of VBRT under such circumstances led many to wonder about the efficacy of VBRT as a stand-alone treatment.

This question about the efficacy of VBRT as a stand-alone treatment was thoroughly addressed in two randomized clinical trials conducted in drug-free clinics in which VBRT was combined with a minimal protocol that protected against suicide and recommended self-help participation but otherwise provided no counseling (Higgins et al., 2003; Rawson et al., 2006). In one of these two trials, VBRT alone was compared to VBRT plus CRA therapy (Higgins et al., 2003) and in the other VBRT alone was compared to cognitive-behavioral therapy (CBT) alone and to VBRT + CBT

TABLE 2.1. Published Articles on VBRT and Cocaine Dependence: January 1999–July 2006

Study	N	Setting	VBRT duration (weeks)	VBRT Target(s)	VBRT schedule type	Total VBRT earnings (max.)	Voucher delivery	Follow-up time points (weeks afer intake)	Positive outcome
Cocaine									
Higgins et al. (2007)	100	DF	12	Abst.	E	$498.75 vs. $1,995.00	I	36, 48, 60, 72, 84, 96	Y
Petry, Martin et al. (2005)	77	MC	12	Abst./Att.	P	$117[a]	I	24	Y
Correia et al. (2005)	47	MC	1	Abst. vs. decr.	F	$100.00 vs $200.00	I	—	Y
Sigmon et al. (2004)[b]	46	MC	24	Abst. vs. decr.	F	$1,200.00	I	—	Y
Jones et al. (2004)[c]	199	DF	12	Abst.	E	$1,155.50	I	—	Y
Higgins et al. (2003)	100	DF	12	Abst.	E	$997.50	I	24, 36, 48, 60, 72, 84, 96	Y
Epstein, Hawkins, Cori, Umbricht, & Preston (2003)	193	MC	12	Abst.	E	$1,155.50	I	24, 36, 60	Y
Correia et al. (2003)	58	MC	5 days	Abst.	F	$200.00	I	—	Y
Rawson et al. (2002)	120	MC	16	Abst.	E	$1,277.50	I	26, 52	Y
Katz, Robles-Soleto et al. (2002)d	40	MC	11 days	Abst.	F	$100.00 vs. $400.00	D	—	Y
Preston et al. (2001)[b]	95	MC	8	Abst. vs. decr.	E	$554.00	D	3, 4, 5	Y
Jones, Silverman, Stitzer, & Svikis (2001)	80	MC	2	Abst./Att.	E	$525.00	I	—	Y
Robles et al. (2000)[d]	72	MC	2 days	Abst.	F	$100.00	D	—	Y
Higgins, Wong, et al. (2000)	70	DF	12	Abst.	E	$997.50	I	24, 36, 48, 60, 72	Y
Silverman, Chatuape, et al. (1999)[d]	29	MC	9	Abst.	E	$382.00 vs. $3480.00	I	-	Y
Cocaine and Opiates									
Poling et al. (2006)	106	MC	25	Abst./Act.	E	$934.00	I	—	Y
Schottenfeld et al. (2005)	162	MC	12	Abst.	E	$997.50	I	—	Y
Oliveto et al. (2005)	140	MC	12	Abst.	E	$738.00	D	—	Y
Silverman, Robles, Mulric, Bigelow, & Stitzer, et al. (2004)	78	MC	52	Abst.	E	$5758.75[e]	I	—	Y
Katz et al. (2004)	211	DF	5 days	Abst.	F	$100.00	I	1	Y
Kosten, Oliveto, et al. (2003)	160	MC	12	Abst.	E	$738.00	D	—	Y

(continued)

TABLE 2.1. (continued)

Study	N	Setting	VBRT duration (weeks)	VBRT Target(s)	VBRT schedule type	Total VBRT earnings (max.)	Voucher delivery	Follow-up time points (weeks after intake)	Positive outcome
Kosten, Poling, & Olivetos (2003)	75	MC	12	Abst.	F	$108.00	D	—	Y
Silverman et al. (2002)	40	MC	78	Abst./Act.	E	$10,530.00[f]	I	—	Y
Petry & Martin (2002)	42	MC	12	Abst.	P	$137[a]	I	24	Y
Katz, Chatuape, Jones, & Stitzer (2002)	52	DF	12	Abst.	E	$1,087.50	I	—	N
Silverman et al. (2001)[f]	40	MC	24	Abst./Act.	E	$2,830.00[f]	I	—	Y
Dallery et al. (2001)[b,d]	11	MC	9	Abst.	E	$374.40 vs. $3,369.60	I	—	Y
Jones, Haug, Stitzer, & Svikis, et al. (2000)	93	MC/DF	1	Abst. or Att.	F	$85.00	I	—	N
Polydrug									
Rawson et al. (2006)	177	DF	16	Abst.	E	$988.75	I	17, 26, 52	Y
Pierce et al. (2006)	388	MC	12	Abst.	P	$120.00	I	—	Y
Petry, Peirce et al. (2005)	415	DF	12	Abst.	P	$203.00	I	—	Y
Petry, Alessi et al. (2005)	142	DF	12	Abst./Act.	E vs. P	$335.00[g], $295.00[a]	I	24, 32	Y
Petry et al. (2004)	120	DF	12	Abst./Act.	P	$36.00[a] vs. $68.00[a]	I	—	Y
Carroll, Sivher, Nich, Babuscio, & Rousaville, et al. (2002)	55	DF	12	Abst./Act.	E	$561.60 vs. $1,152.00	I	16, 24, 36	Y
Carroll et al. (2001)	127	DF	12	Abst./Act.	E	$561.00	I	—	Y
Downey, Helmus, & Schuster (2000)	41	MC	12	Abst.	E	$997.50	D	—	N
Piotrowski, Tusel, et al. (1999)	102	MC	17	Abst.	E	$755.00	D	20, 24	Y
Chatuape, Silverman, & Stitzer, et al. (1999)	14	MC	12	Abst.	F	$900.00	I	—	Y

Note. N, sample size, all groups combined. Setting, setting in which study occurred: DF, drug-free clinic; MC, medication clinic. VBRT target: Abst., abstinence; Att., attendance; Act., involvement in other activities. VBRT schedule type: E, escalating magnitude; P, prize-based; F, fixed magnitude. Total VBRT earnings (max.), the maximum amount that could be earned. Voucher delivery: I, immediate (at the same visit the reinforcement was earned); D, delayed (at a visit after the reinforcement was earned). Follow up time points, point in time after completion of the VBRT intervention at which follow up assessments were conducted, (–) indicates there was no post-VBRT follow-up. Positive Outcome, whether or not a significant change was reported for the behavior targeted by the VBRT intervention: Y, yes; N, no.

[a] This is the average total earnings as reported by the authors of the study, as maximum possible earnings could not be calculated.

[b] Though this study included a maintenance or second phase, only the results of the initial intervention are reported.

[c] VBRT targeted continued abstinence after abstinence was achieved with inpatient treatment.

[d] Within-subjects design.

[e] In addition to VBRT earnings, participants could also earn take-home methadone privileges.

[f] This is the maximum earning for abstinence only, although subjects earned vouchers for other workplace behaviors.

[g] This is the average amount earned by subjects in the VBRT condition.

26

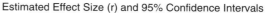

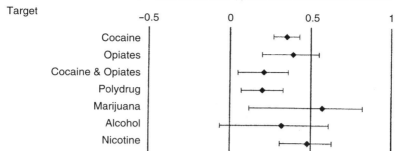

FIGURE 2.1. Weighted average effect sizes and 95% confidence intervals for studies targeting abstinence from cocaine and other substances. Where confidence intervals do not overlap with zero, the intervention is deemed to have produced a treatment effect. From Lussier, Heil, Mongeon, Badger, and Higgins (2006). Copyright 2006 by Blackwell Publishing. Reprinted by permission.

(Rawson et al., 2006). In the trial involving CRA, the combined CRA plus VBRT treatment produced greater cocaine abstinence than VBRT alone during the 12-week period when vouchers were available, but not during the second half of the recommended 24-week course of treatment or during an 18-month posttreatment follow-up period. While differences between treatment conditions were modest with regard to cocaine use, thereby supporting the efficacy of VBRT as a stand-alone treatment the inclusion of CRA made a substantial difference in other areas. Those who received CRA therapy were better retained in treatment, reported less drinking to intoxication during treatment and posttreatment follow-up, a greater number of days of paid employment during treatment and follow-up, fewer depressive symptoms during treatment but not follow-up, and fewer hospitalizations and DUI (driving under the influence) arrests during posttreatment follow-up.

In the trial with CBT, the two abstinence-contingent voucher conditions (VBRT alone and VBRT + CBT) increased retention during the recommended 16-week course of treatment compared to CBT alone as well as the number of stimulant-negative specimens submitted (i.e., negative for cocaine and amphetamines) and the longest duration of continuous abstinence achieved; there also was significantly less psychiatric symptomatology in the VBRT only compared to the other conditions at the end-of-treatment assessment. There were no significant treatment differences through the 1-year follow-up assessment, although cocaine use remained below baseline levels in all treatment conditions throughout the follow-up period.

Overall, then, results from these two trials offer compelling evidence that with regard to cocaine use, VBRT delivered as a stand-alone intervention generally achieves outcomes comparable to those achieved when the intervention is combined with other well-established psychosocial treatments for substance use disorders (CRA and CBT). There is evidence from the trial involving CRA that combining VBRT with other therapy can enhance initial reductions in the frequency of cocaine use, although that was limited to one of the two trials. The trial with CRA offered compelling evidence that combining abstinence-contingent vouchers with an additional intervention that contains elements specifically directed at problem drinking (i.e., monitored disulfiram therapy) and employment (i.e., Job Club) produces clinically important improvements in problem drinking, other substance use, and in selected areas of psychosocial functioning that are not achieved with VBRT alone. The trial with CBT did not demonstrate such additional improvements among patients treated with the combined intervention. However, CBT in that study appeared to be focused specifically on cocaine use whereas CRA focused on a wide range of other areas of functioning.

Sustainability of Treatment Effects

A commonly asked question about VBRT is whether treatment effects are limited to the period while the incentive program is operating. As indicated in the "Follow-up time points" column in Table 2.1, a number of studies report results of assessments completed after the discontinuation of VBRT. Results from several of these studies demonstrate sustained treatment effects after discontinuation of VBRT. A study examining VBRT combined with CRA compared to a noncontingent voucher + CRA control condition demonstrated greater cocaine abstinence among the former during the recommended 24-week course of treatment and during a 15-month posttreatment follow-up period (Higgins, Wong, Badger, Ogden, & Dantona, 2000). Those results systematically replicated and extended earlier findings of sustained treatment effects with CRA + abstinence-contingent vouchers (Higgins et al., 1995).

The study by Rawson and colleagues described above in the section on abstinence-contingent vouchers as a stand-alone intervention also provided an opportunity to examine the sustainability of treatment effects following discontinuation of the voucher interventions (Rawson et al., 2006). While abstinence-contingent vouchers delivered alone or in combination with CBT produced greater during-treatment abstinence compared to CBT alone during the 16-week intervention, there were no significant treatment differences noted during an 8-month follow-up period.

In another study relevant to this topic, patients were randomized to abstinence-contingent vouchers, abstinence-contingent prizes (see description below), or a usual-care treatment condition (Petry, Alessi, Marx, Austin, & Tardif, 2005). Incentives were delivered contingent upon biochemically verified abstinence from cocaine, alcohol, and opiates. Both abstinent-contingent conditions achieved greater during-treatment abstinence than the usual-care condition, but no significant differences between treatment conditions were observed during a 6-month posttreatment follow-up period.

Thus, there is clear and replicable evidence from controlled studies that treatment effects of VBRT remain discernible for a sustained period of time following discontinuation of the incentive program under some conditions. The positive evidence comes mostly from studies in which VBRT was combined with an intensive counseling intervention (e.g., Higgins, Wong, et al., 2000), but not exclusively so (e.g., Rowan-Szal, Bartholomew, Chatham, & Simpson, 2005).

When predictors of posttreatment abstinence have been examined among patients treated with VBRT + CRA, a consistent finding has been that the duration of continuous abstinence achieved during the treatment period is the best predictor (Higgins, Badger, & Budney, 2000). Importantly, that relationship is not specific to the VBRT plus CRA intervention. That same relationship was observed in the study described previously by Petry and colleagues (Petry, Alessi, et al., 2005). Although no statistically significant differences between treatment conditions were observed during the follow-up period in the Petry, Alessi, et al. (2005) study, the incentive conditions produced greater sustained abstinence during treatment than the usual-care condition and sustained abstinence predicted posttreatment abstinence.

Without question, there are a number of studies where no significant treatment effects were discernible once the abstinence-contingent incentives program was discontinued (e.g., Rawson et al., 2002; Rawson et al., 2006). Thus, the evidence indicates that treatment effects obtained with VBRT are sustained in some but certainly not all circumstances, and a distinguishing feature of the most notable instances of sustained effects with VBRT is that the incentive program was delivered in combination with an intensive counseling intervention and generated periods of sustained abstinence during treatment that exceeded levels obtained with the comparison treatments.

A recent study relevant to this topic experimentally tested the notion that a sustained period of during-treatment abstinence was key to obtaining posttreatment abstinence (Higgins et al., 2007). As is discussed further below, increasing the monetary value of vouchers is one effective method for increasing the amount of abstinence achieved during treatment. In this study, 100 cocaine-dependent outpatients were randomly assigned to one of two treatments: CRA therapy combined with VBRT set at twice the conventional value of vouchers and CRA combined with VBRT set at one-half the conventional voucher value. Consistent with the main hypothesis, high-value VBRT significantly increased cocaine abstinence during the 24-week treatment period as well as during an 18-month posttreatment follow-up period (Figure 2.2).

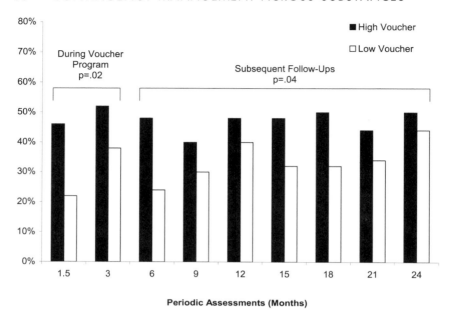

FIGURE 2.2. Percentages of patients abstinent from cocaine at periodic assessments conducted during treatment and posttreatment follow-up. Data points represent point-prevalence abstinence at the respective assessments. Abstinence was defined as self-report of no cocaine use in past 30 days and cocaine-negative urine toxicology results. Data points for the high-value and low-value voucher conditions are represented by closed and open symbols, respectively. Brackets show how the periodic assessments were divided in a categorical modeling analysis and associated significance levels. From Higgins et al. (2007). Copyright 2007 by Blackwell Publishing. Reprinted by permission.

VBRT with Special Populations

The use of VBRT to treat cocaine and other substance use disorders among special populations is an important area within the development of the VBRT. Detailed reviews of the use of VBRT to treat substance use disorders among the homeless, pregnant women, those with serious mental illness, and adolescents can be found in Chapters 9–12 (this volume). One of the most impressive applications of VBRT to reduce cocaine use in a special population has been the development of the therapeutic workplace and its use with pregnant and recently postpartum women (Silverman, Svikis, Robles, Stitzer, & Bigelow, 2001; Silverman et al., 2002; see Heil, Yoon, & Higgins, Chapter 10, Donlin, Knealing, & Silverman, Chapter 17, this volume, for more details). In this arrangement, patients are paid in vouchers to participate in vocational training and, following proper training, a data entry job. Salary is linked to abstinence by requiring objective evidence of abstinence from cocaine and opioid use in order to gain access to the workplace. In the seminal study on this model, 40 methadone-maintained pregnant or recently post-partum women were randomly assigned to the therapeutic workplace or to a usual-care control condition. Cocaine and opioid abstinence levels among patients enrolled in the workplace were significantly greater than those in the control condition. At a 3-year assessment, for example, 30% of therapeutic-workplace patients had had sustained continuous cocaine and opiate abstinence during the past 18 months (period covered by the assessment) versus only 5% of patients treated with usual care. This intervention has tremendous potential for application on a broader scale to combat the terrible problems of chronic unemployment, few employment skills, and chronic drug abuse among many young mothers.

Combining Medications and VBRT

Understanding better how VBRT and medications for substance use inter-act is an important priority in the development of this treatment approach and the focus of some important recent research. Chapter 8 (Rounsaville, Rosen, & Carroll, this volume), for example, provides an insightful review of the potential of VBRT for increasing medication compliance among those with substance use disorders.

An important practice that has been experimentally investigated is the influence of the dose of opioid-replacement therapy when using VBRT to treat cocaine dependence among patients dependent on opioids and cocaine. Logically, a prudent approach is to place patients on a suffi-ciently high dose of the substitute medication to maximize efficacy before pursuing the use of the VBRT adjunct treatment. One would not expect the substitution medication to directly affect cocaine use, but a more sta-ble patient with regard to opioid withdrawal and related problems should be more likely to respond to the adjunct VBRT intervention. Oliveto et al. (2005) experimentally tested these notions using varying doses of levo-alpha-acetylmethadol (LAAM), a long-acting opioid agonist medication, in a 12-week randomized clinical trial. Opioid- and cocaine-dependent patients were randomly assigned to the following four conditions: low-dose LAAM (30, 30, 39 mg/Monday, Wednesday, and Friday [MWF]) with VBRT; low-dose LAAM with non-contingent VBRT control; high-dose LAAM (100, 100, 130 mg/MWF) with VBRT; high-dose LAAM with noncontingent VBRT control. In the two VBRT conditions, voucher delivery was contingent upon abstinence from both opioids and cocaine. Abstinence from opioids was highest in the high-dose LAAM conditions with no differences between the VBRT and noncontingent control condi-tions. However, abstinence from cocaine and from both opioids and cocaine was highest in the high-dose LAAM with VBRT condition (Fig-ure 2.3).

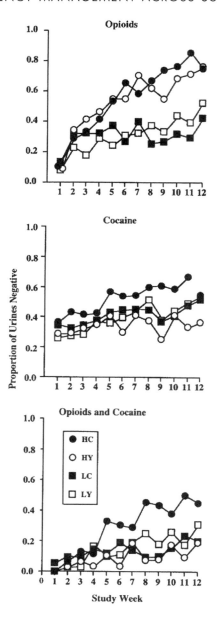

FIGURE 2.3. Weekly proportion of specimens negative in urine toxicology testing for opioids (upper panel), cocaine (middle panel), and opioids and cocaine in four different 12-week treatment conditions: high-dose LAAM with VBRT (HC, filled circles), high-dose LAAM only (HY, open circles), low-dose LAAM with VBRT (LC, filled squares), and low-dose LAAM only (LY, open squares). From Oliveto et al. (2005). Copyright 2005 by Elsevier Ireland, Ltd. Reprinted by permission.

Results consistent with those of Oliveto et al. (2005) were obtained in a study in which opioid- and cocaine-dependent patients were exposed to two different values of vouchers under two different methadone doses. Greater abstinence was observed under the high compared to the low voucher values when the methadone dose was high (120 mg) but not when it was low (60 mg dose) (Dallery, Silverman, Chutuape, Bigelow, & Stitzer, 2001).

Another potentially important area of investigation regarding medications is in the use of antidepressant medications and VBRT for opioid- and cocaine- dependent patients. In a study of desipramine and VBRT, opioid- and cocaine-dependent patients were randomized to one of four conditions: combined desipramine and VBRT, placebo and VBRT, desipramine and noncontingent VBRT, or placebo and noncontingent VBRT (Kosten, Oliveto, et al., 2003). Vouchers were delivered contingent upon abstinence from both opioids and cocaine in the VBRT conditions. Abstinence from cocaine alone and from opioids and cocaine increased more in the desipramine and VBRT condition compared to the other three conditions. A subsequent parallel study examining bupropion reported similar findings except that the effects of the combined medication plus VBRT intervention was seen exclusively on cocaine abstinence rather than opioid and cocaine abstinence (Poling et al., 2006). The possibility that antidepressants and VBRT may interact is interesting practically and theoretically and clearly warrants further investigation.

In still another effort to explore the merits of combining VBRT and medication, a trial was conducted examining the combined use of the serotonin precursor L-trytophan and VBRT among cocaine-dependent patients. Results supported the efficacy of VBRT, but its effects were not influenced by whether patients received medication or placebo (Jones et al., 2004).

Increasing Treatment Response in Refractory Patients

Typically about half the patients exposed to VBRT show a discernible increase in cocaine abstinence. That has led investigators to examine methods to improve outcomes among refractory patients. The aforementioned studies on the dose of substitution medication illustrate one effective method. Another method mentioned previously is to increase the monetary value of the vouchers or reinforcer magnitude. In the seminal study on this topic, methadone patients dependent on opioids and cocaine were exposed to the conventional 12-week VBRT intervention (Silverman, Chutuape, Bigelow, & Stitzer, 1999). Those patients who did not respond to the VBRT intervention were subsequently invited to participate in a within-subjects design wherein they could earn $0, $382, or $3,480 across a 9-week intervention contingent upon cocaine-negative urinalysis results. The high-value VBRT condition significantly increased abstinence compared to the two other conditions, with 45% of patients achieving 4 weeks of continuous cocaine abstinence in the high-value condition compared to only one and zero patients doing so in the low- and zero-value VBRT conditions. These results were replicated in a subsequent study with methadone-maintenance patients (Dallery et al., 2001) and in a study with patients enrolled in a drug-free clinic (Higgins et al., 2007). Consistent with these experimental findings, results from the recent meta-analysis of VBRT identified voucher amount as one of only two significant moderators of the effect size of VBRT (Lussier et al., 2006). The other significant moderator was delay in delivering vouchers, with delivery on the same day as abstinence is verified increasing effect size relative to later delivery.

Another promising method for increasing treatment response is through "shaping" cocaine abstinence. In the seminal experiment on this topic, cocaine-using methadone patients were randomly assigned to the conventional VBRT intervention for 8 weeks or to a condition where patients had to show objective evidence of at least 25% reductions in cocaine metabolites in urine for the first 3 weeks of the intervention and total abstinence for the last 5 weeks in order to earn vouchers (Preston, Umbricht, Wong, & Epstein, 2001). The rationale for the shaping procedure is to increase the proportion of patients who initially earn a voucher by making the response requirement for doing so relatively easier early on and to increase difficulty over time. Cocaine use was lower in the shaping compared to the conventional conditions during the last 5 weeks when the contingencies were identical in the two conditions, suggesting that the shaping procedure better prepared patients for abstaining than did the conventional procedure. Results from subsequent studies examining the benefits of shaping abstinence over requiring complete abstinence from the start of treatment have shown no advantage for the former (e.g., Correia, Sigmon, Silverman, Bigelow, & Stitzer, 2005; Sigmon, Correia, & Stitzer, 2004). There are still too few data available to make a definitive judgment about the merits of shaping abstinence, but there is sufficient empirical support and intuitive appeal to warrant further investigation of the approach.

Efficacy in Community Clinics

In taking on the challenge of moving the use of VBRT into community substance abuse treatment clinics, a creative variation on the original voucher approach was developed that is referred to as the prize-based or fishbowl approach (Petry, Martin, Cooney, & Kranzler, 2000; see Petry & Alessi, Chapter 14, this volume, for more details). The overarching goal of this modification was to produce a lower-cost intervention that retained efficacy. This prize-based VBRT intervention differs from the conventional VBRT procedure in at least three ways. First, intermittent rather than continuous reinforcement is used. Satisfying the reinforcement contingency results in patients earning opportunities to draw slips of paper from an urn which either has a monetary value designated on it or a message offering praise but no monetary reward. Typically, approximately half or more of the slips of paper have no monetary value, approximately 40% very low value ($1), 8% intermediate ($20), and only approximately 1% or less a relatively high value ($80–$100). In the conventional approach, each negative specimen earns a voucher that is worth a specified monetary value. Second, the feature of patients drawing from the urn is akin to a game of chance and is designed to enhance patient interest. The conventional approach has no such feature. Third, the slips of paper having a monetary value are exchanged for one of a selection of "prizes" that are kept at the clinic. The conventional approach is to exchange vouchers for retail items purchased in the community. The important differences here are that with this alternative method, the retail items are already available in the clinic and thus available for exchange with patients with minimum temporal delay, but the range of potential items is necessarily limited. With the conventional voucher approach there is a greater selection of items for which vouchers can be exchanged, but there is also likely to be greater temporal delay because of shopping time.

This alternative "prize" VBRT procedure has now been investigated in a series of clinical trials conducted in community clinics that support its efficacy (Petry et al., 2000, 2004; Petry, Alessi, et al., 2005), including two large, multisite trials conducted through the National Institute on Drug Abuse's (NIDA) Clinical Trials Network (CTN) (Petry, Peirce, et al., 2005; Peirce et al., 2006). Because these trials are described in detail in two excellent chapters (Stitzer & Kellogg, Chapter 13, and Petry & Alessi, Chapter 14, this volume), in this volume we do not review them in detail here. In brief, results from those trials provide robust evidence that adding VBRT to the usual treatment regimen in community drug-free or methadone clinics significantly reduces stimulant and other drug use compared to usual care alone. The relatively low cost of the prize-based approach makes it attractive to community providers, which should greatly enhance dissemination potential. Cost differences between the prize-based and conventional VBRT procedures may be more apparent than real in that they were equally efficacious when delivered at comparable monetary values in the only direct comparison of the two procedures (Petry, Alessi, et al., 2005). The success of the two multisite trials provides strong support for the potential of the VBRT approach to enhance outcomes in community drug abuse treatment clinics.

CONCLUDING COMMENTS

Cocaine use and cocaine dependence continue to represent a serious public health problem in the United States and many other industrialized countries. Developing efficacious interventions for cocaine dependence has been a daunting challenge. VBRT is one intervention that has demonstrated reliable efficacy in rigorous randomized clinical trials conducted over a 15-year period. VBRT is efficacious as a stand-alone intervention, but combining it with an intensive counseling intervention such as CRA also addresses many of the serious co-occurring substance use and other problems that are common among the cocaine-dependent population that otherwise go untreated. In this same vein, patients dependent on opioids and cocaine should receive an adequate dose of the substitution medication in order to maximize the potential efficacy of VBRT. There is also promising evidence that combining antidepressant medications with VBRT may improve outcomes among patients dependent on opioids and cocaine. There is no longer any question that the effects of VBRT on cocaine use can extend well beyond the period when the incentives are in effect, but, as would be expected, obtaining effects posttreatment is less reliable than during treatment, and much remains to be learned about the conditions in which effects are sustained. Correlational and experimental evidence indicates that obtaining a sustained period of cocaine abstinence during treatment is key to achieving positive longer-term outcomes.

An important feature of VBRT's efficacy is its success with special populations, including pregnant and recently postpartum women and those with co-occurring serious mental illness. These are populations for which efficacious interventions are sorely needed and VBRT holds great promise with them.

Of course, even among the general clinical population of cocaine-dependent patients, not all patients respond to the intervention. Modifications to VBRT such as increasing the monetary value of the incentive and requiring reductions in use rather than complete abstinence before delivering the first voucher hold promise for increasing the proportion of patients who benefit from VBRT.

One of the important questions about VBRT is the feasibility of extending use into community clinics. There is no doubt that VBRT is efficacious in community clinics. The modified prize-based and conventional forms of VBRT have been demeonstrated to be efficacious in community clinics. The positive results from the two large, multisite trials of VBRT in drug-free and methadone-maintenance clinics offer as robust a body of evidence supporting efficacy in community clinics as there is for any behavioral treatment for substance use disorder of which we are aware. Moreover, the cost of the VBRT interventions examined in those multisite trials were quite modest, which may help to reduce at least some of the concerns about the added costs that would be associated with adoption of VBRT into community clinics.

Overall, VBRT is reliably efficacious intervention for outpatient treatment of cocaine dependence. There has been tremendous progress made in the development of this treatment approach, which has been extended in many interesting, important, and unanticipated directions. We are optimistic that VBRT has a bright future as the field of substance abuse treatment continues to evolve toward greater use of empirically based and effective treatments.

ACKNOWLEDGMENTS

Preparation of this chapter was supported in part by Grant Nos. R37DA09378 and T32DA07242 from the National Institute on Drug Abuse.

REFERENCES

Alterman, A. I., O'Brien, C. P., McLellan, A. T., August, D. S., Snider, E. C., Droba, M., et al. (1994). Effectiveness and costs of inpatient versus day hospital cocaine rehabilitation. *Journal of Nervous and Mental Disease, 182*(3), 157–163.

Anker, A. L., & Crowley, T. J. (1982). Use of contingency contracts in specialty clinics for cocaine abuse. *NIDA Research Monographs, 41*, 452–459.

Budney, A. J., & Higgins, S. T. (1998). *National Institute on Drug Abuse therapy manuals for drug addiction: Manual 2. A community reinforcement plus vouchers approach: Treating cocaine addiction* (NIH Publication No. 98-4309). Rockville, MD: National Institute on Drug Abuse.

Byck, R. (1987). Cocaine, marijuana and the meanings of addiction. In R. Hamowy (Ed.), *Dealing with drugs: Consequences of government control* (pp. 221–245). Lexington, MA: Lexington Books.

Carroll, K. M., Ball, S. A., Nich, C., O'Connor, P. G., Eagan, D. A., Frankforter, T. L., et al. (2001). Targeting behavioral therapies to enhance naltrexone treatment of opioid dependence: Efficacy of contingency management and significant other involvement. *Archives of General Psychiatry, 58*, 755–761.

Carroll, K. M., Sinha, R., Nich, C., Babuscio, T., & Rounsaville, B. J. (2002). Contingency management to enhance naltrexone treatment of opioid dependence: A randomized clinical trial of reinforcement magnitude. *Experimental and Clinical Psychopharmacology, 10*(1), 54–63.

Chutuape, M. A., Silverman, K., & Stitzer, M. L. (1999). Contingent reinforcement sustains post-detoxification abstinence from multiple drugs: A preliminary study with methadone patients. *Drug and Alcohol Dependence, 54*, 69–81.

Correia, C. J., Dallery, J., Katz, E. C., Silverman, K., Bigelow, G., & Stitzer, M. L. (2003). Single- versus dual-drug target: Effects in a brief abstinence incentive procedure. *Experimental and Clinical Psychopharmacology, 11*, 302–308.

Correia, C. J., Sigmon, S. C., Silverman, K., Bigelow, G., & Stitzer, M. L. (2005). A comparison of voucher-delivery schedules for the initiation of cocaine abstinence. *Experimental and Clinical Psychopharmacology, 13*(3), 253–258.

Dallery, J., Silverman, K., Chutuape, M. A., Bigelow, G. E., & Stitzer, M. L. (2001). Voucher-based reinforcement of opiate plus cocaine abstinence in treatment-resistant methadone patients: Effects of reinforcer magnitude. *Experimental and Clinical Psychopharmacology, 9*(3), 317–325.

Downey, K. K., Helmus, T. C., & Schuster, C. R. (2000). Treatment of heroin-dependent poly-drug abusers with contingency management and buprenorphine maintenance. *Experimental and Clinical Psychopharmacology, 8*(2), 176–184.

Elk, R. (1999). Pregnant women and tuberculosis-exposed drug abusers: Reducing drug use and increasing compliance. In S. T. Higgins & K. Silverman (Eds.), *Motivating behavior change among illicit-drug abusers* (pp. 123–144). Washington, DC: American Psychological Association.

Epstein, D. H., Hawkins, W. E., Covi, L., Umbricht, A., & Preston, K. L. (2003). Cognitive-behavioral therapy plus contingency management for cocaine use: Findings during treatment and across 12–month follow-ups. *Psychology of Addictive Behaviors, 17*, 73–82.

Haasen, C., Prinzleve, M., Zurhold, H., Rehm, J., Guttinger, F., Fischer, G., et al. (2004). Cocaine use in Europe—A multi-centre study. Methodology and prevalence estimates. *European Addiction Research, 10*(4), 139–146.

Higgins, S. T., Alessi, S. M., & Dantona, R. L. (2002). Voucher-based incentives: A substance abuse treatment innovation. *Addictive Behaviors, 27*(6), 887–910.

Higgins, S. T., Badger, G. J., & Budney, A. J. (2000). Initial abstinence and success in achieving longer term cocaine abstinence. *Experimental and Clinical Psychopharmacology, 8*(3), 377–386.

Higgins, S. T., Budney, A. J., Bickel, W. K., Badger, G. J., Foerg, F. E., & Ogden, D. (1995). Outpatient behavioral treatment for cocaine dependence: One-year outcome. *Experimental and Clinical Psychopharmacology, 3*, 205–212.

Higgins, S. T., Budney, A. J., Bickel, W. K., Foerg, F. E., Donham, R., & Badger, G. J. (1994). Incentives improve outcome in outpatient behavioral treatment of cocaine dependence. *Archives of General Psychiatry, 51*(7), 568–576.

Higgins, S. T., Budney, A. J., Bickel, W. K., Hughes, J. R., Foerg, F., & Badger, G. (1993). Achieving cocaine abstinence with a behavioral approach. *American Journal of Psychiatry, 150*(5), 763–769.

Higgins, S. T., Delaney, D. D., Budney, A. J., Bickel, W. K., Hughes, J. R., Foerg, F., et al. (1991). A behavioral approach to achieving initial cocaine abstinence. *American Journal of Psychiatry, 148*(9), 1218–1224.

Higgins, S. T., Heil, S. H., Dantona, R. L., Donham, R., Matthews, M., & Badger, G. (2007). Effects of varying the monetary value of voucher-based incentives on abstinence achieved during and following treatment among cocaine-dependent outpatients. *Addiction, 102*, 271–281.

Higgins, S. T., Heil, S. H., & Lussier, J. P. (2004). Clinical implications of reinforcement as a determinant of substance use disorders. *Annual Review of Psychology, 55*, 431–461.

Higgins, S. T., Roll, J. M., Wong, C. J., Tidey, J. W., & Dantona, R. L. (1999). Clinic and laboratory studies on the use of incentives to decrease cocaine and other substance use. In S. T. Higgins & K. Silverman (Eds.), *Motivating behavior change among illicit-drug abusers* (pp. 35–56). Washington, DC: American Psychological Association.

Higgins, S. T., Sigmon, S. C., Wong, C. J., Heil, S. H., Badger, G. J., Donham, R., et al. (2003). Community reinforcement therapy for cocaine-dependent outpatients. *Archives of General Psychiatry, 60*(10), 1043–1052.

Higgins, S. T., & Silverman, K. (Eds.). (1999). *Motivating behavior change among illicit-drug abusers: Research on contingency management interventions*. Washington, DC: American Psychological Association.

Higgins, S. T., Wong, C. J., Badger, G. J., Ogden, D. E., & Dantona, R. L. (2000). Contingent reinforcement increases cocaine abstinence during outpatient treatment and 1 year of follow-up. *Journal of Consulting and Clinical Psychology, 68*(1), 64–72.

Jones, H. E., Haug, N., Silverman, K., Stitzer, M. L., & Svikis, D. (2001). The effectiveness of incentives in enhancing treatment attendance and drug abstinence in methadone-maintained pregnant women. *Drug and Alcohol Dependence, 61*, 297–306.

Jones, H. E., Haug, N., Stitzer, M. L., & Svikis, D. (2000). Improving treatment outcomes for pregnant drug-dependent women using low-magnitude voucher incentives. *Addictive Behaviors, 25*(2), 263–267.

Jones, H. E., Johnson, R. E., Bigelow, G. E., Silverman, K., Mudric, T., & Strain, E. C. (2004). Safety and efficacy of L-tryptophan and behavioral incentives for treatment of cocaine dependence: A randomized clinical trial. *American Journal on Addictions, 13*(5), 421–437.

Karch, S. B. (2005). Cocaine cardiovascular toxicity. *Southern Medical Journal, 98*(8), 794–799.

Katz, E. C., Chutuape, M. A., Jones, H., Jasinski, D., Fingerhood, M., & Stitzer, M. (2004). Abstinence incentive effects in a short-term outpatient detoxification program. *Experimental and Clinical Psychopharmacology, 12*(4), 262–268.

Katz, E. C., Chutuape, M. A., Jones, H. E., & Stitzer, M. L. (2002). Voucher reinforcement for heroin and cocaine abstinence in an outpatient drug-free program. *Experimental and Clinical Psychopharmacology, 10*, 136–143.

Katz, E. C., Robles-Sotelo, E., Correia, C. J., Silverman, K., Stitzer, M. L., & Bigelow, G. E. (2002). The brief abstinence test: Effects of continued incentive availability on cocaine abstinence. *Experimental and Clinical Psychopharmacology, 10*, 10–17.

Kosten, T., Oliveto, A., Feingold, A., Poling, J., Sevarino, K., McCance-Katz, E., et al. (2003). Desipramine and contingency management for cocaine and opiate dependence in buprenorphine maintained patients. *Drug and Alcohol Dependence, 70*(3), 315–325.

Kosten, T., Poling, J., & Oliveto, A. (2003). Effects of reducing contingency management values on heroin and cocaine use for buprenorphine- and desipramine-treated patients. *Addiction, 98*, 665–671.

Kruszon-Moran, D., & McQuillan, G. M. (2005). *Seroprevalence of six infectious diseases among adults in the United States by race/ethnicity: Data from the third national health and nutrition examination survey, 1988–1994* (Advance data from vital and health statistics: No. 352). Hyattsville, MD: National Center for Health Statistics.

Lucas, C. E. (2005). The impact of street drugs on trauma care. *Journal of Trauma, 59*(3 Suppl.), S57–S60, S67–S75.

Lussier, J. P., Heil, S. H., Mongeon, J. A., Badger, G. J., & Higgins, S. T. (2006). A meta-analysis of voucher-based reinforcement therapy for substance use disorders. *Addiction, 101*(2), 192–203.

Mendelson, J. H., & Mello, N. K. (1996). Management of cocaine abuse and dependence. *New England Journal of Medicine, 334*(15), 965–972.

Nnadi, C. U., Mimiko, O. A., McCurtis, H. L., & Cadet, J. L. (2005). Neuropsychiatric effects of cocaine use disorders. *Journal of the National Medical Association, 97*(11), 1504–1515.

Oliveto, A., Poling, J., Sevarino, K. A., Gonsai, K. R., McCance-Katz, E. F., Stine, S. M., et al. (2005). Efficacy of dose and contingency management procedures in LAAM-maintained cocaine-dependent patients. *Drug and Alcohol Dependence, 79*(2), 157–165.

Peirce, J. M., Petry, N. M., Stitzer, M. L., Blaine, J., Kellogg, S., Satterfield, F., et al. (2006). Effects of lower-cost incentives on stimulant abstinence in methadone maintenance treatment: A national drug abuse treatment Clinical Trials Network study. *Archives of General Psychiatry, 63*(2), 201–208.

Petry, N. M., Alessi, S. M., Marx, J., Austin, M., & Tardif, M. (2005). Vouchers versus prizes: Contingency management treatment of substance abusers in community settings. *Journal of Consulting and Clinical Psychology, 73*(6), 1005–1014.

Petry, N. M., & Martin, B. (2002). Low-cost contingency management for treating co-caine- and opioid-abusing methadone patients. *Journal of Consulting and Clinical Psychology, 70*(2), 398–405.

Petry, N. M., Martin, B., Cooney, J. L., & Kranzler, H. R. (2000). Give them prizes, and they will come: Contingency management for treatment of alcohol dependence. *Journal of Consulting and Clinical Psychology, 68*(2), 250–257.

Petry, N. M., Martin, B., & Simcic, F., Jr. (2005). Prize reinforcement contingency management for cocaine dependence: Integration with group therapy in a methadone clinic. *Journal of Consulting and Clinical Psychology, 73*(2), 354–359.

Petry, N. M., Peirce, J. M., Stitzer, M. L., Blaine, J., Roll, J. M., Cohen, A., et al. (2005). Effect of prize-based incentives on outcomes in stimulant abusers in outpatient psychosocial treatment programs: A national drug abuse treatment Clinical Trials Network study. *Archives of General Psychiatry, 62*(10), 1148–1156.

Petry, N. M., Tedford, J., Austin, M., Nich, C., Carroll, K. M., & Rounsaville, B. J. (2004). Prize reinforcement contingency management for treating cocaine users: How low can we go, and with whom? *Addiction, 99*(3), 349–360.

Piotrowski, N. A., & Hall, S. M. (1999). Treatment of multiple drug abuse in the methadone clinic. In S. T. Higgins & K. Silverman (Eds.), *Motivating behavior change among illicit-drug abusers* (pp. 183–202). Washington, DC: American Psychological Association.

Piotrowski, N. A., Tusel, D. J., Sees, K. L., Reilly, P. M., Banys, P., Meek, P., et al. (1999). Contingency contracting with monetary reinforcers for abstinence from multiple drugs in a methadone program. *Experimental and Clinical Psychopharmacology, 7*(4), 399–411.

Poling, J., Oliveto, A., Petry, N., Sofuoglu, M., Gonsai, K., Gonzalez, G., et al. (2006). Six-month trial of bupropion with contingency management for cocaine dependence in a methadone-maintained population. *Archives of General Psychiatry, 63*(2), 219–228.

Preston, K. L., Umbricht, A., Wong, C. J., & Epstein, D. H. (2001). Shaping cocaine abstinence by successive approximation. *Journal of Consulting and Clinical Psychology, 69*(4), 643–654.

Prinzleve, M., Haasen, C., Zurhold, H., Matali, J. L., Bruguera, E., Gerevich, J., et al. (2004). Cocaine use in Europe—A multi-centre study: Patterns of use in different groups. *European Addiction Research, 10*(4), 147–155.

Rawson, R. A., Huber, A., McCann, M., Shoptaw, S., Farabee, D., Reiber, C., et al. (2002). A comparison of contingency management and cognitive-behavioral approaches during methadone maintenance treatment for cocaine dependence. *Archives of General Psychiatry, 59*(9), 817–824.

Rawson, R. A., McCann, M. J., Flammino, F., Shoptaw, S., Miotto, K., Reiber, C., et al. (2006). A comparison of contingency management and cognitive-behavioral approaches for stimulant-dependent individuals. *Addiction, 101*(2), 267–274.

Robles, E., Silverman, K., Preston, K. L., Cone, E. J., Katz, E., Bigelow, G. E., et al. (2000). The brief abstinence test: Voucher-based reinforcement of cocaine abstinence. *Drug and Alcohol Dependence, 58*, 205–212.

Rowan-Szal, G. A., Bartholomew, N. G., Chatham, L. R., & Simpson, D. D. (2005). A combined cognitive and behavioral intervention for cocaine-using methadone clients. *Journal of Psychoactive Drugs, 37*(1), 75–84.

Schiller, C., & Allen, P. J. (2005). Follow-up of infants prenatally exposed to cocaine. *Pediatric Nursing, 31*(5), 427–436.

Schottenfeld, R. S., Chawarski, M. C., Pakes, J. R., Pantalon, M. V., Carroll, K. M., & Kosten, T. R. (2005). Methadone versus Buprenorphine with contingency management or performance feedback, for cocaine and opioid dependence. *American Journal of Psychiatry, 162*(2), 340–349.

Schumacher, J. E., Milby, J. B., McNamara, C. L., Wallace, D., Michael, M., Popkin, S., et al. (1999). Effective treatment of homeless substance abusers: The role of contingency management. In S. T. Higgins & K. Silverman (Eds.), *Motivating behavior change among illicit-drug abusers* (pp. 77–94). Washington, DC: American Psychological Association.

Shaner, A., Tucker, D. E., Roberts, L. J., & Eckman, T. A. (1999). Disability income, cocaine use, and contingency management among patients with cocaine dependence and schizophrenia. In S. T. Higgins & K. Silverman (Eds.), *Motivating behavior change among illicit-drug abusers* (pp. 95–122). Washington, DC: American Psychological Association.

Sigmon, S. C., Correia, C. J., & Stitzer, M. L. (2004). Cocaine abstinence during methadone maintenance: Effects of repeated brief exposure to voucher-based reinforcement. *Experimental and Clinical Psychopharmacology, 12*(4), 269–275.

Silverman, K., Chutuape, M. A., Bigelow, G. E., & Stitzer, M. L. (1999). Voucher-based reinforcement of cocaine abstinence in treatment-resistant methadone patients: Effects of reinforcement magnitude. *Psychopharmacology, 146*(2), 128–138.

Silverman, K., Preston, K. L., Stitzer, M. L., & Schuster, C. R. (1999). Efficacy and versatility of voucher-based reinforcement in drug abuse treatment. In S. T. Higgins & K. Silverman (Eds.), *Motivating behavior change among illicit-drug abusers* (pp. 168–182). Washington, DC: American Psychological Association.

Silverman, K., Robles, E., Mudric, T., Bigelow, G. E., & Stitzer, M. L. (2004). A randomized trial of long-term reinforcement of cocaine abstinence in methadone-maintained patients who inject drugs. *Journal of Consulting and Clinical Psychology, 72*(5), 839–854.

Silverman, K., Svikis, D., Robles, E., Stitzer, M. L., & Bigelow, G. E. (2001). A reinforcement-based therapeutic workplace for the treatment of drug abuse: Six-month abstinence outcomes. *Experimental and Clinical Psychopharmacology, 9*(1), 14–23.

Silverman, K., Svikis, D., Wong, C. J., Hampton, J., Stitzer, M. L., & Bigelow, G. E. (2002). A reinforcement-based therapeutic workplace for the treatment of drug abuse: Three-year abstinence outcomes. *Experimental and Clinical Psychopharmacology, 10*(3), 228–240.

Silverman, K., Wong, C. J., Higgins, S. T., Brooner, R. K., Montoya, I. D., Contoreggi, C., et al. (1996). Increasing opiate abstinence through voucher-based reinforcement therapy. *Drug and Alcohol Dependence, 41*(2), 157–165.

Silverman, K., Wong, C. J., Umbricht-Schneiter, A., Montoya, I. D., Schuster, C. R., & Preston, K. L. (1998). Broad beneficial effects of cocaine abstinence reinforcement among methadone patients. *Journal of Consulting and Clinical Psychology, 66*(5), 811–824.

Stitzer, M. L., Iguchi, M. L., & Felch, L. J. (1992). Contingent take-home incentive: Effects on drug use of methadone maintenance patients. *Journal of Consulting and Clinical Psychology, 60*, 927–934.

Substance Abuse and Mental Health Services Administration. (1999). *National Household Survey on Drug Abuse: Population estimates, 1998.* Retrieved August 22, 2006, from *www.oas.samhsa.gov/nhsda/Pe1998/TOC.htm.*

Substance Abuse and Mental Health Services Administration. (2005). *Results from the 2004 National Survey on Drug Use and Health: National findings (NSDUH Series H-28, DHHS Publication No. SMA 05-406).* Rockville, MD: Office of Applied Studies.

Van Horn, D. H. A., & Frank, A. F. (1998). Psychotherapy for cocaine addiction. *Psychology of Addictive Behaviors, 12*(1), 47–61.

CHAPTER 3

OPIOIDS

David H. Epstein
and Kenzie L. Preston

BACKGROUND

The availability of both agonist and antagonist treatments for opiate-use disorders provides a seemingly rich selection of cost-effective and reasonably safe pharmacological approaches to the problem. Why is it necessary to consider contingency management (CM) in this context?

In nearly every agonist-maintenance program, some patients persist in using illicit opiates (Ball & Ross, 1991). Such behavior could theoretically be suppressed by high-dose methadone maintenance (Donny, Walsh, Bigelow, Eissenberg, & Stitzer, 2002), but some patients might require heroic doses that would increase the risk of side effects or meet with patient resistance due to detoxification phobia (Milby et al., 1986). Many patients have misgivings about agonist maintenance and choose detoxification; for them, relapse rates are high (Kornor & Waal, 2005). Compliance with antagonist regimens is notoriously poor (Greenstein, Fudala, & O'Brien, 1997). For these reasons, CM approaches remain clinically important even in the context of pharmacological treatment—which is actually where they were developed (Stitzer, Bigelow, & Liebson, 1979).

CM TO COMPLEMENT AGONIST MEDICATIONS

CM during Maintenance

Clinic-Based Reinforcers (Take-Homes and Other Clinic Privileges)

The methadone clinic is a natural laboratory for CM: Each patient must come in every day to get the dose of medication that he or she needs, along with various ancillary services, and all these things can be adjusted in ways that reinforce or punish behavior. Not surprisingly, clinic privileges, including take-home doses of methadone (henceforth *take-homes*), were the first reinforcers to be studied as a basis for CM in opiate dependence (for a review, see Kidorf & Stitzer, 1999).

To our knowledge, the first formal studies of take-homes as reinforcers involved target behaviors such as disulfiram ingestion for alcoholic methadone patients (Liebson, Bigelow, & Flamer, 1973) and counseling attendance (Stitzer et al., 1977). Soon after that, Milby, Garrett, English, Fritschi, and Clarke (1978) targeted urine-verified abstinence from illicit drugs, randomly assigning 69 participants to abstinence-contingent take-homes (with a response requirement of seven consecutive negative urines) or a wait-list control condition. The effect was modest but promising: There was no group difference in overall percentages of negative urines, but the CM group produced more *consecutive* negative urines than did the control group.

Most subsequent studies of abstinence-contingent take-homes seem to have confirmed this initial finding—and the modest size of the effect. These studies tended to have high overall rates of drug-positive urines or large numbers of nonresponsive participants (Chutuape, Silverman, & Stitzer, 1999b; Saxon, Calsyn, Wells, & Stanton, 1998; Schmitz et al., 1998; Stitzer, Iguchi, & Felch, 1992). This may have been partly due to the fact that the response requirement was usually abstinence from multiple drugs simultaneously (an issue discussed later in the section "Targeting Multiple Drugs"). But it also reflects heterogeneity in participant preferences for reinforcers, as shown in a survey in which 36% of patients preferred other services to take-homes (Chutuape, Silverman, & Stitzer, 1998) and in studies in which participants responded to a reinforcer of $30 cash rather than take-homes (Stitzer et al., 1979) or in which $15 cash was chosen over take-homes on 95% of reinforcement occasions (Stitzer, Bigelow, & Liebson, 1980). While contingent take-homes can help motivate abstinence, the need remains for reinforcers that are more individualizable.

Voucher-Based CM

Readers of this volume are probably familiar with the escalating-reinforcement procedure developed by Higgins and colleagues (Higgins et al., 1993, 1991). In this procedure, the reinforcers are vouchers redeemable for goods and services chosen by the participant, and therefore are almost completely tailorable to individual preferences. A similar approach had been used with cash reinforcers in some of the studies cited previously (Stitzer et al., 1979, 1980), but Higgins's substitution of vouchers for cash permitted considerable escalation of the magnitude of reinforcement while largely avoiding the possibility of iatrogenic, cash-triggered relapses.

The first studies of voucher-based CM targeted cocaine abuse in non-opiate-abusing patients (Higgins et al., 1993, 1991), but they were soon followed by similar studies in methadone-maintained patients with persistent use of illicit opiates. In our treatment–research clinic, 13 participants were enrolled in a within-subjects study in which we targeted a possible $1,155 in escalating vouchers toward opiate-negative urine specimens; rates of opiate-negative urines were 22% during a 5-week baseline, 76% during 12 weeks of CM, and 59% during an 8-week return-to-baseline condition (Silverman, Wong, et al., 1996). Each of these percentages was significantly different from the others. We then randomly assigned 120 patients to 8 weeks of a similarly escalating contingent-voucher condition (maximum possible earnings, $554) or to a non-contingent-voucher control condition (Preston, Umbricht, & Epstein, 2000). In the contingent-voucher condition, the overall percentage of opiate-negative urines was 49% (vs. 35% in the noncontingent condition), and the mean maximum duration of opiate abstinence was 3 weeks (vs. 1.8 weeks in the noncontingent condition). These results, although not overwhelming, demonstrate that opiate use in methadone-maintained patients can respond to contingent vouchers. Of the 120 participants in that study, 110 continued in a 12-week follow-up study in which they were immediately rerandomized to receive vouchers (and take-homes) at a fixed value of $10 per opiate-negative urine, or noncontingent vouchers (and noncontingent take-homes) (Preston, Umbricht, & Epstein, 2002). The results showed that a modest, fixed-value maintenance contingency can be effective even in patients who have been exposed to an escalating-reinforcer contingency—a finding that bodes well for the use of CM as a maintenance treatment.

Prize-Based CM

Another approach to individually tailorable CM, described at greater length by Petry and Alessi (Chapter 14, this volume) is to reinforce target behaviors with prize draws rather than vouchers. This approach, technically *variable-ratio reinforcement*, or less technically the *fishbowl procedure* (because slips or tokens may be drawn from a fishbowl), retains many of the advantages of voucher-based CM. The escalating component can be retained by giving increasing numbers of draws; the individualization can be retained by stocking a wide variety of prizes onsite or by including retail gift certificates among the prizes. Unique advantages are that participants can, by chance, contact a high-magnitude reinforcer early in treatment, that prizes are visibly displayed and awarded on the spot, and that each participant can see other participants win. For clinics, the main advantage is that in the prize-based approach, abstinence from drug use is reinforced intermittently rather than continuously as is done in the original voucher arrangement and thus has the potential to be less expensive.

To our knowledge, prize-based CM has not yet successfully targeted opiate use alone. In one study, prize-based CM independently targeted the use of both opiates and cocaine in 42 methadone-maintained patients (Petry & Martin, 2002). The prize procedure increased the rate of cocaine-negative urines but not of opiate-negative urines; one barrier to detecting treatment effects was that the baseline rate of negative urines had been fairly high. Prize-based CM for opiate-use disorders seems likely to be effective but requires further study.

CM during Detoxification

In an early attempt to harness CM in the context of methadone detoxification, McCaul, Stitzer, Bigelow, and Liebson (1984) randomized 20 patients with initial reductions in opiate use to one of two conditions: $10 cash and a take-home for each opiate-negative urine, or $10 noncontingently. Treatment retention was better in the CM condition, but as the dose of methadone got below 15 mg/day, all participants relapsed. The challenge thus appears to be how to counteract the symptoms of physical withdrawal that inevitably occur toward the end of the detoxification. Two approaches have been investigated.

One approach is to combine the motivational effect of CM with the direct pharmacological effect of methadone. This approach was used successfully by Higgins, Stitzer, Bigelow, and Liebson (1986), who randomly assigned 39 patients with initial reductions in opiate use to one of three conditions during an 8-week detoxification: temporary methadone dose supplements contingent upon opiate-negative urines, a control condition in which dose supplements were given noncontingently, and a control condition with no dose supplements. The respective rates of opiate-negative urines were 86%, 62%, and 50%, suggesting that the contingency had effects over and above the direct effects of methadone. Still, when the contingency was removed, half the participants in the contingent group immediately relapsed.

Another approach is to use an escalating schedule of voucher-based reinforcement so that maximum earnings are available toward the end of the detoxification, when withdrawal symptoms and relapse risk are greatest. This approach has been used successfully with maximum possible earnings of $658 during the last 22 weeks of a 26-week buprenorphine detoxification (Bickel, Amass, Higgins, Badger, & Esch, 1997) or $2,232 during 22 weeks *before, during, and after* a 13-week methadone detoxification

(Robles, Stitzer, Strain, Bigelow, & Silverman, 2002). In the latter study, CM continued for 3 weeks after methadone was discontinued, and the effect of CM on opiate abstinence remained significant for those 3 weeks. The results are compromised by a high rate of dropout in both the CM group and a noncontingent control group, but nonetheless they suggest that contingencies should be timed in accordance with the period of greatest risk. The authors suggested that the schedule of CM should be adjusted for maximum effect as the dose of methadone falls below 40 mg/day.

CM after Detoxification

To our knowledge, CM has rarely been studied in opiate-dependent participants who have already completed detoxification. There have been three reports on the use of a CM-like procedure called reinforcement-based outpatient treatment (RBT) (Gruber, Chutuape, & Stitzer, 2000), in which abstinence is reinforced by payments toward drug-free housing, recreational activities, and job-skills training. An initial randomized trial in 52 participants showed that RBT reduced the likelihood of return to drug use during the 4 weeks that the contingencies were in place, but that the rate of dropout was high during a subsequent counseling-only phase (Gruber et al., 2000). A follow-up study in 37 new participants showed that dropout was reduced (at least compared to historical controls) when 4 weeks of RBT was augmented with 12 weeks of vouchers ($890 targeted toward opiates and cocaine simultaneously, on a nonescalating schedule) (Katz, Gruber, Chutuape, & Stitzer, 2001). Another study in 130 participants extended RBT itself to 3 months (in which up to $2,294 in rent payments and other benefits were contingent upon simultaneous abstinence from opiates and cocaine), with continuing non-RBT treatment for 6 months; compared to a usual-care control, RBT produced more abstinence from opiates and cocaine during the 3 months it was in effect (42% vs. 15% abstinent at month 1; 38% vs. 17% abstinent at month 3), but not at months 6 and 12, during which both groups appeared to regress to the mean (i.e., the control group improved) (Jones, Wong, Tuten, & Stitzer, 2005). Taken together, these studies show that drug use in heroin-dependent individuals remains responsive to contingencies after detoxification, but more studies are needed to determine which procedures are most effective and how their effects can be maintained.

CM TO REINFORCE ADHERENCE
TO ANTAGONIST REGIMENS

In an early attempt to address the problem of low adherence to oral-naltrexone regimens with CM, Meyer and Mirin (1979) offered participants $1 per day over 12 weeks to ingest prescribed naltrexone, with a $5 bonus for each 7 consecutive days of ingestion. Nearly all participants dropped out. Subsequent studies showed greater success rates, with escalating voucher payments of $1,155 over 12 weeks (Preston et al., 1999) or $561 over 12 weeks (Carroll et al., 2001). Even in these studies, 12-week dropout rates for reinforced groups were on the order of 50%—but this should be contrasted with dropout rates of, for example, 75% for a noncontingently reinforced group and 95% for a nonreinforced group (Preston et al., 1999).

CM TO REINFORCE BEHAVIORS OTHER THAN ABSTINENCE IN OPIATE-DEPENDENT PATIENTS

Studies targeting treatment goals other than abstinence have been limited and had mixed results. In two pilot studies (involving nine and two patients, respectively), Elk et al. (1993) enhanced adherence to an isoniazid regimen in tuberculosis-positive patients by making methadone contingent upon isoniazid ingestion. Magura, Casriel, Goldsmith, Strug, and Lipton (1988) targeted contingent take-homes to a variety of individual behaviors such as counseling attendance and applying to trade school; five of the seven poly-drug-abusing methadone-maintained patients responded to the contingencies—a success rate of roughly 70%, exceeding the success rate in 33 other patients whose contracts directly involved drug abstinence. Iguchi and colleagues reinforced nondrug behaviors (attending group sessions or other tailored treatment goals) with low-value incentives with the goal of reducing drug use indirectly while avoiding the cost of frequent urinalyses. An initial study with 66 patients showed no decrease in drug use through reinforcement of group therapy attendance (Iguchi et al., 1996), though a second study that targeted completion of specific treatment plan tasks showed increased drug abstinence (Iguchi, Belding, Morral, Lamb, & Husband, 1997).

CM IN OPIATE-DEPENDENT PATIENTS WHO ABUSE OTHER DRUGS

In many geographical regions, polydrug abuse is the norm for opiate-dependent individuals. CM has been applied to this problem in two ways: targeted solely toward one nonopiate drug of abuse, or targeted toward multiple drugs of abuse. The former approach has usually been more successful (Lussier, Heil, Mongeon, Badger, & Higgins, 2006).

Targeting One Drug Alone

Alcohol, Benzodiazepines, Nicotine, and Cannabis

Some of the earliest CM studies in methadone-maintained patients took advantage of the fact that disulfiram can be directly mixed into each dose of liquid methadone; alcoholic patients who wanted methadone had no choice but to take the coadministered disulfiram (or find another program). This contingency, applied after inpatient detoxification from alcohol, reduced alcohol use and rarely resulted in dropout or transfer (Bickel et al., 1988; Liebson et al., 1973; Liebson, Tommasello, & Bigelow, 1978). Another early CM study successfully reduced benzodiazepine abuse in 10 methadone-maintained patients (Stitzer, Bigelow, Liebson, & McCaul, 1984).

More recent studies have targeted tobacco and cannabis smoking. The first published attempt to target tobacco smoking with CM reinforced decreases in exhaled carbon monoxide with $5 in cash (with a maximum payment of $40 over 4 weeks) in five participants; self-reported smoking rates decreased, but the decrease in carbon monoxide did not reach significance, presumably reflecting either inaccurate self-reports or compensatory inhalation (Schmitz, Rhoades, & Grabowski, 1995). Subsequent attempts with slightly larger reinforcers (Shoptaw, Jarvik, Ling, & Rawson, 1996) or substantially larger reinforcers combined with nicotine patches (Shoptaw et al., 2002) have been more successful, though as with smoking cessation in the general population, relapse rates after the intervention ended were high. In a naturalistic study targeting abstinence from cannabis use, eight cannabis-using methadone patients were required to stop using cannabis in order to maintain their clinic privilege of two take-homes per week; four of the eight patients complied (Calsyn & Saxon, 1999).

Cocaine

A large body of literature exists showing that cocaine use is reduced by high-magnitude reinforcers in patients in agonist-maintenance therapy. The reinforcers have generally consisted of escalating-value vouchers, and the magnitudes shown effective are $1,155–$1,950 over 12 weeks (Epstein, Hawkins, Covi, & Preston, 2003; Rawson et al., 2002; Silverman, Higgins, et al., 1996; Silverman et al., 1998), $525 over 2 weeks (Jones, Haug, Silverman, Stitzer, & Svikis, 2001), or $100 over 2 days (Katz, Robles-Sotelo, et al., 2002; Robles et al., 2000). In most of the longer studies, approximately 50% of participants achieve several consecutive weeks of abstinence. Of those who fail to do so, 45% may respond to even larger incentives, such as $3,480 over 9 weeks (Silverman, Chutuape, Bigelow, & Stitzer, 1999).

The obvious question is whether abstinence from cocaine can be achieved without such large monetary outlays. The most promising data involve the prize-based CM discussed earlier. In one study, 77 methadone-maintained participants were randomly assigned to standard treatment or prize-based CM targeting cocaine use. Average winnings over 12 weeks amounted to only $117, but the CM group showed a greater percentage of cocaine-negative urines (35% vs. 17%) and longer continuous abstinence from cocaine (2.9 ± 0.6 weeks vs. 0.8 ± 0.3 weeks) (Petry, Martin, & Simcic, 2005).

Targeting One Drug, Hitting Several: Response Generalization

Up to this point, we have been defining success as abstinence from the single drug being targeted. What about patients who are abusing two or more drugs at once?

In reporting the results of one of the first CM studies from our clinic, we emphasized "broad beneficial effects" of targeting cocaine alone: Participants reduced their rates of illicit opiate use along with their rates of cocaine use, despite there being no formal contingency upon illicit opiate use (Silverman et al., 1998). A similar sort of response generalization has been observed in other studies; reductions in nicotine use were accompanied by reductions in cocaine use (Shoptaw et al., 1996) or opiate and cocaine use (Shoptaw et al., 2002); reductions in cocaine use were accompanied by reductions in opiate use (Jones et al., 2001; Silverman, Higgins, et al., 1996). Unfortunately, this effect is not reliable; in at least four other studies targeting cocaine, reductions in illicit opiate use were tested for and not found (Epstein, Hawkins, et al., 2003; Petry et al., 2005; Rawson et al., 2002; Silverman et al., 1999). There is no clear explanation for the discrepancy across studies, but the studies that showed generalization to illicit opiate use tended to involve lower doses of methadone (mean 42–65 mg/day) than the ones that did not (mean 70–82 mg/day). Thus, generalization from cocaine-targeted CM to illicit opiate use may not occur when methadone dosage is already adequate.

Generalization in the opposite direction, from opiate-targeted vouchers to a reduction in cocaine use, has been observed in one study, conducted during a methadone detoxification (Robles et al., 2002). However, no such generalization occurred in another detoxification study (Bickel et al., 1997) or in a maintenance study (Preston et al., 2000). Presently, we must conclude that vouchers targeted toward one drug cannot be counted on to reduce use of other drugs.

Targeting Multiple Drugs

How, or even whether, to target multiple drugs of abuse simultaneously in a clinical trial remains a contentious question (O'Brien & Lynch, 2003; Rounsaville, Petry, & Carroll, 2003; Strain, 2003), but there is little question that practicing clinicians wish to do it (Petry & Simcic, 2002). It is tempting to try an all-or-nothing approach in which reinforcement is given when patients demonstrate simultaneous abstinence from two or more targeted drugs.

Most attempts to do so have yielded negative or only modest results. When methadone-maintained patients were offered $1,155 in vouchers for heroin and cocaine abstinence over 12 weeks, most never earned a voucher (Downey, Helmus, & Schuster, 2000). In a similar study in an outpatient drug-free program, with $1,087 in vouchers available, the overall rate of drug-free urine specimens was only about 20%, and there was no significant difference between the CM condition and a control condition (Katz, Chutuape, Jones, & Stitzer, 2002). Another study tested a stepwise approach in which the initial response requirement was abstinence from cocaine and heroin, then from all illicit drugs, for a possible $755 in vouchers over 16 weeks. The effect of CM was small (almost 50% of CM patients never provided a negative specimen), slow to develop (significant differences during treatment weeks 12–16 only), and dissipated immediately upon cessation of the contingency (Piotrowski et al., 1999). Negative or modest results of all-or-nothing contingencies have been reported in at least 7 other studies (Calsyn et al., 1994; Chutuape et al., 1999b; Kosten et al., 2003; Oliveto et al., 2005; Rowan-Szal, Joe, Chatham, & Simpson, 1994; Schottenfeld et al., 2005; Stitzer et al., 1992).

A few such studies have yielded positive results, but only in the context of an intensive psychosocial intervention (Silverman, Svikis, Robles, Stitzer, & Bigelow, 2001), with a highly motivated sample (Carroll, Sinha, Nich, Babuscio, & Rounsaville, 2002), in the absence of a control group (Katz et al., 2001), or with high-magnitude vouchers ($3,369 over 9 weeks) (Dallery, Silverman, Chutuape, Bigelow, & Stitzer, 2001) or very long durations of voucher availability ($5,800 over 52 weeks) (Silverman, Robles, Mudric, Bigelow, & Stitzer, 2004). The positive results with high-magnitude or long-duration CM help support the argument that voucher-based CM can almost always be efficacious, but these are not practical adjustments to a treatment whose primary drawback is usually said to be its cost.

In other studies showing positive results of an all-or-nothing contingency, participants tended to be using benzodiazepines rather than cocaine (Chutuape, Silverman, & Stitzer, 1999a; Iguchi, Stitzer, Bigelow, & Liebson, 1988). However, even this does not seem sufficient to guarantee response to such a contingency (Stitzer et al., 1992).

One alternative to the all-or-nothing contingency, still being explored, is to reinforce abstinence from multiple drugs on independent schedules so that patients who use one targeted drug will still have an incentive to abstain from the others. This approach was used in a study of prize-based reinforcement mentioned earlier, with equivocal results (Petry & Martin,

2002). Another successful approach was to combine reinforcement with take-home doses targeted to simultaneous cocaine and heroin abstinence and high-magnitude vouchers targeted to cocaine abstinence; opiate and cocaine abstinence increases were more robust and longer lasting than usual care or the take-home contingency alone (Silverman et al., 2004). Preliminary data from our clinic suggest that reinforcement of multiple-drug abstinence on independent schedules requires an increase in total overall magnitude of reinforcers (Epstein, Schmittner, Schroeder, & Preston, 2003).

PREDICTORS OF EFFECTIVENESS
OF CM IN OPIATE-DEPENDENT PATIENTS

Patient Characteristics

The general principle that past behavior predicts future behavior encounters no exception in CM. To our knowledge, the only robust predictor of responsiveness to CM is the degree of drug use at baseline (Preston et al., 1998; Stitzer et al., 1992). Specifically, we found that responsiveness to cocaine-targeted CM was predicted by cocaine abstinence toward the end of a 5-week baseline phase immediately preceding the intervention (Preston et al., 1998). We speculate that this reflects a preparatory reduction in use.

Intervention Characteristics

In a direct comparison of two different methadone doses, we found that random assignment to a methadone dose increase from 50 to 70 mg/day produced benefits complementing those of opiate-targeted CM: The dose increase enhanced overall abstinence while CM specifically enhanced continuous abstinence (Preston et al., 2000).

A broader range of intervention characteristics has been examined in two recent meta-analyses. In a meta-analytic review of CM in outpatient methadone treatment, combining data from 30 studies with a total of 1,569 participants, Griffith, Rowan-Szal, Roark, and Simpson (2000) found an overall effect size for CM, expressed as a Pearson r, of .25 (small–medium). Lussier et al. (2006) examined voucher-based reinforcement therapy in a meta-analysis of 30 studies conducted in either agonist-maintenance or drug-free settings; they found a similar estimated average effect size (r) of .32. Other significant intervention characteristics demonstrated in either or both meta-analyses were more rapid delivery of the reinforcer, more frequent urine screening, longer duration of treatment, higher methadone dosage, single (vs. multiple) drug targets, and higher incentive values.

IMPLEMENTATION OF CM IN NONRESEARCH CLINICS

The distal aim of nearly every study cited here is to move CM from research clinics to community clinics. One step toward doing so is to understand the current barriers.

A Technical Barrier: Monitoring Opiate Use

Unlike some other commonly abused drugs, such as cocaine, opiates are a diverse class of compounds that produce similar pharmacological effects and substitute for one another in dependent individuals. For example, the synthetic compound methadone and the naturally occurring compound morphine produce effects that are practically indistinguishable, yet they have few chemical similarities. Opioids also vary in potency and usual route of administration. This diversity of chemical entities and potency presents a challenge in opiate-targeted CM because it complicates detection of drug use. Fortunately, the drug-testing industry has developed a wide range of urine screen products that are generally up to the task (Katz & Fanciullo, 2002).

The most practical and commonly used assays in opiate-targeted CM are immunoassays. Immunoassay products range from automated, high-volume systems capable of semiquantitative measurements (such as enzyme-multiplied immunoassay technique [EMIT] and fluorescence polarization immunoassay [FPIA]) to single-use dipstick-type tests (such as the OnTrak) that require almost no equipment and nearly anyone can be trained to perform. Immunoassays do, however, have some weaknesses. Each is sensitive to only a subset of substances. Different immunoassays vary in their sensitivities to frequently targeted analytes such as morphine and codeine, and performance can change when antibody lots are changed (Cone, Dickerson, Paul, & Mitchell, 1992). The EMIT assay for morphine has poor cross-reactivity with oxycodone (Oxycontin) and oxymorphone (Numorphan) (Cone et al., 1992), opiates commonly found on the black market; these drugs may not be detected in standard screens (Von Seggern, Fitzgerald, Adelman, & Adelman, 2004). Potent drugs, such as buprenorphine, can be particularly difficult to detect because of the low concentrations present in urine. Fortunately, assays for buprenorphine have recently been developed (Cirimele, Etienne, Villain, Ludes, & Kintz, 2004). Because most clinics do not conduct the multiple tests that would be necessary to detect all opiates, patients can avoid detection by switching to an opiate that is not readily picked by the particular assay used by their treatment clinic, and those on methadone maintenance can use street methadone in place of heroin, as urine screens cannot distinguish between licit and illicit methadone.

There is also error inherent in testing. Ferrara et al. (1994) have calculated the rate of false negatives and false positives (respectively) at 8.4 and 2.2% for EMIT and 4.9 and 6.2% for OnTrak. Food (e.g., poppyseeds), other drugs, and some medical conditions can produce false positives (elSohly, elSohly, & Stanford, 1990; Fucci, 2005; Lancelin, Kraoul, Flatischler, Brovedani-Rousset, & Piketty, 2005). At the onset of abstinence, excretion of opiates can take more than a week, with fluctuations above and below cutoff concentrations (Taracha, Habrat, Chmielewska, & Baran-Furga, 2005).

Failure to detect opiate use can result in inadvertent reinforcement of the wrong behaviors while false positives can cause inappropriate withholding of incentives. Any technical problem that reduces the systematic relationship between behaviors and consequences is likely to reduce the effectiveness of CM.

Other Barriers

The most obvious barriers to widespread implementation of CM are financial. Onsite analysis of urine specimens two or three times per week is exceedingly rare in community methadone clinics (Calsyn, Saxon, & Barndt, 1991). Perhaps this problem can be addressed by targeting behaviors that can be verified without urine testing (Iguchi et al., 1997).

Another barrier is the ability to provide reinforcers. Financial barriers to voucher-based or prize-based CM have been discussed elsewhere, and some promising responses have been tested (Amass & Kamien, 2004). Perhaps less often appreciated is the fact that take-home incentives, which cost relatively little, are limited by federal regulation: In community methadone clinics, take-homes can be given only once weekly for the first 90 days of treatment, twice weekly for the next 90 days, and thrice weekly for the 90 days after that (Certification of Opioid Treatment Programs, 2006). States may impose additional restrictions. Such restrictions would obviously hamper clinics' ability to enact escalating schedules of reinforcement for the patients who may be most in need of an intervention.

In some cases, clinic staff may have considerable interest in imposing contingencies, but their preferred contingencies may involve response requirements already shown to be too strict. Careful compromise on such points was needed when CM was implemented in the National Institute on Drug Abuse's Clinical Trials Network (Petry & Simcic, 2002).

Finally, the culture of a community clinic is not that of a behavioral science laboratory; systematic implementation of contingencies is rarely a priority. In the above-cited survey of 324 methadone clinics, the use of urine data varied widely. Almost all clinics responded to drug-positive specimens with more counseling (despite prior findings that this has negligible impact on drug use) and revocation of take-home privileges. Other responses included increases in the frequency of urine collection, methadone dose changes (usually increases, but often decreases, perhaps depending which drug was detected), group therapy, eventual discharge, or contingency contracting (but it was not possible to determine how often or how systematically this was done) (Calsyn et al., 1991). It was difficult to determine from these survey results whether any of the clinics had established a system wherein patients' behaviors were quickly, consistently linked to predictable consequences.

A newer study suggests that such systems are rare (Willenbring, Hagedorn, Postier, & Kenny, 2004). Nine opiate-agonist clinics (with a total of 1,179 patients) were chosen to be representative of all 34 clinics in the U.S. Veterans Health Administration. The authors found that only one of the nine clinics had CM policies consistent with evidence-based guidelines. The other eight clinics used take-home doses as incentives but applied them under less than optimal conditions: difficult target behaviors (typically including 90 days of abstinence from all illicit substances); goals that were often unclear to patients; delayed reinforcer delivery (due to the requirement for 90 days of abstinence); and requiring that patients themselves monitor their own performance and request the incentives they earned.

CONCLUDING COMMENTS

CM is an effective adjuvant to pharmacological treatment for opioid dependence, reducing both ongoing opioid use and concurrent use of other drugs. For CM researchers, the task that lies ahead is not only to continue increasing the amount of abstinence that can be elicited with a given amount of testing and reinforcement, but also to bring to community clinics a culture in which our findings can and will be used.

REFERENCES

Amass, L., & Kamien, J. (2004). A tale of two cities: Financing two voucher programs for substance abusers through community donations. *Experimental and Clinical Psychopharmacology, 12*(2), 147–155.

Ball, J. C., & Ross, A. (1991). *The effectiveness of methadone maintenance treatment: Patients, programs, services, and outcomes.* New York: Springer-Verlag.

Bickel, W. K., Amass, L., Higgins, S. T., Badger, G. J., & Esch, R. A. (1997). Effects of adding behavioral treatment to opioid detoxification with buprenorphine. *Journal of Consulting and Clinical Psychology, 65*(5), 803–810.

Bickel, W. K., Rizzuto, P., Zielony, R. D., Klobas, J., Pangiosonlis, P., Mernit, R., et al. (1988). Combined behavioral and pharmacological treatment of alcoholic methadone patients. *Journal of Substance Abuse, 1*(2), 161–171.

Calsyn, D. A., & Saxon, A. J. (1999). An innovative approach to reducing cannabis use in a subset of methadone maintenance clients. *Drug and Alcohol Dependence, 53*(2), 167–169.

Calsyn, D. A., Saxon, A. J., & Barndt, D. C. (1991). Urine screening practices in methadone maintenance clinics: A survey of how the results are used. *Journal of Nervous and Mental Disease, 179*(4), 222–227.

Calsyn, D. A., Wells, E. A., Saxon, A. J., Jackson, T. R., Wrede, A. F., Stanton, V., et al. (1994). Contingency management of urinalysis results and intensity of counseling services have an interactive impact on methadone maintenance treatment outcome. *Journal of Addictive Diseases, 13*(3), 47–63.

Carroll, K. M., Ball, S. A., Nich, C., O'Connor, P. G., Eagan, D. A., Frankforter, T. L., et al. (2001). Targeting behavioral therapies to enhance naltrexone treatment of opioid dependence: Efficacy of contingency management and significant other involvement. *Archives of General Psychiatry, 58*(8), 755–761.

Carroll, K. M., Sinha, R., Nich, C., Babuscio, T., & Rounsaville, B. J. (2002). Contingency management to enhance naltrexone treatment of opioid dependence: A randomized clinical trial of reinforcement magnitude. *Experimental and Clinical Psychopharmacology, 10*(1), 54–63.

Certification of Opioid Treatment Programs. (2006). 42 C.F.R § 8.

Chutuape, M. A., Silverman, K., & Stitzer, M. L. (1998). Survey assessment of methadone treatment services as reinforcers. *American Journal of Drug and Alcohol Abuse, 24*(1), 1–16.

Chutuape, M. A., Silverman, K., & Stitzer, M. L. (1999a). Contingent reinforcement sustains post-detoxification abstinence from multiple drugs: A preliminary study with methadone patients. *Drug and Alcohol Dependence, 54*(1), 69–81.

Chutuape, M. A., Silverman, K., & Stitzer, M. L. (1999b). Use of methadone take-home contingencies with persistent opiate and cocaine abusers. *Journal of Substance Abuse Treatment, 16*(1), 23–30.

Cirimele, V., Etienne, S., Villain, M., Ludes, B., & Kintz, P. (2004). Evaluation of the One-Step ELISA kit for the detection of buprenorphine in urine, blood, and hair specimens. *Forensic Science International, 143*(2–3), 153–156.

Cone, E. J., Dickerson, S., Paul, B. D., & Mitchell, J. M. (1992). Forensic drug testing for opiates. IV. Analytical sensitivity, specificity, and accuracy of commercial urine opiate immunoassays. *Journal of Analytical Toxicology, 16*(2), 72–78.

Dallery, J., Silverman, K., Chutuape, M. A., Bigelow, G. E., & Stitzer, M. L. (2001). Voucher-based reinforcement of opiate plus cocaine abstinence in treatment-resistant methadone patients: Effects of reinforcer magnitude. *Experimental and Clinical Psychopharmacology, 9*(3), 317–325.

Donny, E. C., Walsh, S. L., Bigelow, G. E., Eissenberg, T., & Stitzer, M. L. (2002). High-dose methadone produces superior opioid blockade and comparable withdrawal suppression to lower doses in opioid-dependent humans. *Psychopharmacology, 161*(2), 202–212.

Downey, K. K., Helmus, T. C., & Schuster, C. R. (2000). Treatment of heroin-dependent poly-drug abusers with contingency management and buprenorphine maintenance. *Experimental and Clinical Psychopharmacology, 8*(2), 176–184.

Elk, R., Grabowski, J., Rhoades, H., Spiga, R., Schmitz, J., & Jennings, W. (1993). Compliance with tuberculosis treatment in methadone-maintained patients: Behavioral interventions. *Journal of Substance Abuse Treatment, 10*(4), 371–382.

elSohly, H. N., elSohly, M. A., & Stanford, D. F. (1990). Poppy seed ingestion and opiates urinalysis: A closer look. *Journal of Analytical Toxicology, 14*(5), 308–310.

Epstein, D. H., Hawkins, W., Covi, L., & Preston, K. L. (2003). Cognitive-behavioral therapy plus contingency management for cocaine use: Findings during treatment and across 12–month follow-up. *Psychology of Addictive Behaviors, 17*(1), 73–82.

Epstein, D. H., Schmittner, J., Schroeder, J. R., & Preston, K. L. (2003). *Promoting simultaneous abstinence from cocaine and heroin with a methadone dose increase and a novel contingency.* Paper presented at the 65th annual scientific meeting of the College on Problems of Drug Dependence, Bal Harbour, FL.

Ferrara, S. D., Tedeschi, L., Frison, G., Brusini, G., Castagna, F., Bernardelli, B., et al. (1994). Drugs-of-abuse testing in urine: Statistical approach and experimental comparison of immunochemical and chromatographic techniques. *Journal of Analytical Toxicology, 18*(5), 278–291.

Fucci, N. (2005). EMIT dau: Methadone false positive with creatinine interference. *Forensic Science International, 148*(1), 81.

Greenstein, R. A., Fudala, P. J., & O'Brien, C. P. (1997). Alternative pharmacotherapies for opiate addiction. In J. H. Lowinsohn, P. Ruiz, R. B. Millman, & J. G. Langrod (Eds.), *Comprehensive textbook of substance abuse* (3rd ed., pp. 415–425). New York: Williams & Wilkins.

Griffith, J. D., Rowan-Szal, G. A., Roark, R. R., & Simpson, D. D. (2000). Contingency management in outpatient methadone treatment: A meta-analysis. *Drug and Alcohol Dependence, 58*(1–2), 55–66.

Gruber, K., Chutuape, M. A., & Stitzer, M. L. (2000). Reinforcement-based intensive outpatient treatment for inner city opiate abusers: A short-term evaluation. *Drug and Alcohol Dependence, 57*(3), 211–223.

Higgins, S. T., Budney, A. J., Bickel, W. K., Hughes, J. R., Foerg, F., & Badger, G. (1993). Achieving cocaine abstinence with a behavioral approach. *American Journal of Psychiatry, 150*(5), 763–769.

Higgins, S. T., Delaney, D. D., Budney, A. J., Bickel, W. K., Hughes, J. R., Foerg, F., et al. (1991). A behavioral approach to achieving initial cocaine abstinence. *American Journal of Psychiatry, 148*(9), 1218–1224.

Higgins, S. T., Stitzer, M. L., Bigelow, G. E., & Liebson, I. A. (1986). Contingent methadone delivery: Effects on illicit-opiate use. *Drug and Alcohol Dependence, 17*(4), 311–322.

Iguchi, M. Y., Belding, M. A., Morral, A. R., Lamb, R. J., & Husband, S. D. (1997). Reinforcing operants other than abstinence in drug abuse treatment: An effective alternative for reducing drug use. *Journal of Consulting and Clinical Psychology, 65*(3), 421–428.

Iguchi, M. Y., Lamb, R. J., Belding, M. A., Platt, J. J., Husband, S. D., & Morral, A. R. (1996). Contingent reinforcement of group participation versus abstinence in a methadone maintenance program. *Experimental and Clinical Psychopharmacology, 4*(3), 315–321.

Iguchi, M. Y., Stitzer, M. L., Bigelow, G. E., & Liebson, I. A. (1988). Contingency management in methadone maintenance: Effects of reinforcing and aversive consequences on illicit polydrug use. *Drug and Alcohol Dependence, 22*(1–2), 1–7.

Jones, H. E., Haug, N., Silverman, K., Stitzer, M. L., & Svikis, D. (2001). The effectiveness of incentives in enhancing treatment attendance and drug abstinence in methadone-maintained pregnant women. *Drug and Alcohol Dependence, 61*(3), 297–306.

Jones, H. E., Wong, C. J., Tuten, M., & Stitzer, M. L. (2005). Reinforcement-based therapy: 12–month evaluation of an outpatient drug-free treatment for heroin abusers. *Drug and Alcohol Dependence, 79*(2), 119–128.

Katz, E. C., Chutuape, M. A., Jones, H. E., & Stitzer, M. L. (2002). Voucher reinforcement for heroin and cocaine abstinence in an outpatient drug-free program. *Experimental and Clinical Psychopharmacology, 10*(2), 136–143.

Katz, E. C., Gruber, K., Chutuape, M. A., & Stitzer, M. L. (2001). Reinforcement-based outpatient treatment for opiate and cocaine abusers. *Journal of Substance Abuse Treatment, 20*(1), 93–98.

Katz, E. C., Robles-Sotelo, E., Correia, C. J., Silverman, K., Stitzer, M. L., & Bigelow, G. (2002). The brief abstinence test: Effects of continued incentive availability on cocaine abstinence. *Experimental and Clinical Psychopharmacology, 10*(1), 10–17.

Katz, N., & Fanciullo, G. J. (2002). Role of urine toxicology testing in the management of chronic opioid therapy. *Clinical Journal of Pain, 18*(4 Suppl.), S76–S82.

Kidorf, M., & Stitzer, M. L. (1999). Contingent access to clinic privileges reduces drug abuse in methadone maintenance patients. In S. T. Higgins & K. Silverman (Eds.), *Motivating behavior change among illicit-drug abusers* (pp. 221–241). Washington, DC: American Psychological Association.

Kornor, H., & Waal, H. (2005). From opioid maintenance to abstinence: A literature review. *Drug and Alcohol Review, 24*(3), 267–274.

Kosten, T., Oliveto, A., Feingold, A., Poling, J., Sevarino, K., McCance-Katz, E., et al. (2003). Desipramine and contingency management for cocaine and opiate dependence in buprenorphine maintained patients. *Drug and Alcohol Dependence, 70*(3), 315–325.

Lancelin, F., Kraoul, L., Flatischler, N., Brovedani-Rousset, S., & Piketty, M. L. (2005). False-positive results in the detection of methadone in urines of patients treated with psychotropic substances. *Clinical Chemistry, 51*(11), 2176–2177.

Liebson, I. A., Bigelow, G. E., & Flamer, R. (1973). Alcoholism among methadone patients: A specific treatment method. *American Journal of Psychiatry, 130*(4), 483–485.

Liebson, I. A., Tommasello, A., & Bigelow, G. E. (1978). A behavioral treatment of alcoholic methadone patients. *Annals of Internal Medicine, 89*(3), 342–344.

Lussier, J. P., Heil, S. H., Mongeon, J. A., Badger, G. J., & Higgins, S. T. (2006). A metaanalysis of voucher-based reinforcement therapy for substance use disorders. *Addiction, 101*(2), 192–203.

Magura, S., Casriel, C., Goldsmith, D. S., Strug, D. L., & Lipton, D. S. (1988). Contingency contracting with polydrug-abusing methadone patients. *Addictive Behaviors, 13*(1), 113–118.

McCaul, M. E., Stitzer, M. L., Bigelow, G. E., & Liebson, I. A. (1984). Contingency management interventions: Effects on treatment outcome during methadone detoxification. *Journal of Applied Behavior Analysis, 17*(1), 35–43.

Meyer, R., & Mirin, S. (1979). Community outcome on narcotic antagonists. In R. Meyer & S. Mirin (Eds.), *The heroin stimulus: Implications for a theory of addictions* (pp. 215–230). New York: Plenum Medical.

Milby, J. B., Garrett, C., English, C., Fritschi, O., & Clarke, C. (1978). Take-home methadone: Contingency effects on drug-seeking and productivity of narcotic addicts. *Addictive Behaviors, 3*(3–4), 215–220.

Milby, J. B., Gurwitch, R. H., Wiebe, D. J., Ling, W., McLellan, A. T., & Woody, G. E. (1986). Prevalence and diagnostic reliability of methadone maintenance detoxification fear. *American Journal of Psychiatry, 143*(6), 739–743.

O'Brien, C. P., & Lynch, K. G. (2003). Can we design and replicate clinical trials with a multiple drug focus? *Drug and Alcohol Dependence, 70*(2), 135–137.

Oliveto, A., Poling, J., Sevarino, K. A., Gonsai, K. R., McCance-Katz, E. F., Stine, S. M., et al. (2005). Efficacy of dose and contingency management procedures in LAAM-maintained cocaine-dependent patients. *Drug and Alcohol Dependence, 79*(2), 157–165.

Petry, N. M., & Martin, B. (2002). Low-cost contingency management for treating cocaine- and opioid-abusing methadone patients. *Journal of Consulting and Clinical Psychology, 70*(2), 398–405.

Petry, N. M., Martin, B., & Simcic, F., Jr. (2005). Prize reinforcement contingency management for cocaine dependence: Integration with group therapy in a methadone clinic. *Journal of Consulting and Clinical Psychology, 73*(2), 354–359.

Petry, N. M., & Simcic, F., Jr. (2002). Recent advances in the dissemination of contingency management techniques: Clinical and research perspectives. *Journal of Substance Abuse Treatment, 23*(2), 81–86.

Piotrowski, N. A., Tusel, D. J., Sees, K. L., Reilly, P. M., Banys, P., Meek, P., et al. (1999). Contingency contracting with monetary reinforcers for abstinence from multiple drugs in a methadone program. *Experimental and Clinical Psychopharmacology, 7*(4), 399–411.

Preston, K. L., Silverman, K., Higgins, S. T., Brooner, R. K., Montoya, I., Schuster, C. R., et al. (1998). Cocaine use early in treatment predicts outcome in a behavioral treatment program. *Journal of Consulting and Clinical Psychology, 66*(4), 691–696.

Preston, K. L., Silverman, K., Umbricht, A., DeJesus, A., Montoya, I. D., & Schuster, C. R. (1999). Improvement in naltrexone treatment compliance with contingency management. *Drug and Alcohol Dependence, 54*(2), 127–135.

Preston, K. L., Umbricht, A., & Epstein, D. H. (2000). Methadone dose increase and abstinence reinforcement for treatment of continued heroin use during methadone maintenance. *Archives of General Psychiatry, 57*(4), 395–404.

Preston, K. L., Umbricht, A., & Epstein, D. H. (2002). Abstinence reinforcement maintenance contingency and one-year follow-up. *Drug and Alcohol Dependence, 67*(2), 125–137.

Rawson, R. A., Huber, A., McCann, M., Shoptaw, S., Farabee, D., Reiber, C., et al. (2002). A comparison of contingency management and cognitive-behavioral approaches during methadone maintenance treatment for cocaine dependence. *Archives of General Psychiatry, 59*(9), 817–824.

Robles, E., Silverman, K., Preston, K. L., Cone, E. J., Katz, E., Bigelow, G. E., et al. (2000). The brief abstinence test: Voucher-based reinforcement of cocaine abstinence. *Drug and Alcohol Dependence, 58*(1–2), 205–212.

Robles, E., Stitzer, M. L., Strain, E. C., Bigelow, G. E., & Silverman, K. (2002). Voucher-based reinforcement of opiate abstinence during methadone detoxification. *Drug and Alcohol Dependence, 65*(2), 179–189.

Rounsaville, B. J., Petry, N. M., & Carroll, K. M. (2003). Single versus multiple drug focus in substance abuse clinical trials research. *Drug and Alcohol Dependence, 70*(2), 117–125.

Rowan-Szal, G., Joe, G. W., Chatham, L. R., & Simpson, D. D. (1994). A simple reinforcement system for methadone clients in a community-based treatment program. *Journal of Substance Abuse Treatment, 11*(3), 217–223.

Saxon, A. J., Calsyn, D. A., Wells, E. A., & Stanton, V. V. (1998). The use of urine toxicology to enhance patient control of take-home doses in methadone maintenance: Effects on reducing illicit drug use. *Addiction Research, 6*(3), 203–214.

Schmitz, J. M., Rhoades, H. M., Elk, R., Creson, D., Hussein, I., & Grabowski, J. (1998). Medication take-home doses and contingency management. *Experimental and Clinical Psychopharmacology, 6*(2), 162–168.

Schmitz, J. M., Rhoades, H., & Grabowski, J. (1995). Contingent reinforcement for reduced carbon monoxide levels in methadone maintenance patients. *Addictive Behaviors, 20*(2), 171–179.

Schottenfeld, R. S., Chawarski, M. C., Pakes, J. R., Pantalon, M. V., Carroll, K. M., & Kosten, T. R. (2005). Methadone versus buprenorphine with contingency management or performance feedback for cocaine and opioid dependence. *American Journal of Psychiatry, 162*(2), 340–349.

Shoptaw, S., Jarvik, M. E., Ling, W., & Rawson, R. A. (1996). Contingency management for tobacco smoking in methadone-maintained opiate addicts. *Addictive Behaviors, 21*(3), 409–412.

Shoptaw, S., Rotheram-Fuller, E., Yang, X., Frosch, D., Nahom, D., Jarvik, M. E., et al. (2002). Smoking cessation in methadone maintenance. *Addiction, 97*(10), 1317–1328.

Silverman, K., Chutuape, M. A., Bigelow, G. E., & Stitzer, M. L. (1999). Voucher-based reinforcement of cocaine abstinence in treatment-resistant methadone patients: Effects of reinforcement magnitude. *Psychopharmacology, 146*(2), 128–138.

Silverman, K., Higgins, S. T., Brooner, R. K., Montoya, I. D., Cone, E. J., Schuster, C. R., et al. (1996). Sustained cocaine abstinence in methadone maintenance patients through voucher-based reinforcement therapy. *Archives of General Psychiatry, 53*(5), 409–415.

Silverman, K., Robles, E., Mudric, T., Bigelow, G. E., & Stitzer, M. L. (2004). A randomized trial of long-term reinforcement of cocaine abstinence in methadone-maintained patients who inject drugs. *Journal of Consulting and Clinical Psychology, 72*(5), 839–854.

Silverman, K., Svikis, D., Robles, E., Stitzer, M. L., & Bigelow, G. E. (2001). A reinforcement-based therapeutic workplace for the treatment of drug abuse: Six-month abstinence outcomes. *Experimental and Clinical Psychopharmacology, 9*(1), 14–23.

Silverman, K., Wong, C. J., Higgins, S. T., Brooner, R. K., Montoya, I. D., Contoreggi, C., et al. (1996). Increasing opiate abstinence through voucher-based reinforcement therapy. *Drug and Alcohol Dependence, 41*(2), 157–165.

Silverman, K., Wong, C. J., Umbricht-Schneiter, A., Montoya, I. D., Schuster, C. R., & Preston, K. L. (1998). Broad beneficial effects of cocaine abstinence reinforcement among methadone patients. *Journal of Consulting and Clinical Psychology, 66*(5), 811–824.

Stitzer, M. L., Bigelow, G. E., Lawrence, C., Cohen, J., D'Lugoff, B., & Hawthorne, J. (1977). Medication take-home as a reinforcer in a methadone maintenance program. *Addictive Behaviors, 2*(1), 9–14.

Stitzer, M. L., Bigelow, G. E., & Liebson, I. A. (1979). Reinforcement of drug abstinence: A behavioral approach to drug abuse treatment. *NIDA Research Monograph, 25*, 68–90.

Stitzer, M. L., Bigelow, G. E., & Liebson, I. A. (1980). Reducing drug use among methadone maintenance clients: Contingent reinforcement for morphine-free urines. *Addictive Behaviors, 5*(4), 333–340.

Stitzer, M. L., Bigelow, G. E., Liebson, I. A., & McCaul, M. E. (1984). Contingency management of supplemental drug use during methadone maintenance treatment. *NIDA Research Monograph, 46*, 84–103.

Stitzer, M. L., Iguchi, M. Y., & Felch, L. J. (1992). Contingent take-home incentive: Effects on drug use of methadone maintenance patients. *Journal of Consulting and Clinical Psychology, 60*(6), 927–934.

Strain, E. C. (2003). Single versus multiple drug focus in substance abuse clinical trials research: The devil is in the details. *Drug and Alcohol Dependence, 70*(2), 131–134.

Taracha, E., Habrat, B., Chmielewska, K., & Baran-Furga, H. (2005). Excretion profile of opiates in dependent patients in relation to route of administration and type of drug measured in urine with immunoassay. *Journal of Analytical Toxicology, 29*(1), 15–21.

Von Seggern, R. L., Fitzgerald, C. P., Adelman, L. C., & Adelman, J. U. (2004). Laboratory monitoring of OxyContin (oxycodone): Clinical pitfalls. *Headache, 44*(1), 44–47.

Willenbring, M. L., Hagedorn, H. J., Postier, A. C., & Kenny, M. (2004). Variations in evidence-based clinical practices in nine United States Veterans Administration opioid agonist therapy clinics. *Drug and Alcohol Dependence, 75*(1), 97–106.

CHAPTER 4

MARIJUANA

Alan J. Budney *and* Catherine Stanger

THE CANNABIS PROBLEM

Cannabis remains the most widely used illicit drug among adults and adolescents in the United States, Australia, and numerous European countries (European Monitoring Center for Drugs and Drug Addiction, 2003; Hall, Johnston, & Donnelly, 1999; Substance Abuse and Mental Health Services Administration [SAMHSA], 2003a). An estimated 14.6 million people in the United States are current (past month) cannabis users (SAMHSA, 2005a). Recent estimates of adolescent cannabis use indicate that 6%, 16%, and 20% of 8th-, 10th-, and 12th-graders, respectively, used cannabis during the previous month (Johnston, O'Malley, Bachman, & Schulenberg, 2005). Although some may consider cannabis a "soft drug" with few consequences associated with its use, regular cannabis use has been linked to impairment in cognitive functioning, motivation, health, employment, and psychiatric functioning (Kalant, Corrigall, Hall, & Smart, 1999; Kandel, 1984) Regular use among adolescents is associated with greater risk of experiencing delinquency, school failure, and health and psychological problems (Dennis, Godley, & Titus, 1999).

Lifetime and past-year prevalence of cannabis disorder (abuse or dependence) far exceed that of any other illicit substance use disorder (Compton, Conway, Sinson, Colliver, & Grant, 2005). Rates of conditional dependence (i.e., the risk of developing dependence among those who have used the drug) suggest that the "dependence potential" of cannabis is substantial (9%), albeit lower than alcohol (15%), cocaine (17%), or heroin (23%) (Anthony, Warner, & Kessler, 1994). More frequent use results in greater risk for dependence, with some estimates indicating that the rate of dependence is 20–30% among those using at least five times (Hall et al., 1999).

Most relevant to this chapter, those who develop cannabis-related problems do enroll in treatment. In the United States and Australia, treatment admissions for cannabis increased since the early 1990s such that they occur at a rate comparable with admissions for cocaine and heroin (SAMHSA, 2005b; Torres, Mattik, Chen, & Baillie, 1995). Note that individuals under the age of 20 comprise about 45% of all cannabis-related admissions. The severity and specificity of the problems have been well documented. The great majority of adult patients have been using cannabis for over 10 years, use marijuana on a daily basis, use multiple times per day, clearly meet DSM-dependence criteria, report experiencing withdrawal symptoms and repeated unsuccessful attempts to stop using, and perceive themselves as unable to quit (Budney, Hughes, Moore, & Vandrey, 2004; Budney, Moore, Higgins, & Rocha, 2006; Stephens, Babor, Kadden, Miller, & Marijuana Treatment Project Research Group, 2002) The most common marijuana-related consequences reported are feeling bad/guilty, procrastination, low productivity, low self-confidence, interpersonal/family problems, memory problems, and financial difficulties.

During the past 12 years, a handful of clinical trials targeting cannabis abuse and dependence suggest that treatment efficacy appears comparable to that observed with other substance-dependence disorders (McRae, Budney, & Brady, 2003). Cognitive-behavioral and motivational interventions such as relapse prevention, behavioral coping-skills therapy, and motivational enhancement therapy appear efficacious. However, many participants who enroll in these treatments do not have positive outcomes. That is, many never achieve abstinence or substantial reductions in cannabis use, and many of those who are initially successful relapse. Thus, as with treatments for all types of substance dependence, the development and testing of more potent interventions remain a priority.

WHY CONTINGENCY MANAGEMENT FOR CANNABIS DEPENDENCE?

Because contingency management (CM) interventions represent a treatment approach with great potential to effectively motivate and facilitate change, it may be particularly useful for treating individuals for cannabis abuse or dependence, as their motivation to change their cannabis use may not be as great as those seeking treatment for other types of drug abuse (Budney, Radonovich, Higgins, & Wong, 1998). Perhaps because cannabis abusers do not typically experience the type of acute crises or severity of consequences that often drive alcohol-, cocaine-, or heroin-dependent individuals into treatment, their motivation and commitment to change may be more capricious than that of persons seeking treatment for other types of substance problems. CM interventions targeting abstinence from cannabis might enhance motivation to initiate abstinence and facilitate sustained efforts not to use.

ABSTINENCE-BASED VOUCHERS FOR CANNABIS DEPENDENCE

Borrowing from the CM model developed for treatment of cocaine dependence (Higgins, Heil, Rogers, & Chivers, Chapter 2, this volume; Higgins et al., 1991), we sought to develop an abstinence-based voucher program that could increase rates of initial abstinence among adults seeking treatment for cannabis dependence. The basic concept behind this CM intervention is to reinforce documented abstinence by providing monetary-based vouchers that can be used to increase participation in alternative healthy-lifestyle activities. We describe this CM procedure for cannabis dependence here, highlighting the modifications to the original voucher program for cocaine dependence.

Objective Measure of Abstinence (Urine Toxicology)

Urinalysis testing provides the usual and typically best method for obtaining the documented evidence needed to effectively administer a CM program targeting drug abstinence. With cannabis, such testing poses some unique issues that deserve comment. First, regular, heavy cannabis users are likely to test positive for cannabis use for 1–3 weeks after cessation at detection levels of 50 or 100 ng/ml, which are the accepted cutoff levels for documenting recent abstinence. Thus, in our voucher program for cannabis, we provide a 2-week notice prior to initiating the voucher program that informs clients that it will take 2 weeks of abstinence from cannabis for them to achieve a cannabis-negative urinalysis result. Thus, reinforcement for abstinence must be delayed. Note that some clinical agencies and researchers have begun to use quantitative or semiquantitative testing for cannabinoid levels as a means to differentiate abstinence from residual cannabinoids. These methods could potentially reduce the need for delaying reinforcement. However, the accuracy of these procedures depends heavily on more frequent testing in the early weeks of abstinence and can be much costlier than the qualitative tests that rely on standardized cutoffs.

A second related concern much less frequently encountered is the possibility that a participant can provide a urine specimen that is negative for cannabis use on one day and then positive for cannabis the next day. This may occur because cannabinoid metabolites are stored in the fat cells and the rate of their release can vary depending on things such as exercise. We have observed this only a handful of times, but it is worth noting. A third concern is that urinary cannabinoid levels are affected by the dilution factor of the urine specimen provided. Many clients either intentionally or inadvertently drink large quantities of liquid that dilute a urine specimen such that a false-negative test result is obtained. If possible, a method to screen for diluted urine specimens should be used as part of the urine-toxicology program. Measurement of creatinine is one method to objectively test for the dilution factor.

Notwithstanding these issues, the methods to detect recent cannabis use described here have been used effectively and without substantial problems in multiple clinical trials. A comprehensive understanding of the urine-toxicology process can facilitate implementation of an effective program.

Voucher Schedule

Our voucher schedule designed for cannabis abstinence does not commence until the third week of treatment because of the aforementioned issue with the prolonged presence of cannabinoids in the urine. Therapists provide comprehensive information about the urine-toxicology program and the voucher system to help participants understand, accept, and comply with the program. During the 2 weeks prior to initiating the voucher program, participants are provided with a voucher ($5 value) each time they provide a valid urine specimen. This procedure serves multiple functions: (1) reinforces the provision of the urine specimen, (2) serves as a priming reinforcer to demonstrate what can be gained via the voucher program, and (3) reinforces abstinence in those who have already initiated cannabis abstinence.

A second modification involves the frequency of urine testing and therefore frequency of reinforcement delivery. We conduct urine tests and deliver vouchers on a twice-per-week rather than three-times-per-week schedule as had been used in the original voucher program for cocaine. Our decision to modify the schedule was twofold. First, we felt it was more practical for participants to make two rather than three visits to the clinic per week. Second, we were concerned that a single instance of cannabis use would carryover to multiple urine tests with the more frequent schedule. The twice-a-week schedule should be sufficient to detect most cannabis use without exacerbating the potential for carryovers. In summary, we believe that the practical advantages and reduction in the carryover problem gained with the twice-per-week schedule outweigh the potential benefits that might come from using a voucher delivery schedule that would reinforce abstinence more frequently.

Third, overall magnitude (value) of the reinforcement schedule used in our cannabis voucher programs was reduced by almost 50% compared with what had been used in the cocaine programs ($590 vs. $1,030 potential earnings over 12 weeks). Again, we felt it was more practical (less costly) to use lower-magnitude vouchers. Second, we thought that the use of lower-magnitude vouchers might be sufficient to effectively engender abstinence in cannabis-dependent adults. Although the lower magnitude turned out to be effective (Budney, Higgins, Radonovich, & Novy, 2000; Budney et al., 2006), we expect that using a higher-magnitude voucher program would further enhance the effects of the voucher program we have tested to date.

All other aspects of the voucher reinforcement schedule are similar to the original cocaine program. Table 4.1 illustrates the schedule. Voucher earnings escalate with each consecutive cannabis-negative specimen provided. A documented week of abstinence (two consecutive negative specimens) earns a $10 voucher bonus. Cannabis-positive specimens or missed specimens result in no voucher earnings, and the value of the next cannabis-negative specimen is reset to the amount that was provided for the first negative specimen. If following a cannabis-positive specimen, three consecutive negative specimens are provided, the value of the vouchers returns to the level achieved prior to the submission of the positive specimen. Each time participants provide a urine specimen negative for cannabis they are given a slip of paper (voucher) indicating current and cumulative earnings. Voucher earnings can then be redeemed at any time for retail goods or services chosen by the participant and agreed on by his or her therapist. Research staff make all purchases.

Implementation

Effective implementation of a voucher program requires a clear understanding of the rationale for the program, good communication with the participant, and awareness of and preparation for clinical issues that are critical to its success. We have discussed these factors in more detail elsewhere (Budney & Higgins, 1998; Budney, Sigmon, & Higgins, 2001). Here we briefly review a few important aspects of implementation.

Most clients are expecting individual or group counseling when they seek treatment for cannabis. Hence, therapists must foster understanding, interest, and compliance with a voucher program that is likely unfamiliar to clients, and which may give rise to skepticism or mistrust. For example, embracing urine testing as an essential element of the treatment process may foster resistance from many clients. Even therapists may be hesitant about the need for urine testing and how it may affect the client's willingness to participate. Similarly, the idea of "rewarding" abstinence will likely be novel and perplexing to all involved. Therapists and staff must also be

TABLE 4.1. Voucher Earnings Schedule for Cannabis Abstinence

	Test 1	Test 2	Bonus	Total
Weeks 1–2	(vouchers are provided independent of test results)			
	$5.00	$5.00	—	$10.00
	$5.00	$5.00	—	$10.00
Week 3	$1.50	$3.00	$10.00	$14.50
Week 4	$4.50	$6.00	$10.00	$20.50
Week 5	$7.50	$9.00	$10.00	$26.50
Week 6	$10.50	$12.00	$10.00	$32.50
Week 7	$13.50	$15.00	$10.00	$38.50
Week 8	$16.50	$18.00	$10.00	$44.50
Week 9	$19.50	$21.00	$10.00	$50.50
Week 10	$22.50	$24.00	$10.00	$56.50
Week 11	$25.50	$27.00	$10.00	$62.50
Week 12	$28.50	$30.00	$10.00	$68.50
Week 13	$31.50	$33.00	$10.00	$74.50
Week 14	$34.50	$36.00	$10.00	$80.50
Total				$590.00

Note. Voucher earnings for participants who provide all cannabis-negative urine specimens.

prepared to deal with issues such as the participant's denial of cannabis use in the face of a cannabis-positive urine test. Effective clinical responses to these types of issues are important for retention and advancement of treatment progress.

EFFICACY OF ABSTINENCE-BASED VOUCHERS

Cannabis-Dependent Adults

As discussed previously, cognitive-behavioral and motivational treatment approaches have demonstrated efficacy for cannabis abuse and dependence. However, as with treatments for other types of substance dependence, room remains for improved success rates. Two trials have now examined whether an abstinence-based voucher program can enhance cannabis-abstinence outcomes (Budney et al., 2000; Budney et al., 2006).

Trial 1

Three outpatient treatments were compared: a brief motivational therapy (M); brief motivational therapy combined with cognitive-behavioral coping-skills therapy (MBT); and a combination of the brief motivational therapy, the coping-skills therapy, and an abstinence-based voucher program (MBTV) (Budney et al., 2006). Sixty adults (43 men and 17 women) seeking treatment for cannabis dependence were randomly assigned to one of the three treatment conditions. All participants met DSM-III-R criteria for current cannabis dependence. Exclusion criteria included dependence on alcohol or any other drug except nicotine. Most participants used cannabis on an almost daily basis, smoked multiple times per day, and had been regular cannabis users for 10–15 years. Most participants were Caucasian (83%) with an average age of 32 (SD = 8.5) years.

All three treatments lasted 14 weeks and were manual driven. All participants provided urine specimens on a twice-weekly schedule throughout treatment. The M treatment was adapted from the motivational enhancement therapy used in the Project Match alcohol treatment study (Project Match Research Group, 1998). Participants received four individual motivational interviewing sessions spaced throughout the treatment period. The MBT treatment combined motivational enhancement therapy with an adapted version of the behavioral coping-skills therapy also used in Project Match. The coping-skills component involved once-weekly individual therapy sessions focused on increasing motivation, developing skills to help achieve and maintain cannabis abstinence, and setting lifestyle-change goals. The MBTV treatment integrated the abstinence-based voucher program described above with MBT. In addition to providing MBT, therapists regularly reviewed and discussed voucher earnings and purchases with the goal of using the vouchers to promote abstinence and to facilitate healthy-lifestyle-change goals.

Rates of treatment acceptability (attended more than one session) and treatment completion did not significantly differ across the three treatments. The primary treatment outcome variable was the longest period of documented continuous cannabis abstinence based on the urinalysis testing. Missing urinalysis specimens were considered positive for cannabis. The MBTV group achieved significantly longer periods of continuous cannabis abstinence (M = 4.8 ± 4.9 weeks) than the MBT (M = 2.3 ± 3.0 weeks) or M group (1.6 ± 2.4 weeks). A significantly greater percentage of participants in the MBTV group were able to achieve specific periods of cannabis abstinence (i.e., at least 4, 6, or 10 weeks) than in the MBT or M groups, and a greater percentage of MBTV participants were abstinent at the end of treatment (35% vs. 10% vs. 5%). No treatment group differences were detected on other drug use or psychosocial outcome measures. However, significant improvement from intake to treatment completion was noted within all groups on the self-reported days of cannabis use and multiple measures of psychosocial functioning.

This study clearly demonstrated that the addition of an abstinence-based voucher program to previously documented effective therapies enhanced abstinence during treatment for cannabis dependence. Of note, the specific effect of the voucher program was to increase continuous periods of abstinence, which was the hypothesized outcome based on the design of the reinforcement schedule.

Trial 2

Many unanswered questions emanated from this initial study. First, because the voucher component was integrated with MBT, we could not determine how MBT contributed to the effects of the voucher program. Second, we had no information on whether the voucher program is effective if delivered without MBT. Third, we did not know whether the positive effects of the voucher program would be maintained posttreatment. A second study was designed to address these issues (Budney et al., 2006).

Ninety cannabis-dependent adults (69 men, 21 women) with similar sociodemographics as in Trial 1 were enrolled in a randomized clinical trial comparing one of three treatments. MBTV was provided as in Trial 1. MBT was provided as in Trial 1 with one exception: Participants received a $5 voucher for each urine specimen provided (scheduled twice weekly) independent of the test results to encourage compliance with the monitoring program and help equate retention across groups. The third condition was vouchers alone (V). This involved the same abstinence-based voucher program delivered in the MBTV condition. An initial 20–30-minute meeting with a clinical research staff member provided the participant with the rationale for and details of the voucher program. The program was described as a method to enhance and maintain initial motivation to abstain from marijuana use by providing a structure (urine monitoring) and incentive (vouchers) for doing so. The details of the program were provided in a written abstinence contract discussed thoroughly with staff. V participants (as well as those in the other two conditions) received a guide-to-quitting pamphlet and information on local self-help groups. Contact with staff following this initial meeting was limited to twice-per-week urine-toxicology testing. At each visit, staff conducted a brief interview to assess for clinical crises and asked if the participant wanted to make a purchase with his or her voucher earnings.

Rates of treatment acceptability were again high (85%) and did not differ across the three treatments. This was an important finding as we were initially concerned that those offered V alone might reject the idea of not receiving some type of counseling. However, very few participants expressed disappointment when they received their assignment to V, and the rate of treatment retention did not differ between the treatment conditions.

Results observed during the abstinence period provided a partial replication of Trial 1. During the treatment period, MBTV engendered more abstinence than MBT, but the difference was not statistically significant. Interestingly, V alone clearly engendered longer periods of continuous abstinence than MBT. V also produced longer periods of abstinence than MBTV but not significantly so. A similar pattern of results was observed with a dichotomous measure of cannabis abstinence (i.e., percentage of participants who achieved specified periods of abstinence). These findings indicated a positive effect of vouchers on rates of initial abstinence and did not demonstrate an enhancement effect of adding MBT to the voucher program.

Posttreatment findings showed that the positive effects observed with MBTV during the active treatment period were maintained during the 12-month follow-up (i.e., MBTV engendered significantly greater posttreatment abstinence levels than MBT) (see Figure 4.1). Results also suggested that adding MBT to the vouchers enhanced posttreatment outcome. That is, MBTV evidenced a trend toward higher abstinence rates than V alone, despite V showing higher rates of abstinence during treatment. Abstinence rates for V alone and MBT did not differ during the follow-up period, suggesting that the positive effects of V alone in comparison with MBT did not maintain once treatment had ended. However, the "equivalence" of V and MBT across the posttreatment period also suggests that V alone is a viable treatment alternative that might be considered for adults seeking treatment for cannabis dependence.

In sum, these two studies suggest that the integration of V and MBT provided overall better abstinence outcomes over time than either intervention delivered alone. Findings from Trial 2 also suggest that the voucher program appears to be a potent intervention for engendering initial abstinence, even when delivered without any type of counseling services. The MBT component (motivational enhancement and coping-skills training) may be particularly beneficial for maintaining the positive effects of the vouchers. Note that a recent study by another research group found similar results in a more diverse (40% minority) and larger sample ($N = 240$) using a modified voucher program (Kadden, Litt, Kabela-Cormier, & Petry, 2007).

A few comments regarding the limitations of these studies are warranted. Other than abstinence outcomes, few outcome differences were observed between treatment groups. The clinical importance of various in dices of change and improvement is not clear. Moreover, outcomes achieved even with the combined treatment conditions leave much room for improvement. Related to these issues is the relative cost of the various treatment combinations. It appears clear that vouchers can enhance the efficacy of standard cognitive-behavioral treatments, and cognitive-behavioral treatments may help maintain abstinence effects achieved with vouchers. However, are the costs related to integrating these treatment components the most cost-effective way to provide services to outpatients in need of treatment for cannabis dependence? The evaluation of cost-effectiveness in the context of future testing of interventions that manipulate parameters such as type, frequency, intensity, and magnitude of both CM and counseling interventions is needed to develop optimal cost-effective interventions for cannabis dependence.

CANNABIS-ABUSING ADOLESCENTS

Cannabis is being used at increasingly younger ages, and use by adolescents is twice as high as in 1991 (SAMHSA, 2005a). Such use is associated with

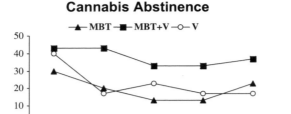

FIGURE 4.1. Point-prevalence abstinence rates as determined by urine toxicology results at the end of treatment and at each 3-month posttreatment assessment. Adapted from Budney, Moore, Higgins, and Rocha (2006). Copyright 2006 by the American Psychological Association. Adapted by permission.

emotional, health, and behavioral problems, and marijuana is the leading illicit drug mentioned in emergency room admissions and autopsies (SAMHSA, 2004). Adolescents are also more likely to meet criteria for cannabis dependence than for alcohol dependence (Young et al., 2002). The number of adolescents receiving treatment for primary cannabis abuse or dependence increased 350% from 1992 to 2002, and the majority of adolescent substance abuse admissions report cannabis as the primary substance (SAMHSA, 2005b).

Despite a growing need for adolescent marijuana abuse treatment, little consensus exists on how to best treat this clinical population. Family-based and cognitive-behavioral treatments appear to hold promise (Liddle, 2004; Waldron & Kaminer, 2004). Most recently, a large multisite study demonstrated positive effects across five empirically based interventions for cannabis-abusing teens: (1) multidimensional family therapy, (2) community reinforcement approach, (3 and 4) 5- and 12-session versions of motivational enhancement therapy (MET) combined with cognitive-behavioral therapy (CBT), and (5) MET/CBT combined with family support network (Dennis et al., 2004). Across groups, significant improvement in drug use and decreases in symptoms of dependence were observed. While promising and offering multiple alternatives for treatment, the majority of teens across these treatments did not report positive outcomes. As with treatment for adults, room remains to enhance the effects of adolescent interventions for cannabis.

Chapter 12 (Krishnan-Sarin, Duhig, & Cavallo, this volume) provides an in-depth discussion of CM approaches with adolescent substance abusers. Here, we briefly describe a multicomponent CM intervention that we have developed for adolescent cannabis abusers in an effort to enhance rates of positive outcomes in this clinical population (Kamon, Budney, &

Stanger, 2005). The 14-week treatment comprises weekly 90-minute counseling sessions that integrate individual CBT with the adolescent, with two CM components: an abstinence-based voucher program and behavioral parent training for the parent(s).

The adolescent CBT sessions follow the MET/CBT 5 + 7 curriculum (Webb, Scudder, Kaminer, & Kadden, 2001). The abstinence-based voucher program (V) uses the same reinforcement schedule described for our trials with adult cannabis abusers. The major modification to this program is that the reinforcement contingency is on abstinence from cannabis, alcohol, and other drugs, not just cannabis. Documentation of abstinence is based on urine toxicology, parent-administered breathalyzers, and parent reports. Note that targeting multiple drugs has generally decreased the efficacy of CM interventions (Lussier, Higgins, Heil, Badger, & Mongeon, 2006). Nonetheless, we chose to target all substances for the following reasons. First, although cannabis is the primary drug of abuse for these youth, they quite frequently use alcohol, and occasionally other drugs such as opiates, cocaine, or amphetamines. One concern with such other substance use, particularly with alcohol intoxication, was that it would impair judgment and potentially prompt cannabis use even among those committed to abstaining. Second, and perhaps most important, we felt that parents would not be receptive to a treatment that provides reinforcement for cannabis abstinence in situations in which we know that their child has been using other substances typically considered more harmful than marijuana. Our experience to date using this procedure suggests that placing voucher contingencies on all drugs of abuse with these adolescent marijuana abusers is not problematic. Little other drug use is usually observed, attrition is low, and the majority of adolescents earn incentives for drug abstinence during the intervention.

The other CM intervention, behavioral parent training, involves teaching the parents to effectively use CM procedures. We felt that parent involvement was crucial with adolescents for several reasons. First, adolescents rarely seek treatment on their own but are brought to treatment by their parents. Accordingly, they frequently do not perceive their cannabis use as a problem, and motivation is low to quit using and remain abstinent. Second, parents typically consider their youths' cannabis use a problem, are motivated to take action, but do not necessarily have the knowledge or skills to effectively change their adolescents' behavior. Hence, we designed our parent interventions to motivate adolescents and provide parents with tools and strategies to manage substance abuse and related conduct problems.

The parent-directed contingency management (PCM) has two primary components, a substance monitoring contract (SMC) and behavioral parent training. The SMC uses a behavioral contract among the therapist, parent(s), and youth that focuses on substance use or abstinence. The contract specifies positive and negative consequences to be delivered by the parents in response to documented abstinence or use (based on the aforementioned monitoring procedures). The consequences are determined via a collaborative process between therapist, parent(s), and adolescent and revaluated each week during weekly counseling sessions.

The second CM component is a behavioral parent training program delivered to the parents during the weekly sessions. The Family Management Curriculum of the Adolescent Transitions program was used to teach parents basic principles and skills designed to decrease problem behaviors and increase prosocial behaviors (Dishion et al., 2003). This program, designed to target youth conduct problems seemed likely to yield broad benefits because conduct problems, are highly comorbid with and strong predictors of poor outcomes among treated adolescent substance abusers (Randall, Henggeler, Pickrel, & Brondino, 1999; Young et al., 2002). We also utilized a CM intervention to enhance parent participation and compliance. The fishbowl technique (Petry, Martin, Cooney, & Kranzler, 2000) was used to reward parents for completing therapeutic activities (e.g., attendance, homework, and SMC). Last, an additional 12 weeks of once-weekly urine testing following the treatment program were provided to encourage parents to continue using the SMC. Continued monitoring and implementation of the SMC were hypothesized to improve maintenance of abstinence and reduce relapse rates during the immediate posttreatment period.

An initial pilot study of this CM-based intervention evaluated outcomes for 19 youth who received this multicomponent intervention: individual CBT + PCM + V (Kamon et al., 2005). Adolescents attended an average of 10.4 (SD = 4.5) of 14 sessions and at least one parent attended an average of 10.7 (SD = 4.7) sessions. Over the course of treatment, youth showed significant reductions in cannabis use. Twice as many adolescents provided cannabis-negative urine specimens at the end of treatment compared with intake (37% vs. 74%), and days of cannabis use reported during the last month of treatment significantly decreased from intake (M = 14.37 [SD = 11.5] vs. 4.47 [SD = 9.2]). Significant improvements in internalizing and externalizing psychopathology were observed as measured by the Child Behavior Checklist and Youth Self-Report (Achenbach & Rescorla, 2001). Indicators of positive changes in parenting behavior as measured by the Alabama Parenting Questionnaire also showed significant improvement (Wells et al., 2000). Overall, this initial uncontrolled trial suggested that CBT + PCM + V was acceptable to parents and adolescents, produced substantial reductions in cannabis use and conduct problems, and produced improvements in parenting.

We have recently completed a randomized trial testing the efficacy of this CM intervention for adolescent marijuana abuse. We hypothesized that PCM + V will (1) engender longer periods of cannabis abstinence when added to CBT and (2) enhance maintenance of abstinence following treatment. Preliminary findings provide support for this intervention (Budney,

2005). Future analyses and studies are planned to determine the unique effects of the two CM components and to test for behavioral mechanisms of action.

CANNABIS ABUSE IN PROBATION-REFERRED YOUNG ADULTS

A substantial proportion of those seeking treatment for cannabis are under the age of 25 and report involvement with the criminal justice system (SAMHSA, 2005a). Like the adolescent population described previously, many outpatients with this profile are not highly motivated to quit using cannabis use and do not engage well in treatment. Sinha, Easton, Renee-Aubin, and Carroll (2003) conducted a randomized trial to determine whether adding a modified voucher program to a three-session MET treatment would improve outcomes among probation-referred young adults referred to outpatient treatment for cannabis abuse. The voucher program was designed to reinforce attendance at counseling sessions rather than abstinence from cannabis. Voucher earnings escalated from a $25 voucher for attendance at session one, $35 for session two, and $45 for the third, and a $5 voucher was provided for arriving within 5 minutes of the appointment time for each session. Vouchers could be redeemed for prosocial items or services. The voucher program was successful in that those who received vouchers were more likely to complete treatment (64% vs. 39%), attend sessions (2.3 vs. 1.8), and continue with treatment after completing the three sessions. The voucher program enhanced treatment attendance and engagement as hypothesized; however, no concomitant effects were observed for cannabis use or other psychosocial outcome measures.

CANNABIS USE IN INDIVIDUALS WITH SEVERE PSYCHIATRIC ILLNESS

Cannabis is the most common illicit drug used among individuals with schizophrenia (Kandel, Chen, Warner, Kessler, & Grant, 1997; Zisook et al., 1992), and it has been associated with numerous adverse consequences such as earlier or more abrupt onset of symptomatology, poor medication compliance, increasing risk for recurrent symptoms, or relapse (Dixon, Haas, Weiden, Sweeney, & Frances, 1991; Negrete & Gill, 1999). However, this clinical population does not typically identify cannabis use as problematic and self-refer for treatment. CM strategies therefore might offer a method for enhancing motivation and prompting quit attempts.

Sigmon, Steingard, Badger, Anthony, and Higgins (2000) conducted an initial feasibility study with adults diagnosed with schizophrenia or another serious mental illness who were not seeking treatment for cannabis. Participants were recruited with newspaper advertisements and posters in a local mental health clinic. A within-subjects experimental design examined the effects of three abstinence-incentive conditions during which participants received either $25, $50, or $100 in cash (not vouchers) each time they provided a specimen that was negative for cannabis use. Abstinence engendered in these incentive conditions was compared with two baseline conditions during which participants received $25 independent of urinalysis results each time they submitted a urine specimen. Each condition involved twice-per-week urinalysis testing, lasted one week, and did not include any counseling. Results clearly showed that the three incentive conditions effectively engendered greater periods of cannabis abstinence than did the baseline conditions. Surprisingly, no differences were observed among incentive conditions. These findings provided initial evidence that cannabis use among severely mentally ill individuals is sensitive to CM reinforcement interventions.

A second within-subjects study examined abstinence-based vouchers rather than cash incentives (Sigmon & Higgins, 2006). A 12-week voucher program similar to that used in the original cocaine studies was evaluated. Results again clearly showed that the voucher program effectively engendered cannabis abstinence. As reviewed in Chapter 11 (Tidey & Ries, this volume), similar findings have been reported with cigarette smoking in individuals with schizophrenia. Moreover, examples of the effective use of innovative CM-based interventions to reduce substance use in clinical samples of severely mentally ill adults have begun to appear in the literature.

CANNABIS AS A SECONDARY DRUG OF ABUSE

Cannabis tends to be the most common other drug used by individuals seeking treatment for other types of drug dependence (Budney, Bickel, & Amass, 1998; Budney, Higgins, & Wong, 1996). Such cannabis use is commonly viewed as a significant risk factor for relapse or treatment failure, although the empirical support for this is equivocal (Epstein & Preston, 2003). This issue presents a significant challenge for treatment providers because the majority of these individuals do not consider their cannabis use problematic, and their readiness to change is significantly lower for cannabis use than for their primary substance of abuse. Hence, CM interventions may offer a promising approach for addressing cannabis use in these difficult clinical populations.

The Opiate Clinic

The majority of adults enrolled in clinics that provide methadone or buprenorphine maintenance programs for opiate dependence report cannabis use (Calsyn & Saxon, 1999). The clinical importance of such use is many times minimized because the problems and consequences related to cannabis use are usually considered minimal compared with those associated with opiate dependence. Accordingly, many clinics do not conduct regular urinalysis testing for cannabis, and if they do, many do not have any negative consequences associated with the detection of cannabis use. Such lack of consequences may give the impression that such use is condoned. In response to this issue, a number of studies have explored the effects of CM-based approaches targeting cannabis use in these clinics.

Calsyn and Saxon (1999) capitalized on the well-documented positive effects of using take-home medication privileges to engender positive behaviors in this clinical population. They devised a cannabis CM program to function as an adjunct to an existing CM program that required 6 months of drug-negative urinalysis tests (except for cannabis) in order to earn twice-a-week methadone-dose take-home privileges (i.e., had to attend the clinic twice per week to pick up their medication). The cannabis CM intervention increased the requirement for obtaining twice-weekly take-home status to include cannabis-negative urinalysis test results. This quasi-experimental study involved eight adults who had already earned the twice-per-week take-home under the usual clinic CM program but were still using cannabis regularly. A 6-month notice informed these participants about the new cannabis requirement. Three of the eight cannabis users achieved abstinence during this 6-month period. The other five lost their take-home privilege when the new program began due to cannabis-positive urine tests. One of these subsequently initiated cannabis abstinence and earned back the privilege. The other four remained at the lower-privilege status (thrice-weekly take-homes) for the remainder of the 1-year study. This study demonstrated how a CM program targeting cannabis in this population can be implemented without having significant adverse effects on other aspects of treatment.

Primary Cocaine Dependence

Many in treatment for cocaine dependence use cannabis regularly, and many of those who stop using cocaine continue to use cannabis (Budney et al., 1996). As in the opiate clinic, this poses a clinical dilemma regarding how best to address the issue without adversely affecting cocaine use outcomes. We conducted a small-n demonstration study to explore a sequential strategy of initially targeting abstinence from cocaine with a voucher program and subsequently targeting cannabis after cocaine abstinence has been achieved (Budney, Higgins, Delaney, Kent, & Bickel, 1991). The experience of achieving cocaine abstinence and its associated positive effects might increase awareness of the negative impact of cannabis use on a prosocial lifestyle and enhance motivation to quit. Moreover, an initial positive experience with a voucher program for cocaine might motivate participation in a similar program that targets cannabis abstinence.

Using a multiple-baseline design, a 12-week voucher program first engendered cocaine abstinence in two participants, but both continued to use cannabis regularly despite counseling that encouraged cannabis abstinence. At the end of the 12 weeks, both participants were offered a second 12-week voucher program at staggered time intervals that involved a modified contingency requiring abstinence from *both* cocaine and cannabis. Both participants achieved abstinence from both drugs with initiation of cannabis abstinence coinciding with initiation of the modified voucher program. Unfortunately, following discontinuation of the program, both participants resumed cannabis use. They did, however, remain abstinent from cocaine. This small study illustrated that voucher programs offer an effective method for initiating cannabis abstinence in multiple drug users who are ambivalent about their cannabis use, but it also suggested that additional intervention may be needed to obtain enduring effects.

CONCLUDING COMMENTS

Although only a few carefully controlled studies have examined the effects of CM on clinical samples of cannabis abusers, the findings clearly demonstrate that these approaches can be effective and should be considered a viable treatment alternative. With cannabis, the usual questions surrounding the cost-effectiveness of CM programs arise, perhaps with even more concern than with other substance-dependence treatments. Some might question whether or not cannabis dependence is a substantial problem in need of more potent and perhaps more costly treatments. Historically, cannabis dependence has not been viewed as a significant problem, and it was questioned whether cannabis dependence existed at all (Stephens & Roffman, 1993). More recently, however, an empirical base of knowledge has accumulated demonstrating the significant impact of cannabis abuse and dependence on a substantial number of youth and adults. The large number of persons who enroll in treatment with cannabis use disorders clearly indicates the clinical and public health importance of this problem. Effective dissemination of information about the adverse impact of cannabis may need to occur simultaneously with efforts to disseminate effective treatments like CM that require additional resources or modifications to existing treatment programs. The practical and clinical obstacles to these efforts have been discussed in depth elsewhere (Kirby, Amass, & McLellan, 1999).

REFERENCES

Achenbach, T. M., & Rescorla, L. A. (2001). *Manual for ASEBA School-Age Forms and Profiles*. Burlington: University of Vermont, Research Center for Children, Youth, and Families.

Anthony, J. C., Warner, L. A., & Kessler, R. C. (1994). Comparative epidemiology of dependence on tobacco, alcohol, controlled substances and inhalants: Basic findings from the National Comorbidity Survey. *Experimental and Clinical Psychopharmacology, 2*, 244–268.

Budney, A. J. (2005). *Novel behavioral treatments for adolescent marijuana abusers and their parents.* Paper presented at the College on Problems of Drug Dependence, Orlando, FL.

Budney, A. J., Bickel, W. K., & Amass, L. (1998). Marijuana use and treatment outcome among opioid-dependent patients. *Addiction, 93*(4), 493–503.

Budney, A. J., & Higgins, S. T. (1998). *Treating cocaine dependence: A community reinforcement plus vouchers approach.* Rockville, MD: National Institute on Drug Abuse.

Budney, A. J., Higgins, S. T., Delaney, D. D., Kent, L., & Bickel, W. K. (1991). Contingent reinforcement of abstinence with individuals abusing cocaine and marijuana. *Journal of Applied Behavior Analysis, 24*, 657–665.

Budney, A. J., Higgins, S. T., Radonovich, K. J., & Novy, P. L. (2000). Adding voucher-based incentives to coping skills and motivational enhancement improves outcomes during treatment for marijuana dependence. *Journal of Consulting and Clinical Psychology, 68*, 1051–1061.

Budney, A. J., Higgins, S. T., & Wong, C. J. (1996). Marijuana use and treatment outcome in cocaine-dependent patients. *Experimental and Clinical Psychopharmacology, 4*, 396–403.

Budney, A. J., Hughes, J. R., Moore, B. A., & Vandrey, R. G. (2004). A review of the validity and significance of the cannabis withdrawal syndrome. *American Journal of Psychiatry, 161*(11), 1967–1977.

Budney, A. J., Moore, B. A., Higgins, S. T., & Rocha, H. L. (2006). Clinical trial of abstinence-based vouchers and cognitive-behavioral therapy for cannabis dependence. *Journal of Consulting and Clinical Psychology, 74*, 307–316.

Budney, A. J., Radonovich, K. J., Higgins, S. T., & Wong, C. J. (1998). Adults seeking treatment for marijuana dependence: A comparison to cocaine-dependent treatment seekers. *Experimental and Clinical Psychopharmacology, 6*(4), 419–426.

Budney, A. J., Sigmon, S. C., & Higgins, S. T. (2001). Implementing contingency management programs: Using science to motivate change. In R. Coombs (Ed.), *Addiction recovery tools: A practical handbook* (pp. 147–172). Thousand Oaks, CA: Sage.

Calsyn, D. A., & Saxon, A. J. (1999). An innovative approach to reducing cannabis use in a subset of methadone clients. *Drug and Alcohol Dependence, 53*, 167–169.

Compton, W. M., Conway, K. P., Sinson, F. S., Colliver, J. D., & Grant, B. F. (2005). Prevalence, correlates, and comorbidity of DSM-IV antisocial personality syndromes and alcohol and specific drug use disorders in the United States: Results from the National Epidemiologic Survey on Alcohol and Related Conditions. *Journal of Clinical Psychiatry, 66*, 677–685.

Dennis, M., Godley, S. H., Diamond, G., Tims, F. M., Babor, T., Donaldson, J., et al. (2004). The Cannabis Youth Treatment (CYT) study: Main findings from two randomized trials. *Journal of Substance Abuse Treatment, 27*, 197–213.

Dennis, M. L., Godley, S., & Titus, J. (1999). *Co-occurring psychiatric problems among adolescents: Variations by treatment, level of care and gender* (TIE communique). Available at *www.treatment.org/communique/CHIPtreatment.pdf.*

Dishion, T. J., Kavanagh, K., Veltman, M., McCartney, T., Soberman, L., & Stormshak, E. A. (2003). *Family Management Curriculum V2.0: Leader's guide.* Eugene, OR: Child and Family Center Publications.

Dixon, L., Haas, G., Weiden, P. J., Sweeney, J., & Frances, A. J. (1991). Drug abuse in schizophrenic patients: Clinical correlates and reasons for use. *American Journal of Psychiatry, 148*, 224–230.

Epstein, D. H., & Preston, K. L. (2003). Does cannabis use predict poor outcome for heroin-dependent patients on maintenance treatment? Past findings and more evidence against. *Addiction, 98*(3), 269–279.

European Monitoring Center for Drugs and Drug Addiction. (2003). *Annual report 2003: The state of the drugs problem in the acceding and candidate countries to the European Union.* Luxembourg: Office of the Official Publications of the European Communities.

Hall, W., Johnston, L., & Donnelly, N. (1999). Epidemiology of cannabis use and its consequences. In H. Kalant, W. A. Corrigall, W. Hall, & R. Smart (Eds.), *The health effects of cannabis* (pp. 69–126). Toronto, Ontario, Canada: Centre for Addiction and Mental Health.

Higgins, S. T., Delaney, D. D., Budney, A. J., Bickel, W. K., Hughes, J. R., Foerg, F., et al. (1991). A behavioral approach to achieving initial cocaine abstinence. *American Journal of Psychiatry, 148*, 1218–1224.

Johnston, L. D., O'Malley, P. M., Bachman, J. G., & Schulenberg, J. E. (2005). *Monitoring the Future national survey results on drug use, 1975–2004. Volume I: Secondary school students* (NIH Publication No. 05-5727). Bethesda, MD: National Institute on Drug Abuse.

Kadden, R. M., Litt, M. D., Kabela-Cormier, E., & Petry, N. M. (2007). Abstinence rates following behavioral treatments for marijuana dependence. *Addictive Behaviors, 32*(6), 1220–1236.

Kalant, H., Corrigall, W., Hall, W., & Smart, R. (Eds.). (1999). *The health effects of cannabis.* Toronto: Centre for Addiction and Mental Health.

Kamon, J., Budney, A., & Stanger, C. (2005). A contingency management intervention for adolescent marijuana abuse and conduct problems. *Journal of the American Academy of Child and Adolescent Psychiatry, 44*, 513–521.

Kandel, D., Chen, K., Warner, L. A., Kessler, R. C., & Grant, B. (1997). Prevalence and demographic correlates of symptoms of dependence on cigarettes, alcohol, marijuana and cocaine in the U.S. population. *Drug and Alcohol Dependence, 44*, 437–442.

Kandel, D. B. (1984). Marijuana users in young adulthood. *Archives of General Psychiatry, 41*, 200–209.

Kirby, K. C., Amass, L., & McLellan, A. T. (1999). Disseminating contingency management research to drug abuse treatment practitioners. In S. T. Higgins & K. Silverman (Eds.), *Motivating behavior change among illicit-drug abusers* (pp. 327–344). Washington, DC: American Psychological Association.

Liddle, H. A. (2004). Family-based therapies for adolescent alcohol and drug use: Research contributions and future research needs. *Addiction, 99*, 76–92.

Lussier, J., Higgins, S., Heil, S., Badger, G., & Mongeon, J. (2006). Voucher-based reinforcement therapy for substance use disorders: A quantitative review. *Addiction, 101*, 192–203.

McRae, A. L., Budney, A. J., & Brady, K. T. (2003). Treatment of marijuana dependence: A review of the literature. *Journal of Substance Abuse Treatment, 24*, 369–376.

Negrete, J. C., & Gill, K. (1999). Cannabis and schizophrenia: An overview of the evidence to date. In G. G. Nahas (Ed.), *Marihuana and medicine* (pp. 671–681). Totowa, NJ: Humana Press.

Petry, N. M., Martin, B., Cooney, J. L., & Kranzler, H. R. (2000). Give them prizes, and they will come: Contingency management for treatment of alcohol dependence. *Journal of Consulting and Clinical Psychology, 68*, 250–257.

Project Match Research Group. (1998). Matching alcoholism treatments to client hetergeneity:

Treatment main effects and matching effects on drinking during treatment. *Journal of Studies on Alcohol, 59*, 631–639.

Randall, J., Henggeler, S. W., Pickrel, S. G., & Brondino, M. J. (1999). Psychiatric comorbidity and the 16-month trajectory of substance-abusing and substance-dependent juvenile offenders. *Journal of the American Academy of Child and Adolescent Psychiatry, 38*, 1118–1124.

Sigmon, S. C., & Higgins, S. T. (2006). Voucher-based contingent reinforcement of marijuana abstinence among individuals with serious mental illness. *Journal of Substance Abuse Treatment, 30*(4), 291–295.

Sigmon, S. C., Steingard, S., Badger, G. J., Anthony, S. L., & Higgins, S. T. (2000). Contingent reinforcement of marijuana abstinence among individuals with serious mental illness: A feasibility study. *Experimental and Clinical Psychopharmacology, 8*, 509–517.

Sinha, R., Easton, C., Renee-Aubin, L., & Carroll, K. M. (2003). Engaging young probation-referred marijuana-abusing individuals in treatment: A pilot trial. *American Journal on Addictions, 12*, 314–323.

Stephens, R. S., Babor, T. F., Kadden, R., Miller, M., & Marijuana Treatment Project Research Group. (2002). The marijuana treatment project: Rationale, design, and participant characteristics. *Addiction, 97*(S1), 109–124.

Stephens, R. S., & Roffman, R. A. (1993). Adult marijuana dependence. In J. S. Baer, G. A. Marlatt, & R. J. McMahon (Eds.), *Addictive behaviors across the lifespan: Prevention, treatment, and policy issues* (pp. 243–273). Newbury Park, CA: Sage.

Substance Abuse and Mental Health Services Administration. (2005a). *Summary of findings from the 2002 National Household Survey on Drug Abuse.* Rockville, MD: U.S. Department of Health and Human Services. Available at *www.oas.samhsa.gov/msduh.htm.*

Substance Abuse and Mental Health Services Administration. (2005b). *Treatment episode data set.* Available at *www.oas.samhsa.gov/tx.htm.*

Substance Abuse and Mental Health Services Administration. (2004). *DAWN, 2003 interim national estimates of drug-related emergency department visits. http://dawninfo.samhsa.gov.*

Torres, M. L., Mattik, R. P., Chen, R., & Baillie, A. (1995). *Clients of treatment service agencies: March 1995 census findings.* Canberra, Australia: Commonwealth Department of Health and Human Services.

Waldron, H. B., & Kaminer, Y. (2004). On the learning curve: The emerging evidence supporting cognitive behavioral therapies for adolescent substance abuse. *Addiction, 99*, 93–105.

Webb, C., Scudder, M., Kaminer, Y., & Kadden, R. (2001). *The motivational enhancement therapy and cognitive behavioral therapy for adolescent cannabis users* (Vol. 2). Rockville, MD: Center for Substance Abuse Treatment, Substance Abuse and Mental Health Services Administration.

Wells, K. C., Epstein, J. N., Hinshaw, S. P., Conners, C. K., Klaric, J., Abikoff, H. B., et al. (2000). Parenting and family stress treatment outcomes in attention deficit hyperactivity disorder (ADHD): An empirical analysis in the MTA study. *Journal of Abnormal Child Psychology, 28*, 543–553.

Young, S. E., Corley, R. P., Stallings, M. C., Rhee, S. H., Crowley, T. J., & Hewitt, J. K. (2002). Substance use, abuse and dependence in adolescents: Prevalence, symptoms profiles and correlates. *Drug and Alcohol Dependence, 68*(3), 309–322.

Zisook, S., Heaton, R., Moranville, J., Kuck, J., Jernigan, T., & Braff, D. (1992). Past substance abuse and clinical course of schizophrenia. *American Journal of Psychiatry, 149*, 552–553.

CHAPTER 5

METHAMPHETAMINES

John M. Roll *and* Thomas Newton

BACKGROUND

(Methamphetamine manufacture, trafficking, and use represent a serious public health and criminal justice problem (e.g., Anglin, Burke, Perrochet, Stamper, & Dawud-Nouri, 2000; Clark, 2000)). Methamphetamine is abused throughout the world. In the United States, methamphetamine use has historically been encountered most commonly in the western and midwestern states, but use appears to be increasing east of the Mississippi River (Rawson, Gonzales, & Brethen, 2002). Methamphetamine use has been reported in all types of communities from large cities to rural settings, although its most severe impact is often observed in rural areas and moderately sized urban communities (Rawson et al., 2002).

[Methamphetamine abuse[1] is associated with a number of medical consequences, including increased HIV (human immunodeficiency virus) risk and HCV (hepatitis C virus) infection (e.g., Beyrer et al., 2004; Cherner et al., 2005; Frosch, Shoptaw, Huber, Rawson, & Ling, 1996; Shoptaw, Reback, & Freese, 2002; Freese, Miotto, & Reback, 2002; Tominaga, Garcia, Dzierba, & Wong, 2004) and psychiatric comorbidity (Zweben et al., 2004)./

---

[1]Throughout this chapter, the term *methamphetamine abuse* is used to describe problematic methamphetamine use unless specific DSM criteria are being discussed.

In addition to the risks associated with use, the manufacture and distribution of methamphetamine pose serious medical risks such as fire and accidental poisoning (Danks et al., 2004; Kashani & Ruha, 2004). Fortunately, treatment of methamphetamine use disorders appears to ameliorate some of the medical risks associated with its continued use (e.g., Shoptaw, Reback, Peck, et al., 2005; Reback, Larkins, & Shoptaw, 2004).

Methamphetamine abuse is also associated with neuropsychiatric and neurocognitive impairment that persists even during the early stages of abstinence (e.g., Kalechstein, Newton, & Green, 2003; Simon et al., 2004). Recent data suggest that prolonged abstinence ameliorates some, but perhaps not all, of this impairment (Newton, Kalechstein, Duran, Vansluis, & Ling, 2004; Wang et al., 2004). Some have suggested that methamphetamine-abusing individuals do not perform as well during treatment as do individuals addicted to other types of stimulants because of these neurocognitive deficits, which make it difficult for the individual in treatment to attend to, comprehend, and act on treatment material. The presence of this neurocognitive impairment during treatment for methamphetamine use disorders argues for a treatment plan that does not tax the participant's cognitive capability, such as contingency management (CM). CM is based on principles of learning that have been found to operate independently of an organism's verbal ability; thus, even though instructional control may influence the rapidity with which a client understands CM, instructions are not necessary for the principles of reinforcement to operate.

Potentially related to the neurocognitive impairment often experienced by methamphetamine abusers is an impulsive pattern of behavior similar to that often observed in substance abusers using other illicit drugs. Impulsive behavior is most frequently observed among injection or heavy methamphetamine users (e.g., Semple, Zians, Grant, & Patterson, 2005; Simons, Oliver, Gather, Ebel, & Brummels, 2005; Semple, Patterson, & Grant, 2004). This impulsive behavior can take many forms, including risky drug use behaviors (e.g., Shoptaw et al., 2005), risky sexual behavior (e.g., Peck et al., 2005), increased levels of criminal behavior (e.g., Cartier, Farabee, & Prendergast, 2006), and decreased compliance with medication regimens (Shoptaw et al., 2005)—all of which can have serious consequences.

Although it is possible that these impulsive behaviors are a result of the neuropharmacological consequences of methamphetamine use, another potential explanation is that they are the result of the methamphetamine abuser's inability to obtain sufficient natural reinforcers from his or her environment. Perhaps methamphetamine abusers tend to live in impoverished environments or have been drug involved for so long that they do not have the requisite skills needed to obtain reinforcers from their environment. In these situations, where a person cannot readily obtain naturalistic reinforcers it may make sense to behave impulsively and abuse drugs as they provide positive reinforcement. Such a situation argues for a treatment approach such as CM designed to remediate this reliance on drug-based reinforcement.

TREATMENT APPROACHES

To a large extent, treatment strategies for methamphetamine use disorders have been based on strategies shown to be effective in treating cocaine use disorders, as the two share many commonalities (e.g., Copeland & Sorensen, 2001; Cretzmeyer, Sarrazin, Huber, Block, & Hall, 2003). However, some differences between the use of cocaine and the use of methamphetamine do exist, and these may be of clinical importance in developing efficacious treatment interventions. Perhaps the most important difference is that cocaine has a relatively short half-life relative to methamphetamine.

Methamphetamine may be used in a more periodic fashion than cocaine, which is often used in a pattern characterized by a binge followed by a crash (e.g., Rawson et al., 2000; Simon et al., 2002). Thus, the natural periods of abstinence that are seen following a cocaine binge may not be present in a person using methamphetamine. Thus, when treating methamphetamine abuse it may be necessary to initiate abstinence during a time of ongoing regular drug use. CM should be ideally suited to this method as it is often thought of as a procedure specifically designed to initiate abstinence. In addition, although cocaine and alcohol are commonly used together, methamphetamine appears to be preferentially used with marijuana (Rawson et al., 2000).

These differences notwithstanding, some of the psychosocial interventions that have been useful in the treatment of cocaine use disorders also appear to be promising for treating methamphetamine use disorders, including brief cognitive-behavioral interventions (Yen, Wu, Yen, & Ko, 2004) and the Matrix model of substance abuse treatment (Rawson et al., 2004). In a large randomized, multi-site trial, the Matrix model of treatment was shown generally to produce better treatment outcomes than any other psychosocial intervention to which it was compared (e.g., Rawson et al., 2004). Other approaches are being investigated, including pharmacotherapy (e.g., Galloway, Newmeyer, Knapp, Stalcup, & Smith, 1994) and immunotherapy (Haney & Kosten, 2004).

CONTINGENCY MANAGEMENT

CM has proven useful in treating cocaine and other types of substance use disorders. CM interventions are based on an extensive basic science literature supporting the position that drug use is a form of operant behavior (e.g., Bigelow & Silverman, 1999; Higgins, 1997, Higgins, Heil, & Plebani-Lussier, 2004). Thus, the salient alternative nondrug reinforcers that are available contingent upon verified periods of abstinence generally decrease drug use (Carroll, Lac, & Nygaard, 1989; Higgins, Bickel, & Hughes, 1994; Nader & Woolverton, 1991). These observations form the conceptual basis for the CM approaches to drug abuse treatment. Several recent meta-analyses have supported the efficacy of CM in reducing illicit drug use (Lussier, Heil, Mongeon, Badger, & Higgins, 2006; Prendergast, Podus, Finney, Greenwell, & Roll, 2007).

The most common type of CM intervention in current use for treating stimulant use disorders (primarily cocaine) was developed by Higgins and colleagues (e.g., Higgins et al., 1991, 1993; Higgins, Budney, et al., 1994). In this procedure patients receive "vouchers" for the provision of biological samples (urine or breath) that indicate no recent drug use. Hence, the procedure is often called voucher-based reinforcement therapy (VBRT). These vouchers are withheld when the biological sample indicates recent drug use. As originally conceived, these vouchers were to be for goods or services that would help the patient initiate or reestablish behavior that resulted in non-drug-based reinforcement. For example, if, prior to becoming dependent on cocaine, a person had an appreciation for poetry, he or she might use any vouchers earned in treatment to purchase poetry books or to attend a poetry reading. Thus, the vouchers could be conceptualized as tools for acquainting or reacquainting individuals in treatment to nondrug sources of reinforcement available in their environment, which might then serve to compete with drug use.

VBRT has proven to be successful at initiating periods of abstinence (Higgins et al., 1991, 1993; Higgins & Silverman, 1999) and has been shown to produce relatively long periods of abstinence (Higgins, Badger, & Budney, 2000; Higgins, Wong, Badger, Ogden, & Dantona, 2000; Silverman et al., 1996). Many individuals achieve some period of sobriety using this technique.

Another CM technique was developed by Petry (e.g., Petry, Martin, & Finocche, 2001; Petry, Martin, Cooney, & Kranzler, 2000; Petry & Martin, 2002; Petry et al., 2004) and has been variously referred to as the fishbowl procedure, prize-based CM, or the variable-magnitude-of-reinforcement procedure. This technique has many similarities to VBRT. Participants receive draws, often from a number of slips of paper kept in a fishbowl, for providing a biological specimen that indicates no recent drug use. Provision of a sample indicating recent drug use results in the withholding of draws. Each draw has a chance of winning a "prize," the size of which varies. Typically, about half the draws result simply in the participant receiving a slip of paper that says "good job!" Approximately half the draws, though, result in the earning of a prize. The majority of the prizes are "small" and are valued at about $1, some prizes are large and are worth about $20, and typically there is one "jumbo" prize, which is worth about $80. Each time a participant draws a prize, he or she has a small chance of winning a jumbo prize, a moderate chance of winning a large prize, and an approximately 50% chance of winning a small prize.

The main impetus for developing the variable-magnitude-of-reinforcement procedure was a desire to minimize the cost of the CM interventions, which can appear prohibitive to community-based treatment providers (Petry et al., 2000). Early results suggest that VBRT and variable-magnitude-of-reinforcement procedures are approximately equivalent in their ability to initiate and maintain abstinence if reinforcement schedules are kept comparable (Petry et al., 2005).

With regard to methamphetamine abuse, one treatment approach is to utilize CM in combination with psychosocial and/or pharmacotherapeutic interventions. We favor this approach over any approach that uses only CM, as we believe that psycho- and/or pharmacotherapy may be needed to address the psychiatric comorbidity that often occurs with methamphetamine abuse.

There are several reasons to expect that the addition of CM will enhance methamphetamine treatment outcomes. First, CM has been rigorously developed in a logical progression from very basic to applied research over the course of the last 75 years (e.g., Skinner, 1938; Higgins, Bickel, & Hughes, 1994; Silverman et al., 1996). Thus, one can have high levels of confidence in the procedure, as it is based on principles gleaned from the field of behavior analysis that have been replicated and refined repeatedly.

In addition, CM has proven useful in the treatment of many types of substance use disorders. Includes opioids (Higgins, Stitzer, Bigelow, & Liebson, 1986), marijuana, (Budney, Higgins, Radonovich, & Novy, 2000), benzodiazepines (Stitzer, Bigelow, & Liebson, 1979), alcohol (Petry et al., 2000), nicotine (Roll, 2005), and cocaine (Higgins, Budney, et al., 1994). It has been identified as one of the most effective behavioral treatment approaches available for treating drug abuse (Carroll & Onken, 2005).

LABORATORY STUDY

Given the desirability of a programmatic approach to the science of substance abuse treatment, we were interested to see if methamphetamine use could be moderated via the presentation of alternative sources of reinforcement. Because this modulation is central to the efficacy of CM, we believe that it represents a pragmatic use of resources (money and participant and investigator time) to first demonstrate this efficacy in a laboratory setting. We believe it is also the most ethical course to pursue because it provides the greatest likelihood of developing effective treatment strategies that will maximally benefit the treatment-seeking participants who enroll in those studies.

To investigate this belief, we recruited seven Caucasian participants who were diagnosed with a methamphetamine use disorder and were not interested in receiving treatment. These individuals were enrolled in a study that was approved by the appropriate institutional review boards. All were in good health and none met diagnostic criteria for other current substance abuse or Axis I disorders. Participants resided in a hospital research ward for the approximate 15-day duration of the study. Four of the participants (one female and three male) withdrew for reasons unrelated to the study, primarily related to adhering to rules on the research ward. All withdrawals happened prior to Phase 2 (described later).

The study was divided into two phases. During all sessions participants' vital signs were monitored, a physician was present for actual drug administration, and additional medical personnel were continuously available. Sessions were conducted at the same time each day, 7 days a week. Participants were monitored intensively for 6 hours following drug administration and periodically after that. During the first phase participants sampled 0.42 mg/kg of oral methamphetamine and placebo on consecutive days in a double-blind fashion. On the following 3 days participants elected to receive methamphetamine, placebo, or nothing. Only those participants who selected methamphetamine on all 3 days were eligible to proceed to Phase 2. Participants were not informed about this relationship between Phase 1 preferences and eligibility for Phase 2. During Phase 2 participants made repeated choices between methamphetamine and money. Each day the dose of methamphetamine they had previously sampled was divided into tenths and they made 10 choices between the drug and money. The amount of money varied across sessions but was constant during sessions. Monetary values were $0.05, $1, and $5 per choice. Choices were registered by completing an FR 10 response on a computer keyboard (10 keystrokes). Participants responded every 5 minutes for 50 minutes. Participants were also informed that they were free not to respond, though none elected to do so. The order in which the various magnitudes of the monetary alternative were presented was randomly determined for each participant. Money and drugs were made available to the participant after all choices had been registered. Each participant experienced each condition twice. Table 5.1 shows the results for each participant.

These results suggest that methamphetamine self-administration, the hallmark of methamphetamine addiction, is amenable to alteration via the presentation of alternative sources of reinforcement. Specifically, as the magnitude of the alternative source of reinforcement increased, the likelihood of self-administering methamphetamine decreased. This was shown twice for two of the three participants and once for one of the participants. The participant who selected money on the second set of exposures was re-

TABLE 5.1. Number of Times Methamphetamine Was Selected
in the Laboratory Study

	$0.05		$1.00		$5.00	
	First exposure	Second exposure	First exposure	Second exposure	First exposure	Second exposure
Participant 1	10	10	5	5	0	0
Participant 2	10	10	5	5	0	0
Participant 3	10	0	5	0	1	0
Mean	8.3		4.2		0.2	

sponding to an external pressure, raised by the participant's significant
other, who resented the participant being in the hospital and taking methamphetamine while the significant other was looking for employment. As a
result, this respondent selected money on all of the second-choice sessions.
In our opinion, this does not detract from the results obtained; it merely
points to the difficulties in obtaining good experimental control in studies
of this type with human participants.

These data add to a growing body of literature that suggests that drug
abuse is largely a case of operant behavior and thus is amenable to alteration via changing the environmental context (e.g., Higgins et al., 2004).

Given the similarity of these results to those obtained for other drugs
of abuse, which have been shown to be sensitive to CM-based treatment
(e.g., cocaine; cf. Higgins et al., 1994), it appears that studies investigating
the use of CM in the treatment of methamphetamine addiction are warranted.

TREATMENT STUDIES

To date, very few clinical assessments of CM's efficacy in treating methamphetamine abuse have been published. We describe two trials here, one using the variable-magnitude-of-reinforcement procedure (Roll et al., 2006)
and one using the VBRT procedure (Shoptaw et al., 2005). Following that
we describe two VBRT studies designed to optimize the reinforcement
schedule with which vouchers and/or prizes are distributed in the treatment
of methamphetamine abuse (Roll, Huber, et al., 2006; Roll & Shoptaw,
2006).

Variable Magnitude of Reinforcement

This study was conducted as part of NIDA's Clinical Trials Network initiative. Detailed descriptions of this project may be found in Roll, Huber, et

al. (2006). In the original project, stimulant-dependent participants (cocaine and methamphetamine) were randomized to receive variable-magnitude-of-reinforcement CM + treatment as usual (TAU) (Petry et al., 2000, 2002, 2004) or TAU only at various drug-free clinics around the country. The overall outcomes of that project have been reported elsewhere and suggest that the CM procedure was effective at retaining individuals in treatment and initiating abstinence (Petry et al., 2005). The overall study consisted largely of cocaine-dependent individuals (72%). The remaining 113 individuals were primary methamphetamine abusers.

These 113 methamphetamine-abusing participants were randomized to one of the two study conditions: TAU or CM + TAU. Following randomization, the intervention was in effect for 12 weeks, during which time participants were concurrently enrolled in TAU at their respective clinics. All participants were expected to attend two study visits per week on nonconsecutive days. Study schedules were individualized to make them as convenient as possible and to coincide with clinic attendance. Participants were expected to provide a urine sample at each of the twice-weekly study visits during the 12-week period, for a total of up to 24 samples. If a participant failed to give a valid sample or attend a scheduled visit, the sample was considered missing. Urine samples were tested with OnTrak TesTcup 5® (Roche Diagnostics, Indianapolis, Indiana), which tests for amphetamine, methamphetamine, cocaine, THC, and morphine. Participants also provided a breath sample at each visit that was tested for alcohol using a breathalyzer.

Description of Study Conditions

TREATMENT AS USUAL

Participants received usual care at their clinics, which consisted primarily of group and some individual and family counseling. In addition to usual care, participants provided urine and breath samples twice weekly and received immediate feedback on their results. Research staff congratulated participants whenever they tested negative and encouraged them to stop using whenever they tested positive. If participants reported personal problems or clinical issues, research staff responded in an empathetic manner and encouraged them to discuss concerns with their counselor.

CONTINGENCY MANAGEMENT

In addition to usual care plus drug testing described earlier, participants assigned to this condition earned the chance to win prizes each time they tested negative for methamphetamine. Those who tested negative for all primary target drugs were invited to draw between 1 and 12 square plastic chips from an opaque container containing 500 chips. Each chip was marked with a reward value: 250 (50%) were marked "good job!," 209 (41.8%) were marked "small," 40 (8%) were marked "large," and 1 (0.2%) was marked "jumbo." "Good job!" chips meant no tangible reward was earned. Prizes associated with "Small" chips were worth approximately $1. When such a chip was drawn, participants selected from a variety of prizes in the category; popular small items included toiletries, snacks, bus tokens, and gift certificates to fast-food restaurants. Items available as "large" prizes were worth about $20. Commonly selected ones included kitchen objects, toys, cordless telephones, portable CD players, and gift certificates to retail stores. "Jumbo" prizes were worth $80–$100; popular items were televisions, stereos, and DVD players. Prizes were stored in locked cabinets and replenished regularly. Although prize categories were defined by retail value, each clinic, in consultation with the participants, chose items desirable to the participants.

The number of draws earned was determined by a schedule that was responsive to test outcomes. Specifically, the number of draws increased by one for each week in which all submitted samples tested negative for the primary target drugs. The number of draws earned reset to a single draw after an unexcused absence or submission of a sample positive for one or more primary target drugs. This escalating schedule with a reset contingency has been demonstrated to produce relatively more continuous, in-treatment abstinence than other schedules to which it has been compared (Roll & Higgins, 2000).[2] Participants who provided all scheduled urine and breath samples throughout the study and who were negative for all drugs earned 204 draws, resulting in an average of approximately $400 in prizes. For additional details see Petry et al. (2005) and Roll et al. (2006).

RESULTS

Demographic variables did not differ between the two conditions. Retention was not statistically different between groups. With regard to stimulant use during treatment, participants in the CM condition produced significantly more ($M = 13.9$, SEM = 1.2) stimulant-negative samples than did participants in the TAU condition ($M = 9.9$, SEM = 1.0). Similarly, participants in the incentive condition produced longer mean periods of abstinence ($M = 9.3$, SEM = 1.2) than did participants in the TAU condition ($M = 5.6$, SEM =0.9). Abstinence rates across treatment visits were assessed with generalized estimating equations (GEE) analysis, which indicated that

---

[2]A discussion of reinforcement schedules follows this section.

the CM participants were more likely to submit negative urine samples than TAU participants (see Figure 5.1). In addition, 18% of those individuals in the incentive condition were abstinent throughout the entire trial compared with only 6% in the TAU condition. For additional information, see Roll, Petry, et al. (2006), and Petry et al. (2005).

These results are noteworthy for several reasons. First, they represent the first controlled trial of variable-magnitude-of-reinforcement CM as an adjunct to psychosocial treatment of methamphetamine abuse. The results clearly demonstrate the benefits of adding prize-based CM to standard treatment. Participants receiving a combination of CM and psychosocial treatment were abstinent more often during the 12-week intervention and were abstinent for longer continuous periods during the intervention than participants receiving psychosocial treatment alone.

The results from this study build on a large body of evidence suggesting that most types of substance use disorders are amenable to treatment via CM (e.g., Higgins et al., 2004). This study unequivocally adds methamphetamine dependence to the list of substance use disorders for which CM is an appropriate intervention. The results extend our earlier laboratory work suggesting that methamphetamine use would be amenable to CM interventions. Demonstrating the sensitivity of methamphetamine dependence to CM further strengthens the position that drug abuse can be usefully characterized as operant behavior.

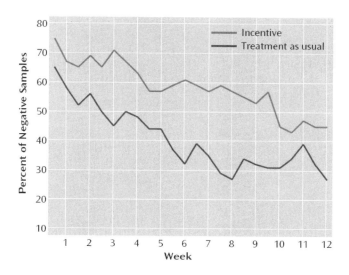

FIGURE 5.1. Methamphetamine use during the course of the 12-week intervention. From Roll et al. (2006). Copyright 2006 by the American Psychiatric Association. Reprinted by permission.

Notably, this study was conducted at multiple locales and in community-based treatment centers as opposed to a single facility designed for research. We believe this speaks to the external validity of the results. We believe that demonstrating the efficacy of CM in a real-world setting shows that the intervention has actual clinical utility.

VOUCHER-BASED REINFORCEMENT THERAPY

Shoptaw et al. (2005) conducted one study examining the efficacy of VBRT CM for the treatment of methamphetamine abuse. This study was conducted with a population of treatment-seeking gay and bisexual men (GBM).

In this study, participants were randomized to one of four conditions (CBT, CM, CM + CBT, or a specific form of CBT designed for GBM, GCBT). The study examined a number of outcomes related to drug use and risky sexual behavior. We limit the discussion in this chapter to the drug use outcomes. A total of 162 participants were randomized (CBT = 40, CM = 42, CBT + CM = 40, GCBT = 40). CM consisted of VBRT (e.g., Higgins et al., 1993). Initial voucher value was $2.50 and each consecutive urine sample that tested negative for methamphetamine increased the value of the voucher by an additional $2.50. The provision of three consecutive methamphetamine-negative samples resulted in the delivery of a "bonus" voucher worth $10 (see discussion of reinforcement schedules below). In addition there was a reset contingency for failure to abstain. Vouchers could be exchanged for goods or services promoting prosocial, nonaddiction lifestyles (groceries, camera equipment, plane fare to go visit relatives, etc.). Urine samples were collected thrice weekly and analyzed with SYVA EMIT (enzyme-multiplied immunoassay technique). Treatment episodes lasted for 16 weeks.

Results

Participants in the conditions receiving CM consistently outperformed participants in the other conditions with regard to continuous abstinence and treatment retention. Participants in the CBT condition were retained for approximately 9 weeks, those in the CM condition for approximately 12 weeks, those in the CM + CBT condition for approximately 13 weeks, and those in the GCBT for approximately 11 weeks. Participants in the CBT condition achieved approximately 2 weeks of consecutive abstinence, participants in the CM condition achieved approximately 5 weeks of continuous abstinence, participants in the CBT + CM condition achieved approximately 7 weeks of continuous abstinence, and participants in the GCBT obtained approximately 3.5 weeks of consecutive abstinence. Overall percentage of methamphetamine-negative samples was high for all conditions (CBT = 75%, CM = 76%, CBT + CM = 78%, and GCBT = 69.7%) and did not significantly differ between conditions. It should be noted that sexual risk behaviors declined during treatment for all conditions but more dramatically for the GCBT condition.

This study demonstrates that methamphetamine use can be addressed clinically with VBRT. This further strengthens our position that methamphetamine use, like most compulsive drug use, is a form of operant behavior. Because this study was conducted with a GBM population, its generality to other populations needs to be considered. Given the laboratory results described earlier, the numerous demonstrations of the applicability of CM in other populations, and the results of the variable-magnitude-of-reinforcement procedure described previously, we suspect that these results are generalizable.

FACTORS INFLUENCING THE EFFICACY OF CM

A number of important factors that may contribute to the success of CM have been studied, including type of reinforcer (e.g., Iguchi, Stitzer, Bigelow, & Liebson, 1988; Petry & Martin, 2002; Schmitz, Rhoades, Elk, Creson, Hussein, & Grabowski, 1998), type of response needed to earn reinforcement (e.g., Petry, Martin, Cooney, & Kranzler, 2000; Stitzer & Bigelow, 1985), type of procedure for distributing reinforcers (Petry, 2002), delay to the delivery of reinforcement (Schwartz, Lauderdal, Montgomery, Burch, & Gallant, 1987; Reilly, Roll, & Downey, 2000), magnitude of reinforcement (e.g., Dallery, Silverman, Chutuape, Bigelow, & Stitzer, 2001; Silverman, Chutuape, Bigelow, & Stitzer, 1999; Stitzer & Bigelow, 1985; Roll, Reilly, & Johanson, 2000), population (Corby, Roll, Ledgerwood, & Schuster, 2000; McNamara, Schumacher, Milby, Wallace, & Usdan, 2001; Roll, Higgins, Steingard, & McGinley, 1998; Shaner et al., 1997), and schedule with which reinforcement is delivered (Kirby, Marlowe, Festinger, Lamb, & Platt, 1998; Roll, Higgins, & Badger, 1996; Roll & Higgins, 2000).

It is our belief that two of these factors, magnitude and reinforcement schedule, are perhaps the most important (see Higgins & Silverman, Chapter 1, this volume for discussion of related issues). Magnitude must be sufficient to combat drug use (e.g., Lussier et al., 2006). If it is not, the CM procedure will likely fail. This suggests that clinicians and researchers have the common task of identifying potential reinforcers (e.g., prizes, vouchers, or other activities or items) that are salient to individual participants.

To date, we believe that the data support the position that the most effective reinforcement schedule for delivering vouchers or prizes is the one initially proposed by Higgins et al. (1991). This schedule incorporates an escalating-reinforcer magnitude for consecutive instances of abstinence, a reset in reinforcer magnitude for failure to abstain, and a bonus for consecutive instances of abstinence. We have demonstrated in several analog studies using cigarette smokers the importance of the combination of the reinforcer escalation and the reset contingencies in promoting continuous, in-treatment abstinence (Roll et al., 1996; Roll & Higgins, 2000). Because the amount of in-treatment abstinence is one of the best predictors of long-term, posttreatment abstinence for several drugs (cocaine, Higgins et al., 2000; marijuana, Moore & Budney, 2002; and methamphetamine, Roll, Petry, et al., 2006), it makes clinical sense to utilize the scheduling procedure that has the greatest likelihood of producing long periods of in-treatment abstinence.

To assess the efficacy of different scheduling arrangements in the treatment of methamphetamine abuse we conducted two studies (Roll, Huber, et al., 2006; Roll & Shoptaw, 2006).

In the first of these studies (Roll, Huber, et al., 2006), participants seeking outpatient behavioral treatment for methamphetamine use disorders were randomly assigned to one of five conditions each of which delivered VBRT for methamphetamine use. The only difference between conditions was the schedule of reinforcement with which the vouchers were delivered. Each schedule delivered approximately the same magnitude of reinforcement (i.e., $990–$1,005). Four schedules were developed by clinicians experienced in the treatment of substance abuse and these were compared to the schedule developed by Higgins. The clinician-generated schedules varied initial rates and escalation of reinforcement values. In all five conditions participants came to our research clinic three times a week. During the first 8–12 weeks of treatment, VBRT procedures were in effect. On every Monday, Wednesday, and Friday participants provided an observed urine specimen, which was immediately analyzed to detect recent methamphetamine use. If the sample indicated no recent use, the participant received a voucher of the specified monetary value. Failure to provide a urine sample was treated the same as the provision of a positive urine sample for reinforcement scheduling purposes.

All five reinforcement schedules engendered considerable abstinence. There was no statistically significant difference between the groups in either mean total number of abstinences during treatment or terms of the mean longest period of continuous abstinence. However, as in our analog studies, the likelihood of maintaining abstinence once it had been initiated was greater when using the schedule developed by Higgins than in any of the other conditions.

In the second study (Roll & Shoptaw, 2006) we further investigated the use of VBRT to treat methamphetamine abuse. In this study participants were randomized to one of two conditions, both of which included an escalating voucher magnitude for consecutive instances of abstinence. However, only one of them included a reset for failure to abstain. Results indicated that the schedule with the reset outperformed the other schedule with regard to total number of abstinences and longest duration of in-treatment abstinence.

These pilot studies suggest that the greatest likelihood for a successful treatment episode using CM will be produced when high-magnitude reinforcers (prizes or vouchers) are disbursed according to a reinforcement schedule that incorporates escalating-reinforcer magnitude for consecutive instances of abstinence and a reset in reinforcer value for a failure to abstain.

CONCLUDING COMMENTS

Methamphetamine use is spreading and becoming a public health problem of considerable importance. We believe that law enforcement, prevention, and treatment efforts will all be needed to successfully combat this problem. While the study of CM for the treatment of methamphetamine abuse is relatively recent, we are encouraged by the results to date.

ACKNOWLEDGMENTS

This research was supported by National Institute on Drug Abuse Grant Nos. R01-017407, R01-017084, and R21-14392.

REFERENCES

Anglin, M. D., Burke, C., Perrochet, B., Stamper, E., & Dawud-Noursi, S. (2000). History of the methamphetamine problem. *Journal of Psychoactive Drugs, 32*, 137–141.

Beyrer, C., Razak, M. H., Jittiwutikar, J., Suriyanon, V., Vongchak, T., Srirak, N., et al. (2004). Methamphetamine users in northern Thailand: Changing demographics and risks for HIV and STD among treatment-seeking substance abusers. *International Journal on the Study of AIDS, 15*, 697–704.

Bigelow, G. E., & Silverman, K. (1999). Theoretical and empirical foundations of contingency management treatments for drug abuse. In S. T. Higgins & K. Silverman (Eds.), *Motivating behavior change among illicit-drug abusers: Research on contingency management interventions* (pp. 15–31). Washington, DC: American Psychological Association.

Budney, A. J., Higgins, S. T., Radonovich, K. J., & Novy, P. L. (2000). Adding voucher-based incentives to coping skills and motivational enhancement improves outcomes during treatment for marijuana dependence. *Journal of Consulting and Clinical Psychology, 68*, 1051–1061.

Carroll, K. M., & Onken, L. S. (2005). Behavioral therapies for drug abuse. *American Journal of Psychiatry, 162,* 1452–1460.

Carroll, M. E., Lac, S. T., & Nygaard, S. L. (1989). A concurrently available nondrug reinforcer prevents the acquisition or decreases the maintenance of cocaine-reinforced behavior. *Psychopharmacology, 97,* 23–29.

Cartier, J., Farabee, D., & Prendergast, M. L. (2006). Methamphetamine use, self-reported violent crime, and recidivism among offenders in California who abuse substances. *Journal of Interpersonal Violence, 21,* 435–445.

Cherner, M., Letendre, S., Heaton, R. K., Durelle, J., Marquie-Beck, J., Gragg, B., et al. (2005). Hepatitis C augments cognitive deficits associated with HIV infection and methamphetamine. *Neurology, 26,* 1328–1329.

Clark, H. W. (2000). The CSAT methamphetamine treatment project. *Journal of Psychoactive Drugs, 32,* 133–134.

Copeland, A. L., & Sorensen, J. L. (2001). Differences between methamphetamine users and cocaine users in treatment. *Drug and Alcohol Dependence, 62,* 91–95.

Corby, C. A., Roll, J. M., Ledgerwood, D., & Schuster, C. R. (2000). Contingency management interventions for treating the substance abuse of adolescents: A feasibility study. *Experimental and Clinical Psychopharmacology, 8,* 371–376.

Cretzmeyer, M., Sarrazin, M. V., Huber, D. L., Block, R. I., & Hall, J. A. (2003). Treatment of methamphetamine abuse: Research findings and clinical directions. *Journal of Substance Abuse Treatment, 24,* 267–277.

Dallery, J., Silverman, K., Chutuape, M. A., Bigelow, G. E., & Stitzer, M. L. (2001). Voucher-based reinforcement of opiate plus cocaine abstinence in treatment-resistant methadone patients: Effects of reinforcer magnitude. *Experimental Clinical Psychopharmacology, 9,* 317–325.

Danks, R. R., Wibbenmeyer, L. A., Faucher, L. D., Sihler, K. C., Kealey, G. P., Chang, P., et al. (2004). Methamphetamine-associated burn injuries: A retrospective analysis. *Journal of Burn Care and Rehabilitation, 25,* 425–429.

Freese, T. E., Miotto, K., & Reback, C. J. (2002). The effects and consequences of selected club drugs. *Journal of Substance Abuse Treatment, 23,* 151–156.

Frosch, D., Shoptaw, S., Huber, A., Rawson, R. A., & Ling, W. (1996). Sexual HIV risk among gay and bisexual male methamphetamine abusers. *Journal of Substance Abuse Treatment, 13,* 483–486.

Galloway, G. P., Newmeyer, J., Knapp, T., Stalcup, S. A., & Smith, D. (1994). Imipramine for the treatment of cocaine and methamphetamine dependence. *Journal of Addictive Disorders, 13,* 201–216.

Haney, M., & Kosten, T. R. (2004). Therapeutic vaccines for substance dependence. *Expert Review of Vaccines, 3,* 11–18.

Hanson, G. (2005). Paper presented at ACNP methamphetamine meeting, Waikoloa, HI.

Higgins, S. T. (1997). The influence of alternative reinforcers on cocaine use and abuse: A brief review. *Pharmacology and Biochemistry of Behavior, 57,* 419–427.

Higgins, S. T., Badger, G. J., & Budney, A. J. (2000). Initial abstinence and success in achieving longer term cocaine abstinence. *Experimental and Clinical Psychopharmacology, 8,* 377–386.

Higgins, S. T., Bickel, W. K., & Hughes, J. R. (1994). Influence of an alternative reinforcer on human cocaine self-administration. *Life Science, 55,* 179–187.

Higgins, S. T., Budney, A. J., Bickel, W. K., Foerg, F. E., Donham, R., & Badger, G. J. (1994). Incentives improve outcome in outpatient behavioral treatment of cocaine dependence. *Archives of General Psychiatry, 51,* 568–576.

Higgins, S. T., Budney, A. J., Bickel, W. K., Hughes, J. R., Foerg, F., & Badger, G. (1993).

Achieving cocaine abstinence with a behavioral approach. *American Journal of Psychiatry, 150,* 763–769.

Higgins, S. T., Delaney, D. D., Budney, A. J., Bickel, W. K., Hughes, J. R., Foerg, F., et al. (1991). A behavioral approach to achieving initial cocaine abstinence. *American Journal of Psychiatry, 148,* 1218–1224.

Higgins, S. T., Heil, S. H., & Plebani-Lussier, J. (2004). Clinical implications of reinforcement as a determinate of substance use disorders. *Annual Review of Psychology, 55,* 431–461.

Higgins, S. T., & Silverman, K. (Eds.). (1999). *Motivating behavior change among illicit drug abusers: Contemporary research on contingency-management interventions.* Washington, DC: American Psychological Association.

Higgins, S. T., Stitzer, M. L., Bigelow, G. E., & Liebson, I. A. (1986). Contingent methadone delivery: Effects on illicit-opiate use. *Drug and Alcohol Dependence, 17,* 311–322.

Higgins, S. T., Wong, C. J., Badger, G. J., Ogden, D. E., & Dantona, R. L. (2000). Contingent reinforcement increases cocaine abstinence during outpatient treatment and 1 year of follow-up. *Journal of Consulting and Clinical Psychology, 68,* 64–72.

Iguchi, M. Y., Stitzer, M. L., Bigelow, G. E., & Liebson, I. A. (1988, October). Contingency management in methadone maintenance: Effects of reinforcing and aversive consequences on illicit polydrug use. *Drug and Alcohol Dependence, 22,* 1–7.

Kalechstein, A. D., Newton, T. F., & Green, M. (2003). Methamphetamine dependence is associated with neurocognitive impairment in the initial phases of abstinence. *Journal of Neuropsychiatry and Clinical Neuroscience, 15,* 215–220.

Kashani, J., & Ruha, A. M. (2004). Methamphetamine toxicity secondary to intravaginal body stuffing. *Journal of Toxicology and Clinical Toxicology, 42,* 987–989.

Kirby, K. C., Marlowe, D. B., Festinger, D. S., Lamb, R. J., & Platt, J. J. (1998). Schedule of voucher delivery influences initiation of cocaine abstinence. *Journal of Consulting and Clinical Psychology, 66,* 761–767.

Lussier, J. P., Heil, S. H., Mongeon, J. A., Badger, G. J., & Higgins, S. T. (2006). A meta-analysis of voucher-based reinforcement therapy for substance use disorders. *Addiction, 101,* 192–203.

McNamara, C., Schumacher, J. E., Milby, J. B., Wallace, D., & Usdan, S. (2001). Prevalence of nonpsychotic mental disorders does not affect treatment outcome in a homeless cocaine dependent sample. *American Journal of Drug and Alcohol Abuse, 27,* 91–106.

Moore, B. A., & Budney, A. J. (2002). Abstinence at intake for marijuana dependence treatment predicts response. *Drug and Alcohol Dependence, 67,* 249–257.

Nader, M. A., & Woolverton, W. L. (1991). Effects of increasing the magnitude of an alternative reinforcer on drug choice on a discrete-trials choice procedure. *Psychopharmacology, 105,* 169–174.

Newton, T. F., Kalechstein, A. D., Duran, S., Vansluis, N., & Ling, W. (2004). Methamphetamine abstinence syndrome: Preliminary findings. *American Journal of Addiction, 13,* 248–255.

Peck, J. A., Shoptaw, S., Rotheram-Fuller, E., Reback, C. J., & Bierman, B. (2005). HIV-associated medical, behavioral, and psychiatric characteristics of treatment-seeking, methamphetamine-dependent men who have sex with men. *Journal of Addictive Disorders, 24,* 115–132.

Petry, N. M. (2002). *Vouchers vs. prizes and the winner is.* Paper presented at the 2002 annual conference of the American Psychological Association.

Petry, N. M., Alessi, S. M., Marx, J., Austin, M., & Tardif, M. (2005). Vouchers versus prizes: Contingency management treatment of substance abusers in community settings. *Journal of Consulting and Clinical Psychology, 73*, 1005–1014.

Petry, N. M., & Martin, B. (2002, April). Low-cost contingency management treatment for treating cocaine- and opioid-abusing methadone patients. *Journal of Consulting and Clinical Psychology, 70*, 398–405.

Petry, N. M., Martin, B., Cooney, J. L., & Kranzler, H. R. (2000). Give them prizes, and they will come: Contingency management for treatment of alcohol dependence. *Journal of Consulting and Clinical Psychology, 68*, 250–257.

Petry, N. M., Martin, B., & Finocche, C. (2001, September). Contingency management in group treatment: A demonstration project in an HIV drop-in center. *Journal of Substance Abuse and Treatment, 21*, 89–96.

Petry, N. M., Peirce, J., Stitzer, M., Blaine, J., Roll, J. M., Cohen, A., et al. (2005). Effect of prize-based incentives on outcomes in stimulant abusers in outpatient psychosocial treatment programs: A national drug abuse treatment Clinical Trials Network Study. *Archives of General Psychiatry, 62*, 1148–1156.

Petry, N. M., Tedford, J., Austin, M., Nich, C., Carroll, K. M., & Rounsaville, B. J. (2004). Prize reinforcement contingency management for treating cocaine users: How low can we go, and with whom? *Addiction, 99*, 349–360.

Prendergast, M., Podus, D., Finney, J., Greenwell, L., & Roll, J. (2006). *Contingency management for treatment of substance use disorders: A meta-analysis.* Manuscript submitted for publication.

Rawson, R., Huber, A., Brethen, P., Obert, J., Gulati, V., Shoptaw, S., et al. (2000). Methamphetamine and cocaine users: Differences in characteristics and treatment retention. *Journal of Psychoactive Drugs, 32*, 233–238.

Rawson, R. A., Gonzales, R., & Brethen, P. (2002, September). Treatment of methamphetamine use disorders: An update. *Journal of Substance Abuse Treatment, 23*, 145–150.

Rawson, R. A., Marinelli-Casey, P., Anglin, M. D., Dickow, A., Frazier, Y., Gallagher, C., et al. (2004). A multi-site comparison of psychosocial approaches for the treatment of methamphetamine dependence. *Addiction, 99*, 708–717.

Rawson, R. A., Marinelli-Casey, P., & Washton, A. M. (1996). Integrating the delivery of privately and publicly funded substance abuse services. *Behavioral Healthcare Tomorrow, 5*, 32–35.

Reback, C. J., Larkins, S., & Shoptaw, S. (2004). Changes in the meaning of sexual risk behaviors among gay and bisexual male methamphetamine abusers before and after drug treatment. *AIDS Behavior, 8*, 87–98.

Reilly, M. P., Roll, J. M., & Downey, K. (2000). Impulsivity and voucher versus money preference in polydrug dependent participants enrolled in a contingency-management based substance abuse treatment program. *Journal of Substance Abuse Treatment, 19*, 253–257.

Roll, J. M., & Higgins, S. T. (2000). A within-subject comparison of three different schedules of reinforcement of drug abstinence using cigarette smoking as an exemplar. *Drug and Alcohol Dependence, 58*, 103–109.

Roll, J. M., Higgins, S. T., & Badger, G. (1996). An experimental comparison of three different schedules of reinforcement of drug abstinence using cigarette smoking as an exemplar. *Journal of Applied Behavior Analysis, 29*, 495–505.

Roll, J. M., Higgins, S. T., Steingard, S., & McGinley, M. (1998). Assessment of the sensitivity of substance use by schizophrenics to contingency-management interventions. *Experimental and Clinical Psychopharmacology, 6*, 157–161.

Roll, J. M., Huber, A., Sodano, R., Chudzynski, J., Moynier, E., & Shoptaw, S. (2006). A comparison of five reinforcement schedules for use in contingency management-based treatment of methamphetamine abuse. *Psychological Record, 56,* 67–81.

Roll, J. M., Petry, N. M., Stitzer, M. L., Brecht, M. L., Peirce, J. M., McCann, M. J., et al. (2006). Contingency management for the treatment of methamphetamine use. disorders. *American Journal of Psychiatry, 163,* 1993–1999.

Roll, J. M., Reilly, M. P., & Johanson, C-E. (2000). A laboratory analog examining the influence of exchange delays on the efficacy of an alternative source of reinforcement in preventing human drugs self-administration using cigarette smoking as an exemplar. *Experimental and Clinical Psychopharmacology, 8,* 366–370.

Roll, J. M., & Shoptaw, S. (2006). Contingency management: Schedule effects. *Psychiatric Research, 144,* 91–93.

Schmitz, J. M., Rhoades, H. M., Elk, R., Creson, D., Hussein, I., & Grabowski, J. (1998). Medication take-home doses and contingency management. *Experimental Clinical Psychopharmacology, 6,* 162–168.

Schwartz, B., Lauderdale, R. M., Montgomery, M. L., Burch, E. A., & Gallant, D. M. (1987). Immediate vs. delayed feedback on urinalysis reports for methadone maintenance patients. *Addictive Behavior, 12,* 293–295.

Semple, S. J., Patterson, T. L., & Grant, I. (2004). Determinants of condom use stage of change among heterosexually-identified methamphetamine users. *AIDS Behavior, 8,* 391–400.

Semple, S. J., Zians, J., Grant, I., & Patterson, T. L. (2005). Impulsivity and methamphetamine use. *Journal of Substance Abuse Treatment, 29,* 293–295.

Shaner, A., Roberts, L. J., Eckman, T. A., Tucker, D. E., Tsuang, J. W., Wilkins, J. N., et al. (1997, June). Monetary reinforcement of abstinence from cocaine among mentally ill patients with cocaine dependence. *Psychiatric Services, 48,* 807–810.

Shoptaw, S., Reback, C. J., & Freese, T. (2002). Patient characteristics, HIV serostatus, and risk behaviors among gay and bisexual males seeking treatment for methamphetamine abuse and dependence in Los Angeles. *Journal of Addictive Diseases, 21,* 91–105.

Shoptaw, S., Reback, C. J., Peck, J. A., Yang, X., Rotheram-Fuller, E., Larkins, S., et al. (2005). Behavioral treatment approaches for methamphetamine dependence and HIV-related sexual risk behaviors among urban gay and bisexual men. *Drug and Alcohol Dependence, 78,* 125–134.

Silverman, K., Chutuape, M. A., Bigelow, G. E., & Stitzer, M. L. (1999, September). Voucher-based reinforcement of cocaine abstinence in treatment-resistant methadone patients: Effects of reinforcement magnitude. *Psychopharmacology, 146,* 128–138.

Silverman, K., Higgins, S. T., Brooner, R. K., Montoya, I. D., Cone, E. J., Schuster, C. R., et al. (1996). Sustained cocaine abstinence in methadone maintenance patients through voucher based reinforcement therapy. *Archives of General Psychiatry, 53,* 409–415.

Simon, S. L., Richardson, K., Dacey, J., Glynn, S., Domier, C. P., Rawson, R. A., et al. (2002). A comparison of patterns of methamphetamine and cocaine use. *Journal of Addictive Disease, 21,* 35–44.

Simons, J. S., Oliver, M. N., Gaher, R. M., Ebel, G., & Brummels, P. (2005). Methamphetamine and alcohol abuse and dependence symptoms: Associations with affect lability and impulsivity in a rural treatment population. *Addictive behaviors, 30,* 1370–1381.

Skinner, B. F. (1938). *The behavior of organisms.* New York: Appleton-Century-Crofts.

Stitzer, M., & Bigelow, G. E. (1985). Contingent reinforcement for carbon monoxide reduction: Within-subject effects of pay amount. *Journal of Applied Behavior Analysis, 17,* 477–483.

Stitzer, M., Bigelow, G. E., & Liebson, I. (1979). Reducing benzodiazepine self-administration with contingent reinforcement. *Addictive Behaviors, 4,* 245–252.

Tominaga, G. T., Garcia, G., Dzierba, A., & Wong, J. (2004). Toll of methamphetamine on the trauma system. *Archives of Surgery, 139,* 844–847.

Wang, G. J., Volkow, N. D., Chang, L., Miller, E., Sedler, M., Hitzeman, R., et al. (2004). Partial recovery of brain metabolism in methamphetamine abusers after protracted abstinence. *American Journal of Psychiatry, 161,* 242–248.

Yen, C. F., Wu, H. Y., Yen, J. Y., & Ko, C. H. (2004). Effects of brief cognitive-behavioral interventions on confidence to resist the urges to use heroin and methamphetamine in relapse-related situations. *Journal of Nervous and Mental Disorders, 192,* 788–791.

Zweben, J. E., Cohen, J. B., Christian, D., Galloway, G. P., Salinardi, M., Parent, D., et al. (2004). Psychiatric symptoms in methamphetamine users. *American Journal of the Addictions, 13,* 181–190.

CHAPTER 6

TOBACCO

Stacey C. Sigmon, Richard J. Lamb,
and Jesse Dallery

Cigarette smoking is the leading cause of preventable death in the United States, causing approximately 440,000 deaths annually (Centers for Disease Control [CDC], 2002) and resulting in 5.6 million years of potential life lost, $75 billion in direct medical costs, and $82 billion in lost productivity (CDC, 2002). An estimated 70.3 million Americans (29.2% of those over 12 years of age) reported past-month tobacco use in 2004, and 35.3 million Americans met criteria for nicotine dependence (Substance Abuse and Mental Health Services Administration [SAMHSA], 2005).

Although there are many therapies for smoking cessation (U.S. Department of Health and Human Services, 2000), the majority of patients eventually relapse (Ahluwalia, Harris, Catley, Okuyemi, & Mayo, 2002; Eisenberg, Stitzer, & Henningfield, 1999; Fiore, Smith, Jorenby, & Baker, 1994; Hurt et al., 1997). A review of controlled studies on nicotine replacement therapies revealed that 78% of treatment-seeking smokers relapsed within 6 months (Fiore et al., 1994). Another challenge for smoking cessation is that many smokers experience significant difficulty initiating abstinence. Up to 80% of smokers express some desire to quit, yet only about 30% actually attempt to quit per year (Eisenberg et al., 1999). Especially problematic are so-called hard-core smokers who may be particularly difficult to help with existing treatments (Eméry, Gilpin, Ake, Farkas, & Pierce, 2000; Seidman & Covey, 1999). These smokers have a heavy pattern of smoking, infrequent and unsuccessful quit attempts, and a low motivation to quit smoking (Emery et al., 2000).

The limitations of current smoking-cessation interventions, as well as the difficulties in reaching hard-core smokers, suggest the need for innovative and more intensive smoking-cessation programs (Fagerstrom et al., 1996; Stitzer, 1999). Indeed, Stitzer (1999) argued that increasing the acceptability and accessibility of behavior therapy is critical: "Greater use of behavior therapy is especially important in view of the research findings that support its dose-related ability to improve cessation" (p. 186).

Contingency management (CM) is one behavioral intervention that could serve as an important complement to established treatments. CM interventions represent a form of empirically based substance abuse treatment which has been demonstrated effective across a wide range of populations and drugs. CM procedures provide incentives and disincentives contingent upon changes in patients' behavior and have been used as stand-alone interventions or as adjuncts to a more comprehensive treatment (for additional details, see Higgins & Silverman, Chapter 1, this volume; Higgins & Silverman, 1999; cf. Higgins, Alessi, & Dantona, 2002). This approach typically involves the delivery of a tangible reward, often voucher-based incentives, contingent upon the patient meeting a predetermined therapeutic target (Higgins et al., 1991; Petry, Martion, Cooney, & Kranzler, 2000). The most common targeted behavior is drug abstinence, wherein the patient earns voucher-based incentives for biochemically verified abstinence from recent drug use (e.g., negative urine sample or breath alcohol level). In the area of smoking cessation, CM treatments typically target smoking abstinence and make delivery of incentives contingent upon biochemically verified abstinence from recent smoking (e.g., negative breath carbon monoxide or urine cotinine samples).

One particularly important role for CM may be facilitating abstinence initiation. Abstinence during first 2 weeks of a quit attempt strongly predicts longer-term success (Garvey et al., 1992; Gourlay, Forbes, Marriner, Pethica, & McNeil, 1994; Kenford et al., 1994; Lamb, Morral, Kirby, Iguchi, & Galbicka, 2004; Yudkin, Jones, Lancaster, & Fowler, 1996). This relationship holds regardless of the presence of a pharmacological treatment. Furthermore, even when smoking status during this key period is manipulated experimentally, long-term outcomes can still be predicted based on initial outcomes (Higgins et al., 2004). Therefore, it may be particularly advantageous to use CM to initiate smoking abstinence during the critical initial weeks of a quit attempt.

MEASURING SMOKING STATUS

An especially important aspect of CM is the method used to monitor smoking status. There are two common approaches to monitoring smoking:

measuring breath carbon monoxide (CO) levels and measuring cotinine levels found in urine, plasma, or saliva. Breath CO levels are typically measured using hand-held meters into which the smoker exhales. These devices are easy to use and require little technical training. Breath CO levels are generally considered the best way to verify smoking abstinence during the initial days of cessation (Jarvis, Tunstall-Pedoe, Feyerabend, Vesey, & Saloojee, 1987). The elimination half-life of CO averages about 4 hours; therefore, abstaining smokers can achieve a CO level in the nonsmoker range within 12–24 hours (SRNT Subcommittee on Biochemical Verification, 2002). This time course is particularly relevant when it comes to choosing a breath CO cutoff level for a smoking cessation intervention.

One's choice of the CO cutoff can be one of the most important determining factors in the effectiveness of a CM intervention. Typical CO readings for smokers are in the range of 20–30 parts per million (ppm). In designing a CM treatment for smoking cessation, it is important to choose a CO cutoff that achieves a balance in sensitivity. That is, the CO cutoff should be low enough to detect very low rates of smoking but not so low that true abstinence is missed. Recent studies suggest that CO cutoffs of 3–6 ppm provide an appropriate level of sensitivity based on the particular goals of the intervention (Higgins et al., 2004, 2007; Javors, Hatch, & Lamb, 2005; Middleton & Morice, 2000; SRNT Subcommittee on Biochemical Verification, 2002).

A relatively intense schedule of monitoring and associated reinforcement also may be needed during the initial days and weeks of the cessation effort. Particularly considering that at least 75% of smokers relapse within 2–3 days following an initial quit attempt (Hughes et al., 1992), a combination of intensive monitoring and frequent reinforcement can help to maximize continuous smoking abstinence during the initial weeks of the cessation effort. When breath CO is used as the primary measure of smoking status, the schedule of monitoring also becomes particularly important. Given the elimination half-life of CO (3–8 hours), smokers can rapidly achieve a criterion CO level within several hours following their last cigarette. Thus, CM interventions using CO levels need to include at least daily CO monitoring in order to be confident of an individual's smoking status. Even with daily CO monitoring, smokers may be able to engage in low levels of smoking that go undetected (Javors et al., 2005). Therefore, some CM studies have required CO monitoring to take place multiple times per day.

Cotinine levels can be collected from a range of bodily fluids (e.g., urine, plasma, and saliva) and are typically analyzed using enzyme-multiplied immunoassay testing (EMIT) or gas chromatography. Cotinine is a metabolite of nicotine and has a half-life of approximately 20 hours. There is good consensus that cotinine is an especially sensitive biomarker for verifying smoking status (Benowitz, 1996; Jarvis et al., 1987; Rebagliato, 2002). As opposed to breath CO testing, in which abstaining smokers can achieve a

CO level in the nonsmoker range within hours of stopping smoking, cotinine testing requires several continuous days of abstinence for smokers to achieve levels in the nonsmoker range (SRNT Subcommittee on Biochemical Verification, 2002).

One advantage of cotinine is that a monitoring schedule of only 2–3 times per week should be sufficient to detect recent smoking. However, because of the relatively long half-life of cotinine, basing incentive delivery on cotinine levels during the early days of a quit attempt can be problematic. For example, an individual smoking approximately 20 cigarettes a day would need about 5 days to meet the commonly used cutoff of 80 ng/ml, which would significantly delay the first opportunity to reward him or her for this early abstinence (SRNT Subcommittee on Biochemical Verification, 2002). An additional complication is that other sources of nicotine, such as nicotine replacement therapies, will elevate cotinine levels and confound cotinine testing.

The considerations for choosing an appropriate cotinine cutoff are similar to those outlined for CO levels (e.g., balancing risks of both false positives and false negatives). Currently, there are no clear published guidelines about the sensitivity of different cotinine cutoffs, though the current literature suggests that a urinary cotinine cutoff of 50 ng/ml is recommended when using gas chromatography to classify smoking status among the general population of smokers (SRNT Subcommittee on Biochemical Verification, 2002).

Considering the foregoing issues, a maximally effective CM intervention might combine both CO and cotinine testing. Indeed, Higgins et al. (2007) recently developed a procedure whereby individuals transition from CO testing during first few days of the cessation attempt to testing using urinary cotinine. This procedure maximizes confidence that the person is not engaging in smoking that goes undetected, while simultaneously minimizing the chance that early efforts at abstinence go unrewarded.

EARLY TREATMENT ANALOGUE STUDIES SUGGESTING THAT CM CAN REDUCE SMOKING

Several early studies provided the initial evidence of the feasibility of using CM to reduce smoking (Elliot & Tighe, 1968; Paxton, 1980, 1981, 1983; Winett, 1973). These studies generally offered rewards, such as the return of monetary deposits, contingent upon self-reports of smoking abstinence and showed that CM could reduce levels of smoking. These studies did suffer from a number of limitations, however, including reliance on self-reports of abstinence versus biochemical verification of abstinence for implementing the contingencies or insufficient monitoring of smoking status.

Subsequent studies, using more rigorous experimental methods, provided persuasive demonstrations that CM could reduce smoking. Stitzer and Bigelow (1982) investigated the use of monetary payments for reduced CO levels in smokers not seeking to quit. That study used a within-subjects, A B A design with each phase lasting 1 week. During the first and third weeks, subjects provided CO samples but received no payments associated with their smoking status. In the second week, payments were available contingent upon breath CO samples demonstrating reduced smoking (i.e., half their average value during the first week). Contingent payments were associated with decreased breath CO levels during the contingent condition compared to the baseline conditions. The efficacy of CM interventions in reducing smoking was later replicated across a variety of settings and populations in subsequent studies by these investigators (Stitzer & Bigelow, 1983, 1985; Stitzer, Rand, Bigelow, & Mead, 1986; Rand, Stitzer, Bigelow, & Mead, 1989).

USING CM TO REDUCE SMOKING AMONG SPECIAL CLINICAL POPULATIONS

Over the past two decades, CM interventions have been widely used to reduce cigarette smoking among a variety of challenging clinical populations. Below we review briefly some of the studies demonstrating CM's effectiveness among these groups of smokers. See Chapters 10–12 (this volume) for more detailed information on the use of CM with pregnant women, individuals with serious mental illness, and adolescents.

Pregnant Women

Smoking during pregnancy is the leading cause of infant morbidity and mortality (U.S. Department of Health and Human Services, 2001). In the first study to apply CM to pregnant smokers, subjects receiving a voucher-based CM intervention achieved greater smoking abstinence compared to those in a control group receiving only educational materials on quitting (Donatelle et al., 2000). Two hundred and twenty pregnant smokers were randomly assigned to the treatment and control groups. Smoking status was verified on a monthly basis during the pregnancy and 2 months postpartum, and incentives were contingent upon providing negative cotinine (≤ 30 ng/ml) samples. Local businesses, foundations, and health care organizations provided funding for the incentives. Each smoker also nominated a "social supporter" to help him or her quit, with the recommendation that the individual be a female nonsmoker, and the social supporter also received vouchers if the smoker was abstinent. At the end of pregnancy, abstinence rates were 32% and 9% in the voucher and control groups, respectively. It is not clear, however, to what extent the social support versus voucher reinforcement produced the relatively high rates of smoking abstinence.

More recently, Higgins et al. (2004) examined the effects of contingent versus noncontingent vouchers in 58 pregnant smokers. Smokers were assigned to each group, and smoking abstinence was defined as CO ≤ 6 ppm or cotinine ≤ 80 ng/ml. Daily CO testing was used to monitor smoking during the initial week of treatment, after which cotinine testing was used at varying intervals until 12 weeks postpartum. At the end of pregnancy, abstinence rates were 37% and 9% in the contingent and noncontingent groups, respectively, and these rates were remarkably maintained at 12 weeks postpartum (33% and 0%). Follow-up at 24 weeks postpartum found that CM also produced long-term gains: 27% of participants in the contingent group were abstinent compared to 0% in the noncontingent group.

While additional efforts to replicate the effectiveness of CM in reducing smoking among pregnant women will be important, these results suggest that CM is a promising tool for promoting the initiation and maintenance of smoking abstinence in the high-risk population of pregnant smokers.

Individuals with Serious Mental Illness

Rates of cigarette smoking among schizophrenics are higher than those in the general population and almost twice as high as those with other psychiatric disorders (Hughes, Hatsukami, Mitchell, & Dahlgren, 1986). Two small outpatient studies have provided evidence that CM is feasible and effective in reducing smoking in individuals with schizophrenia (Roll, Higgins, Steingard, & McGinley, 1998; Tidey, O'Neill, & Higgins, 2002). The first used a within-subjects A B A reversal design with 10 participants completing the 3-week study (Roll et al., 1998). During each of the two, 1-week baseline conditions, participants were visited once per day to measure smoking status using CO and were paid $5 regardless of their CO levels. During the contingent condition, participants were visited three times per day and earned monetary incentives for COs ≤ 11 ppm. Abstinence was increased during the contingent condition compared to the baseline conditions. The second study examined the effects of CM with and without a nicotine patch in schizophrenics (Tidey et al., 2002). Fourteen participants were exposed to three treatment conditions, each lasting 5 days: (1) CM + 21-mg nicotine patch, (2) CM + placebo patch, and (3) noncontingent reinforcement + placebo patch. Contingent delivery of incentives produced the highest rate of abstinence. Interestingly, the addition of the patch did not produce greater gains compared to CM alone.

In summary, cigarette smoking among individuals with schizophrenia is sensitive to contingent incentives for abstinence, providing empirical support for the feasibility of using CM alone or in combination with other treatments to reduce smoking among patients with serious mental illness.

Drug Abusers

Many studies have assessed the ability of CM to reduce smoking in drug abusers. The majority of these were conducted with methadone-maintained (MM) patients. While methadone represents one of the most effective treatments for opioid dependence, the prevalence of cigarette smoking among MM patients is more than threefold that of the general population. The mortality rate of opioid-dependent smokers is estimated to be fourfold greater than that of opioid-dependent nonsmokers (Hser, McCarthy, & Anglin, 1994), and individuals who abuse alcohol and other nonnicotine substances are more likely to die of tobacco-related disorders than problems related to their other drug use (Hurt et al., 1996).

The majority of MM patients recognize the serious health risks associated with smoking and express interest in quitting (Clemmey, Brooner, Chutuape, Kidorf, & Stitzer, 1997; Frosch, Shoptaw, Jarvik, Rawson, & Ling, 1998; Kozlowski, Skinner, Kent, & Pope, 1989; Richter, Gibson, Ahluwalia, & Schmelzle, 2001; Sees & Clark, 1993). Further, the MM treatment modality is uniquely situated for implementing smoking-cessation interventions. Many patients are relatively stable, often achieving prolonged periods of abstinence from illicit drug use and remaining engaged in treatment for relatively long periods. This lends itself to frequent and, if necessary, prolonged clinical contact to ensure success with smoking cessation. In addition, methadone maintenance is one of the only treatment modalities adhering to a uniform set of state and federal regulations. As a result, the development of an effective smoking-cessation intervention among MM patients may hold substantial potential for impacting tobacco use in this population across the country.

An initial report by Schmitz, Rhoades, and Grabowski (1995) sought to replicate in MM patients the early study by Stitzer and Bigelow (1982) wherein monetary payments were delivered CO reductions. Five MM patients provided CO samples twice weekly throughout the 10-week study. Subjects were exposed to alternating 2-week contingent and control phases (four total). During contingent phases, reinforcement was available ($5) for each twice-weekly CO that was $\leq 50\%$ levels during the previous control phase. No reinforcement was available for CO reductions during the control phases. The authors reported no reliable effect of the intervention on smoking rates and raised the possibility that CM interventions for smoking cessation may not generalize to MM patients. Instead of population differences, however, several other shortcomings might have accounted for the poor outcomes in this study. First, the frequency of abstinence monitoring was low (twice weekly) compared to 5 days per week in the Stitzer and Bigelow study. Second, overall reinforcer magnitude (maximum of $10 per week) was modest compared to $25 available per week in the Stitzer and Bigelow study. Magnitude and schedule of reinforcement can be important determinants of the efficacy of CM interventions (Kirby, Marlowe, Festinger, Lamb, & Platt, 1998; Roll, Higgins, & Badger, 1996; Roll & Higgins, 2000; Silverman, Chutuape, Bigelow, & Stitzer, 1999; Stitzer & Bigelow, 1983, 1984).

In the second study on this topic (Shoptaw et al., 1996), 17 MM patients provided thrice-weekly CO samples during a 4-week study and earned voucher-based incentives contingent upon submitting COs ≤ 4 ppm. The magnitude of reinforcement for consecutive negative specimens escalated in value (Higgins et al., 1991), with maximum possible earnings of $73 in vouchers. CO levels decreased significantly during the intervention, but only four patients (23.4%) produced three or more consecutive negative samples; that is, there was little evidence that the intervention produced sustained abstinence. All patients resumed smoking by the end of the trial. It is important to note, however, that while the treatment effects were modest, the improved outcomes in this study provided the first demonstration that smoking in the MM population was sensitive to CM or any other treatment intervention.

In a subsequent study, Shoptaw et al. (2002) randomly assigned MM smokers to one of four treatments: nicotine patch only (21 mg), patch + CM, patch + relapse prevention (RP), and patch + CM + RP (Shoptaw et al., 2002). Throughout the 12-week intervention, CO samples were collected thrice weekly. Participants assigned to the CM conditions earned voucher-based incentives for COs ≤ 8 ppm, using an escalating schedule of reinforcement with maximum possible earnings of $447.50. Participants receiving RP attended weekly counseling focusing on skills to initiate and maintain smoking abstinence. All participants received active nicotine patch throughout the study, which precluded an evaluation of the contribution of the pharmacotherapy to outcome. Participants receiving CM with or without RP achieved significantly higher rates of abstinence throughout much of the intervention compared to those not receiving CM, though there were no significant differences among the four conditions at 6- or 12-month follow-ups.

Results from these studies suggest that CM may be effective in reducing smoking among drug abusers and highlight the importance of further investigation into strategies to produce abstinence that can be sustained after incentives or other interventions are discontinued in this population.

Adolescents

Most cigarette smokers begin smoking during adolescence and approximately 18% of adolescents ages 12–17 are current smokers (CDC, 1998). Thus, offering treatments to this population seems particularly warranted. An initial pilot study demonstrated that CM is feasible and effective in adolescents (Corby, Roll, Ledgerwood, & Schuster, 2000). Eight adolescents were exposed to an A B A reversal design in which no contingencies were placed on smoking during the baseline phases, and monetary payments were made available during a contingent incentive phase for CO samples 8 ppm. Contingent incentives produced greater levels of smoking abstinence, as evidenced by a greater mean number of abstinent COs during the contingent incentive phase than during the noncontingent baselines. These positive results were replicated in a subsequent study, in which 22 adolescents were randomly assigned to one of two conditions: an abstinence condition, wherein they received incentives contingent upon submitting COs < 6 ppm, or a control condition in which they received incentives only for attending the scheduled study visits (Roll, 2005). In that study, adolescents in the contingent group achieved greater smoking abstinence during the 4-week study than those in the control group and were also more likely to be abstinent at the 1-month follow-up. These results provide evidence supporting the use of CM interventions to reduce smoking among adolescents.

General Population of Treatment-Seeking Smokers

One randomized clinical trial has evaluated the effects of monetary incentives in a sample of 179 smokers (Volpp et al., 2006). Smokers in an incentive group received $20 for each of five smoking classes attended and $100 for evidence of abstinence 30 days after treatment. Abstinence was defined as a self-report of no smoking during the past 7 days and a urine cotinine level < 500 ng/ml. Smokers in the non-incentive control group were simply offered the five smoking classes. As expected, attendance rates were higher in the incentive compared to the control group. Quit rates at 30 days after program completion also were significantly higher in the incentive (16.3%) than the control group (4.6%). A 6-month follow-up revealed no significant differences between the groups as measured by self-report of no smoking in the past 7 days. The authors noted that modest financial incentives can increase enrollment and short-term quit rates in a community-based clinical setting. They also suggested that future studies should examine the effects of incentives for long-term success and whether they could result in similar positive outcomes.

CM AS A TOOL TO INVESTIGATE OTHER QUESTIONS RELATED TO SMOKING AND ITS TREATMENT

CM procedures in smokers can be used as a tool to investigate larger scientific questions related to smoking cessation, as well as to investigate the parameters of effective CM treatment in general. While this chapter focuses on studies involving tobacco, these issues are not necessarily limited to smokers and are applicable to CM treatments across a wide range of populations and drugs. CM procedures have been used to experimentally produce periods of abstinence even among smokers without plans to quit (e.g., Alessi, Badger, & Higgins, 2004; Chornock, Stitzer, Gross, & Leischow, 1992; Corby et al., 2000; Lamb, Kirby, Morral, Galbicka, & Iguchi, 2004; Roll et al., 1996; Stitzer & Bigelow, 1983). As a result, these procedures are particularly useful for studying the effects of abstinence on behavior and for studying relapse to smoking following abstinence. Several studies used CM to investigate nicotine withdrawal, including questions about the time course and magnitude of withdrawal. For example, recent studies have demonstrated that tobacco withdrawal increases with abstinence induced by a CM intervention (Heil, Tidey, Holmes, Badger, & Higgins, 2003; Alessi et al., 2004), and that symptoms of withdrawal decrease as the duration of abstinence increases and reach baseline levels at approximately 12 days of abstinence (Alessi et al., 2004). Thus, CM can be used to experimentally manipulate smoking abstinence and study nicotine withdrawal in a real-world setting.

CM interventions may also be used to investigate changes in individuals' motivation to stop smoking. For example, the use of CM to promote smoking abstinence in individuals not initially seeking to quit not only produces abstinence but also may change individuals' assessments of their self-efficacy and readiness to quit. Contrary to earlier concerns that CM may decrease both of these measures (Curry, Wagner, & Grothaus, 1991), both smoking self-efficacy (Alessi et al., 2004; Heil, Alessi, Lussier, Badger, & Higgins, 2004; Lamb, Morral, Galbicka, Kirby, & Iguchi, 2005) and readiness to quit (Lamb et al., 2005) have been shown to increase during CM. Thus, CM can be used to experimentally manipulate abstinence and examine how experiencing abstinence may influence attitudes toward smoking cessation.

CM also can be used to produce a period of initial abstinence and to examine the extent to which this period impacts the likelihood of future success at being abstinent. As discussed previously, early abstinence is a robust predictor of treatment success in all addiction treatments in which it has been studied (Budney, Higgins, Wong, & Bickel, 1996; Higgins, Badger, & Budney, 2000). CM procedures in smokers can be an especially effective tool for experimentally investigating the influences of early abstinence on relapse. For example, a study by Heil et al. (2004) provided the first experimental demonstration of the ability of a prior history of abstinence to directly facilitate later abstinence. In that study, CM was used to produce subjects with two different abstinence histories: Contingent-ALL (C-ALL), subjects who earned monetary incentives contingent upon COs 8 ppm during three 5-day (M–F) experimental periods; or Contingent-LAST (C-LAST), subjects who earned incentives independent of CO level during the first two periods and then contingent upon COs ≤ 8 ppm during the final period. Abstinence levels were significantly greater in the C-ALL than the C-LAST condition during the third 5-day period. These results provided the initial experimental evidence that a prior history of abstinence can directly influence subsequent efforts to abstain from smoking.

Two subsequent studies examined why an initial period of abstinence is associated with increased long-term success. In the first, CM was used to promote abstinence during the initial 2 weeks of a cessation effort and frequent, detailed assessments of nicotine withdrawal, the relative reinforcing effects of smoking, and other measures were collected in order to characterize changes over time (Alessi et al., 2004). Nicotine withdrawal, the relative reinforcing effects of smoking, and ratings of craving decreased over time in the contingent condition, suggesting where in the course of initial abstinence significant decreases in risk for relapse may begin to emerge. The final study examined changes in the reinforcing effects of smoking after experimentally varying duration of abstinence (Lussier, Higgins, & Badger, 2005). CM was used to promote 1, 7, or 14 day(s) of abstinence. At the end of Day 14, all subjects participated in a 3-hour relapse-risk challenge session wherein they could choose among smoking, receiving money, or neither. The percentage of subjects in each condition who chose to smoke during the challenge (i.e., relapsed) was only 19% in the 14-day condition compared to 57% and 62% in the 7-day and 1-day conditions, respectively. These results provided direct experimental evidence that a 2-week period of abstinence is associated with a significant reduction in the relative reinforcing effects of smoking and suggested that the second week of abstinence, in particular, may be critical to longer-term success.

CM procedures in smokers also can be used to produce periods of abstinence and then examine what factors may influence the subsequent likelihood of relapse. For example, Chornock et al. (1992) examined how an experimentally manipulated smoking lapse influenced subsequent abstinence following 3 days of abstinence in smokers without plans to quit. They found that individuals assigned to smoke five cigarettes after the initial abstinence period relapsed to smoking more quickly than those not assigned to smoke. These results provided experimental evidence for the widespread clinical assertion that the probability of a full relapse is increased following an isolated lapse to smoking.

From these studies, one can see that CM can be an effective tool to investigate a variety of questions related to smoking cessation and relapse in smokers. CM also has been used to study parameters related to the effective implementation of CM, including incentive magnitude, escalating-reinforcement schedules, and shaping procedures. Again, while the studies that follow are limited to those conducted with cigarette smokers, these findings likely hold generality to other forms of drug use.

One consistent finding in CM research is that larger-magnitude incentives are more effective than smaller-magnitude incentives. In an early study, Stitzer and Bigelow (1983) directly examined the effects of payment amount on the reduction of breath CO levels using a between-groups design in which participants were required to reduce their CO level to half their baseline level to earn an incentive. They found that success at meeting the CO criterion increased as the payment amount increased. These results were replicated in subsequent studies (Lamb et al., 2005; Stitzer & Bigelow, 1984). Clearly, incentive amount can be an important determinant of CM smoking outcomes, which is consistent with the larger literature of CM and illicit drug use (e.g., Silverman et al., 1999).

Another important characteristic of CM programs is the reinforcement schedule used for delivering incentives. Escalating-payment schedules, for example, reward an individual for achieving continuous abstinence by increasing the value of the incentives earned with each consecutive negative sample. Rather than promoting only brief durations of abstinence, escalating schedules are specifically designed to reinforce the continuous periods of sustained abstinence that we believe are important for longer-term success. To further promote continuous abstinence, escalating schedules often include a reset component wherein voucher values following an instance of drug use are reset back to the initial value (from which they can escalate again with new abstinence). An alternative to escalating schedules is fixed-payment schedules, in which an individual receives the same payment for each negative sample, regardless of how long he or she has been abstinent. Two studies directly examined the contribution of escalating payments and the reset component in promoting abstinence. In the first study, 60 smokers were assigned to one of three groups: an escalating schedule, a fixed-payment schedule, and a yoked control (Roll et al., 1996). Participants in all three groups were asked to refrain from smoking for 1 week. Those in the escalating and fixed groups achieved more smoking abstinence than those in the control group. In addition, participants in the escalating group were less likely to resume smoking when they became abstinent compared to participants in the other groups. The second study directly compared escalating payments with and without a reset contingency to a fixed-payment condition (Roll & Higgins, 2000). Eighteen smokers experienced the three schedules in counterbalanced order, with each schedule in effect for 5 days (M–F). The escalating schedule with the reset contingency was more effective than the other two schedules in sustaining abstinence. The results from these studies demonstrated that escalating schedules with a reset contingency are more effective than fixed-payment conditions. Indeed, escalating payments are now a common feature of many CM programs for drug abuse (e.g., Higgins et al., 1993; Silverman et al., 1996).

While CM is effective in promoting abstinence, there is often a subset of individuals for whom CM as typically implemented does not work. These hard-to-treat patients often do not experience the available incentives because they never meet the abstinence requirement (see Lamb, Morral, et al., 2004). Shaping procedures may help surmount this problem.

Percentile schedules, which set reinforcement criteria so that behavior in the best Xth percentile of recent behavior is reinforced, can be used to shape behavior (Galbicka, 1994). Indeed, Lamb, Kirby, et al. (2004) have demonstrated that CO contingencies set by percentile schedules promote reductions in CO levels. They also investigated two specific parameters of these schedules. First, the authors examined the percentile used (e.g., whether it is better to reinforce the best 10th or the best half of a smoker's behavior). Lamb, Kirby, et al. (2004) compared the effectiveness of four percentile schedules that differed in the percentile criterion used (10th, 30th, 50th, 70th percentiles). The authors found that the most stringent condition (i.e., a condition that required a CO ≤ the lowest of the last nine samples) produced fewer participants delivering a CO < 4 ppm. Further, they found that those participants who achieved abstinence early in the study did well regardless of the shaping procedure. These findings suggest that less stringent shaping procedures may aid individuals who are hard to treat in typical CM interventions. Second, the number of CO samples used for calculating the percentile criterion was investigated, which is an important parameter in percentile schedules (Lamb et al., 2005). When more samples are used to calculate the percentile, for example, the criterion changes less rapidly and is less influenced by recent behavior. When fewer samples are used, the criterion changes more rapidly and is more influenced by recent behavior. In this study, shaping schedules using either four or nine visits to calculate the criterion were studied in smokers with no interest in quitting. Smokers treated with these schedules often had sustained periods in which they consistently delivered COs < 4 ppm. Around half the participants assigned to the four-visit window had 20 sequential visits with COs < 4 ppm. This is comparable to the rate seen examining different percentile values in smokers *seeking* to quit smoking (Lamb, Morral, et al., 2004). Thus, percentile schedules appear to be an effective means for promoting change even in those without plans to quit. Interestingly, the four-visit window was more effective than the nine-visit window at promoting abstinence. This may be because the four-visit window is more responsive to the individual's current behavior than the nine-visit window.

The foregoing studies highlight several elements of CM that may be crucial in optimizing its effectiveness. Overall, results demonstrate that CM in smokers not only serves as an effective intervention but also can provide a powerful way to study a variety of processes related to smoking cessation and CM treatments in general.

DISSEMINATING CM FOR SMOKING CESSATION

Despite the effectiveness of CM, there have been obstacles in transferring CM into clinical practice for smoking cessation. These issues are discussed in detail in Chapters 13–18 (this volume) and are touched on only briefly here. One such obstacle is the cost of implementing CM, particularly the costs associated with the monetary incentives typically used in CM interventions. Fortunately, there are a variety of potential solutions that could either defray or eliminate these costs. Donations could be solicited from businesses, health care groups, and foundations (Donatelle, Prows, Champeau, & Hudson, 2000). Indeed, Amass and Kamien (2004) assessed the effects of soliciting donations for use in a CM program for drug users in two cities. In Toronto, $8,000 was donated over a 2-month period and, in Los Angeles, $161,000 was donated over the course of 34 months. These findings provide support for the feasibility of using community donations to help fund CM in clinical settings.

Smoking-cessation programs at the worksite may offer some advantages (Donatelle et al., 2004; Matson, Lee, & Hopp, 1993), including the possibility of using payroll deductions and refunds for program attendance or abstinence (Jeffrey, Pheley, Forster, Kramer, & Snell, 1988). Employers may be particularly interested in this model because it can reduce the health care costs associated with smoking. Also, the worksite may be a convenient setting in which to offer CM, as it minimizes practical barriers such as travel to treatment. Collection of CO samples at a worksite, for example, can be a relatively easy way to assess smoking status. Results from some studies on incentives in the workplace suggest that these programs can increase participation and increase cessation rates over the short term relative to control groups (Donatelle et al., 2004; Matson et al., 1993; Rand et al., 1989), while other studies have failed to find such an effect (Glasgow, Hollis, Ary, & Boles, 1993; Hennrikus et al., 2002). Overall, worksite settings appear to hold significant potential for disseminating CM for smoking cessation, though more research will be needed to further refine CM interventions in the workplace.

Another solution is to employ a fee-for-treatment model (Paxton, 1980, 1981, 1983). In this model, the fee is set at a level such that participants can earn more in vouchers than they contribute. For example, if the fee is $75, then $100 in vouchers is offered for demonstrating continuous abstinence. This type of CM program can be self-sustaining as some participants would not receive all of the available vouchers. There is also evidence that smokers would consider paying for such a treatment. Busch et al. (2004), for example, assessed smokers' willingness to pay for new, hypothetical treatments. Smokers were told to assume that a standard nicotine patch treatment costs $30 a week for 8 weeks and has a 25% success rate. They were then prompted to imagine a treatment that would double their chances of quitting and were asked if they would pay $50 a week for it. Eighty-four percent of smokers said they would indeed consider such an intervention. These data suggest a strong market for more effective treatments such as CM. Also worth noting is that a sliding scale could be used so that lower-income smokers would not find the initial fee prohibitive.

In another approach to addressing cost-related issues, there have been a number of community-level interventions using "quit and win" strategies (reviewed by Donatelle et al., 2004). The advantage of such programs is that they can target a large number of smokers, up to 70,000 in one program (Puska, Korhonen, Korhonen, & McAlister, 1996), and yet require only limited resources. However, smoking outcomes are typically self-reports of smoking status, and only the winner of the prize is subject to biochemical testing. The prizes are in the form of desirable goods such as bicycles, cars, or vacations. In general, such programs seem to increase motivation and participation, though long-term effects on smoking cessation are often limited (e.g., Croghan et al., 2001; Matson et al., 1993).

An additional obstacle in applying CM to smokers is measuring smoking status on a frequent, sustained basis. In most CM studies, COs are used to assess smoking status and represent an immediate, noninvasive, and simple method. However, as discussed earlier, the short half-life of CO requires a relatively frequent collection of samples to ensure effective implementation of CM. Thus, monitoring can be burdensome and impractical in many settings. Requiring patients to make daily visits to the clinic, for example, may limit the success of and access to the treatment for some individuals. There are at least two ways to circumvent this obstacle. First, one may modify the monitoring procedures to make them more practical for the typical clinical setting. For example, transitioning from CO to cotinine, as described earlier in this chapter, could allow frequent CO monitoring during the early part of the cessation effort and then taper to a less frequent cotinine-based system for continued monitoring (Higgins et al., 2004). There are also new low-cost urinary dipstick techniques becoming available (Parker et al., 2002). Although somewhat early in development, these new products may become useful as a hand-held semiquantitative assessment of urinary cotinine, particularly as issues of sensitivity and specificity become more established with these products.

Another solution would be to employ new technologies to remotely monitor CO collection. Dallery and Glenn (2005) established and tested a home-based CM program for initiating smoking abstinence. Smoking status was verified using Internet technology to observe participants providing CO samples via a web camera. These video recordings were simply emailed to the clinic twice daily, and abstinence was defined as a CO $\leq$ 4 ppm. A study website provided access to cessation techniques, an individualized home page for each participant (which included a graph of the participant's progress), and other resources. Results indicated that the Internet-based program is feasible, and that it may be effective in promoting smoking reductions and abstinence. Computer-based and web-assisted tobacco interventions (WATIs) are receiving increased attention (e.g., Feil, Noell, Lichtenstein, Boles, & McKay, 2003; Riley, Jerome, Behar, & Weil, 2002; Meis et al., 2002; Woodruff, Edwards, Conway, & Elliot, 2001). In conjunction with the study website, CM interventions could be considered an intensive WATI. More work is needed to test the effectiveness of this approach, but it appears to hold significant potential for lowering the response effort associated with daily CO sample collection. Further, such an approach may be particularly useful for special populations such as adolescents, smokers with disabilities, and smokers in rural areas. A disproportionate number of smokers reside in rural areas, where smoking-cessation programs may be held at a considerable distance (Aloise-Young, Wayman, & Edwards, 2002; Epstein, Botvin, & Spoth, 2003).

CONCLUDING COMMENTS

Cigarette smoking continues to be a significant public health concern in the United States and is associated with increased morbidity and mortality. Efforts to develop efficacious interventions to promote smoking cessation are sorely needed. Consistent with the extensive literature showing that CM is effective in reducing illicit drug use, a large body of evidence supports the effectiveness of CM in reducing cigarette smoking. Further, the efficacy of CM for smoking cessation has been demonstrated across a wide range of populations, including adults, adolescents, pregnant women, drug abusers, and patients with serious mental illness. Continued efforts by clinicians and researchers alike are warranted for exploring ways to further disseminate CM for smoking cessation across clinical settings and populations.

REFERENCES

Ahluwalia, J. S., Harris, K. J., Catley, D., Okuyemi, K. S., & Mayo, M. S. (2002). Sustained release bupropion for smoking cessation in african Americans. *Journal of the American Medical Association, 288*, 468–474.

Alessi, S. M., Badger, G. J., & Higgins, S. T. (2004). An experimental evaluation of the initial weeks of abstinence in cigarette smokers. *Experimental and Clinical Psychopharmacology, 12*(4), 276–287.

Aloise-Young, P. A., Wayman, J. C., & Edwards, R. W. (2002). Prevalence of cigarette smoking among rural adolescents in the United States. *Substance Use and Misuse, 37*, 613–630.

Amass, L., & Kamien, J. (2004). A tale of two cities: Financing two voucher programs for substance abusers through community donations. *Experimental and Clinical Psychopharmacology, 12*, 147–155.

Benowitz, N. L. (1996). Cotinine as a biomarker of environmental tobacco smoke exposure. *Epidemiologic Reviews, 18*, 188–204.

Budney, A. J., Higgins, S. T., Wong, C. J., & Bickel, W. K. (1996). Early abstinence predicts outcomes in behavioral treatment for cocaine addiction. In L. S. Harris (Ed.), *NIDA Research Monograph: Problems of Drug Dependence 1995: Proceedings of the 57th annual scientific meeting of the College on Drug Dependence* (p. 98). Rockville, MD: National Institute on Drug Abuse.

Busch, S. H., Falba, T. A., Duchovny, N., Jofre-Bonet, M., O'Malley, S. S., & Sindelar, J. L. (2004). Value to smokers of improved cessation products: Evidence from a willingness-to-pay survey. *Nicotine and Tobacco Research, 6,* 631–639.

Centers for Disease Control and Prevention. (1998). Incidence of initiation of cigarette smoking—United States, 1965–1996. *Morbidity and Mortality Weekly Report, 47,* 837–840.

Centers for Disease Control and Prevention. (2002). Annual smoking-attributable mortality, years of potential life lost, and economic costs—United States 1995–1999. *Morbidity and Mortality Weekly Report, 51,* 300–303.

Chornock, W. M., Stitzer, M. L., Gross, J., & Leischow, S. (1992). Experimental model of smoking re-exposure: Effects on relapse. *Psychopharmacology, 108,* 495–500.

Clemmey, P., Brooner, R., Chutuape, M. A., Kidorf, M., & Stitzer, M. (1997). Smoking habits and attitudes in a methadone maintenance treatment population. *Drug and Alcohol Dependence, 44,* 123–132.

Corby, E. A., Roll, J. M., Ledgerwood, D. M., & Schuster, C. R. (2000). Contingency management interventions for treating adolescents: A feasibility study. *Experimental and Clinical Psychopharmacology, 8,* 371–376.

Croghan, I. T., O'Hara, M. R., Schroeder, D. R., Patten, C. A., Croghan, G. A., Hays, J. T., et al. (2001). A community-wide smoking cessation program: Quit and win in 1998 in Olmstead County. *Preventive Medicine, 33,* 229–238.

Curry, S. J., Wagner, E. H., & Grothaus, L. C. (1991). Evaluation of intrinsic and extrinsic motivation interventions with a self-help smoking cessation program. *Journal of Consulting and Clinical Psychology, 59*(2), 318–324.

Dallery, J., & Glenn, I. M. (2005). Effects of an Internet-based voucher reinforcement program for smoking abstinence: A feasibility study. *Journal of Applied Behavior Analysis, 38,* 349–357.

Donatelle, R., Hudson, D., Dobie, S., Goodall, A., Hunsberger, M., & Oswald, K. (2004). Incentives in smoking cessation: Status of the field and implications for research and practice with pregnant smokers. *Nicotine and Tobacco Research, 6,* S163–S179.

Donatelle, R. J., Prows, S. L., Champeau, D., & Hudson, D. (2000). Randomized controlled trial using social support and financial incentives for high-risk pregnant smokers: Significant other supporter (SOS) program. *Tobacco Control, 9*(3), 67–69.

Eisenberg, T., Stitzer, M. L., & Henningfield, J. E. (1999). Current issues in nicotine replacement. In D. F. Seidman & L. S. Covey (Eds.), *Helping the hard-core smoker: A clinician's guide* (pp. 137–158). Mahwah, NJ: Erlbaum.

Elliott, R., & Tighe, T. (1968). Breaking the cigarette habit: Effects of a technique involving threatened loss of money. *The Psychological Record, 18,* 503–513.

Emery, S., Gilpin, E. A., Ake, C. A., Farkas, A. J., & Pierce, J. P. (2000). Characterizing and identifying "hard-core" smokers: Implications for further reducing smoking prevalence. *American Journal of Public Health, 90,* 387–394.

Epstein, J. A., Botvin, G. J., & Spoth, R. (2003). Predicting smoking among rural adolescents: Social and cognitive processes. *Nicotine and Tobacco Research, 5,* 485–492.

Fagerstrom, K. O., Kunze, M., Schoberberger, R., Breslau, N., Hughes, J. R., Hurt, R. D., et al. (1996). Nicotine dependence versus smoking prevalence: Comparisons among countries and categories of smokers. *Tobacco Control, 5,* 52–56.

Feil, E. G., Noell, J., Lichtenstein, E., Boles, S. M., & McKay, G. H. (2003). Evaluation of an Internet-based smoking cessation program: Lessons learned from a pilot study. *Nicotine and Tobacco Research, 5,* 189–194.

Fiore, M. C., Smith, S. S., Jorenby, D. E., & Baker, T. B. (1994). The effectiveness of nicotine patch for smoking cessation: A meta-analysis. *Journal of the American Medical Association, 271*, 1940–1947.

Frosch, D. L., Shoptaw, S., Jarvik, M. E., Rawson, R. A., & Ling, W. (1998). Interest in smoking cessation among methadone maintained outpatients. *Journal of Addictive Disease, 17*, 9–19.

Galbicka, G. (1994). Shaping in the 21st century: Moving percentile schedules into applied settings. *Journal of Applied Behavioral Analysis, 27*, 739–760.

Garvey, A. J., Bliss, R. E., Hitchcock, J. L., Heinold, J. W., & Rosner, B. (1992). Predictors of smoking relapse among self-quitters: A report from the normative aging study. *Addictive Behaviors, 17*, 367–377.

Glasgow, R. E., Hollis, J. F., Ary, D. V., & Boles, S. M. (1993). Results of a year-long incentives-based worksite smoking-cessation program. *Addictive Behavior, 18*, 455–464.

Gourlay, S. G., Forbes, A., Marriner, T., Pethica, D., & McNeil, J. J. (1994). Prospective study of factors predicting outcome of transdermal nicotine treatment in smoking cessation. *British Medical Journal, 309*, 842–846.

Heil, S. H., Alessi, S. M., Lussier, J. P., Badger, G. J., & Higgins, S. T. (2004). An experimental test of the influence of prior cigarette smoking abstinence on future abstinence. *Nicotine and Tobacco Research, 6*(3), 471–479.

Heil, S. H., Tidey, J. W., Holmes, H. W., Badger, G. J., & Higgins, S. T. (2003). A contingent payment model of smoking cessation: Effects on abstinence and withdrawal. *Nicotine and Tobacco Research, 5*, 205–213.

Hennrikus, D. J., Jeffery, R. W., Lando, H. A., Murray, D. M., Brelje, K., Davidann, B., et al. (2002). The SUCCESS project: The effect of program format and incentives on participation and cessation in worksite smoking cessation programs. *American Journal of Public Health, 92*, 274-279.

Higgins, S. T., Alessi, S. M., & Dantona, R. L. (2002). Voucher-based incentives: A substance abuse treatment innovation. *Addictive Behavior, 27*, 887–910.

Higgins, S. T., Badger, G. J., & Budney, A. J. (2000). Initial abstinence and success in achieving longer term cocaine abstinence. *Experimental and Clinical Psychopharmacology, 8*, 377–386.

Higgins, S. T., Budney, A. J., Bickel, W. K., Hughes, J. R., Foerg, F., & Badger, G. (1993). Achieving cocaine abstinence with a behavioral approach. *American Journal of Psychiatry, 150*, 763–769.

Higgins, S. T., Delaney, D. D., Budney, A. J., Bickel, W. K., Hughes, J. R., Foerg, F., et al. (1991). A behavioral approach to achieving initial cocaine abstinence. *American Journal of Psychiatry, 148*, 1218–1224.

Higgins, S. T., Heil, S. H., Badger, G. J., Mongeon, J. A., Solomon, L. J., McHale, L., et al. (2007). Biochemical verification of smoking status in pregnant and recently postpartum women. *Experimental and Clinical Psychopharmacology, 15*, 58–66.

Higgins, S. T., Heil, S. H., Solomon, L. J., Lussier, J. P., Abel, R. L., Lynch. M. E., et al. (2004). A pilot study on voucher-based incentives to promote abstinence from cigarette smoking during pregnancy and postpartum. *Nicotine and Tobacco Research, 6*, 1015–1020.

Higgins, S. T., & Silverman, K. (Eds.). (1999). *Motivating behavior change among illicit drug abusers*. Washington, DC: American Psychological Association.

Hser, Y. I., McCarthy, W. J., & Anglin, M. D. (1994). Tobacco use as a distal predictor of mortality among long-term narcotic addicts. *Preventive Medicine, 23*, 61–69.

Hughes, J. R., Gulliver, S. B., Fenwick, J. W., Valliere, W. A., Cruser, K., Pepper, S., et al. (1992). Smoking cessation among self-quitters. *Health Psychology, 11*, 331–334.

Hughes, J. R., Hatsukami, D. K., Mitchell, J. E., & Dahlgren, L. A. (1986). Prevalence of smoking among psychiatric outpatients. *American Journal of Psychiatry, 143*, 993–997.

Hurt, R. D., Offord, K. P., Croghan, I. T., Gomez-Dahl, L., Kottke, T. E., Morse, R. M., et al. (1996). Mortality following inpatient addictions treatment: Role of tobacco use in a community-based cohort. *Journal of the American Medical Association, 275*, 1097–1103.

Hurt, R. D., Sachs, D. P., Glover, E. D., Offord, K. P., Johnston, J. A., Dale, L. C., et al. (1997). A comparison of sustained-release bupropion and placebo for smoking cessation. *New England Journal of Medicine, 17*, 1195–1202.

Jarvis, M. J., Tunstall-Pedoe, H., Feyerabend, C., Vesey, C., & Saloojee, Y. (1987). Comparison of tests used to distinguish smokers from nonsmokers. *American Journal of Public Health, 77*, 1435–1438.

Javors, M. A., Hatch, J. P., & Lamb, R. J. (2005). Evaluation of cut-off levels for breath carbon monoxide as a marker for cigarette smoking over the past 24 hours. *Addiction, 100*, 159–167.

Jeffrey, R. W., Pheley, A. M., Forster, J. L., Kramer, F. M., & Snell, M. K. (1988). Payroll contracting for smoking cessation: A worksite pilot study. *American Journal of Preventive Medicine, 4*, 83–86.

Kenford, S. L., Fiore, M. C., Jorenby, D. E., Smith, S. S., Wetter, D., & Baker, T. B. (1994). Predicting smoking cessation: Who will quit with and without the nicotine patch. *Journal of the American Medical Association, 271*, 589–594.

Kirby, K. C., Marlowe, D. B., Festinger, D. S., Lamb, R. J., & Platt, J. J. (1998). Schedule of voucher delivery influences cocaine abstinence. *Journal of Consulting and Clinical Psychology, 66*(5), 761–767.

Kozlowski, L. T., Skinner, W., Kent, C., & Pope, M. A. (1989). Prospects for smoking treatment in individuals seeking treatment for alcohol and other drug problems. *Addictive Behaviors, 14*, 273–278.

Lamb, R. J., Kirby, K. C., Morral, A. R., Galbicka, G., & Iguchi, M. Y. (2004). Improving contingency management programs for addiction. *Addictive Behaviors, 29*, 507–523.

Lamb, R. J., Morral, A. R., Galbicka, G., Kirby, K. C., & Iguchi, M. Y. (2005). Shaping reduced smoking in smokers without cessation plans. *Experimental and Clinical Psychopharmacology, 13*(2), 83–92.

Lamb, R. J., Morral, A. R., Kirby, K. C., Iguchi, M. Y., & Galbicka, G. (2004). Shaping smoking cessation using percentile schedules. *Drug and Alcohol Dependence, 76*, 247–259.

Lussier, J. P., Higgins, S. T., & Badger, G. J. (2005). Influence of the duration of abstinence on the relative reinforcing effects of cigarette smoking. *Psychopharmacology, 181*, 486–495.

Matson, D. M., Lee, J. W., & Hopp, J. W. (1993). The impact of incentives and competitions on participation and quit rates in worksite smoking cessation programs. *American Journal of Health Promotion, 7*, 270–280.

Meis, T. M., Gaie, M. J., Pingree, S., Boberg, E. W., Patten, C. A., Offord, K. A., et al. (2002). Development of a tailored, Internet-based smoking cessation intervention for adolescents. *Journal of Computer-Mediated Communication, 7*(3).

Middleton, E. T., & Morice, A. H. (2000). Breath carbon monoxide as an indication of smoking habit. *Chest, 117*, 758–763.

Parker, D. R., Lasater, T. M., Windsor, R., Wilkins, J., Upegui, D. I., & Heimdal, J. (2002). The accuracy of self-reported smoking status assessed by cotinine test strips. *Nicotine and Tobacco Research, 4*, 305–309.

Paxton, R. (1980). The effects of a deposit contract as a component in a behavioral programme for stopping smoking. *Behaviour Research and Therapy, 18*, 45–50.

Paxton, R. (1981). Deposit contracts with smokers: varying frequency and amount of repayments. *Behaviour Research and Therapy, 19*, 117–123.

Paxton, R. (1983). Prolonging the effect of deposit contracts with smokers. *Behaviour Research and Therapy, 21*(4), 425–433.

Petry, N. M., Martin, B., Cooney, J. L., & Kranzler, H. R. (2000). Give them prizes, and they will come: Contingency management for treatment of alcohol dependence. *Journal of Consulting and Clinical Psychology, 68*, 250–257.

Puska, P., Korhonen, H., Korhonen, T., & McAlister, A. (1996). International quit and win '96: A global compaign to promote smoking cessation. *Tobacco Control, 5*, 342.

Rand, C. S., Stitzer, M. L., Bigelow, G. E., & Mead, A. M. (1989). The effects of contingent payment and frequent workplace monitoring on smoking abstinence. *Addictive Behaviors, 14*, 121–128.

Rebagliato, M. (2002). Validation of self-reported smoking. *Journal of Epidemiology and Community Health, 56*, 167–170.

Richter, K. P., Gibson, C. A., Ahluwalia, J. S., & Schmelzle, K. H. (2001). Tobacco use and quit attempts among methadone maintenance clients. *American Journal of Public Health, 91*, 296–299.

Riley, W., Jerome, A., Behar, A., & Weil, J. (2002). Computer and manual self-help behavioral strategies for smoking reduction: Initial feasibility and one-year follow-up. *Nicotine and Tobacco Research, 4*, S183–S188.

Roll, J. M. (2005). Assessing the feasibility of using contingency management to modify cigarette smoking by adolescents. *Journal of Applied Behavior Analysis, 38*, 463–467.

Roll, J. M., & Higgins, S. T. (2000). A within-subject comparison of three different schedules of reinforcement of drug abstinence using cigarette smoking as an exemplar. *Drug and Alcohol Dependence, 58*, 103–109.

Roll, J. M., Higgins, S. T., & Badger, G. J. (1996). An experimental comparison of three different schedules of reinforcement of drug abstinence using cigarette smoking as an exemplar. *Journal of the Experimental Analysis of Behavior, 29*, 495–505.

Roll, J. M., Higgins, S. T., Steingard, S., & McGinley, M. (1998). Use of monetary reinforcement to reduce the cigarette smoking of persons with schizophrenia: A feasibility study. *Experimental and Clinical Psychopharmacology, 6*, 157–161.

Schmitz, J. M., Rhoades, H., & Grabowski, J. (1995). Contingent reinforcement for reduced carbon monoxide levels in methadone maintenance patients. *Addictive Behaviors, 20*, 171–179.

Sees, K. L., & Clark, H. W. (1993). When to begin smoking cessation in substance abusers. *Journal of Substance Abuse Treatment, 10*, 189–195.

Seidman, D. F., & Covey, L. S. (1999). *Helping the hard-core smoker: A clinician's guide.* Mahwah, NJ: Erlbaum.

Shoptaw, S., Jarvik, M. E., Ling, W., & Rawson, R. A. (1996). Contingency management for tobacco smoking in methadone-maintained opiate addicts. *Addictive Behaviors, 21*, 409–412.

Shoptaw, S., Rotheram-Fuller, E., Yang, X., Frosch, D., Nahom, D., Jarvick, M. E., et al. (2002). Smoking cessation in methadone maintenance. *Addiction, 97*, 1317–1328.

Silverman, K., Chutuape, M. A., Bigelow, G. E., & Stitzer, M. L. (1999). Voucher-based reinforcement of cocaine abstinence in treatment-resistant methadone patients: Effects of reinforcement magnitude. *Psychopharmacology, 146*, 128–138.

Silverman, K., Higgins, S. T., Brooner, R. K., Montoya, I. D., Cone, E. J., Schuster, C. R., et al. (1996). Sustained cocaine abstinence in methadone maintenance patients through voucher-based reinforcement therapy. *Archives of General Psychiatry, 53*, 409–415.

SRNT Subcommittee on Biochemical Verification. (2002). Biochemical verification of tobacco use and cessation. *Nicotine and Tobacco Research, 4*, 149–159.

Stitzer, M. L. (1999). Combined behavioral and pharmacological treatments for smoking cessation. *Nicotine and Tobacco Research, 1*, S181–S187.

Stitzer, M. L., & Bigelow, G. E. (1982). Contingent reinforcement for reduced carbon monoxide levels in cigarette smokers. *Addictive Behaviors, 7*, 403–412.

Stitzer, M. L., & Bigelow, G. E. (1983). Contingent payment for carbon monoxide reduction: Effects of pay amount. *Behavior Therapy, 14*, 647–656.

Stitzer, M. L., & Bigelow, G. E. (1984). Contingent reinforcement for carbon monoxide reduction: Within-subject effects of pay amount. *Journal of Applied Behavioral Analysis, 17*, 477–483.

Stitzer, M. L., & Bigelow, G. E. (1985). Contingent reinforcement for carbon monoxide reduction: Target-specific effects on cigarette smoking. *Addictive Behaviors, 10*, 345–349.

Stitzer, M. L., Rand, C. S., Bigelow, G. E., & Mead, A. M. (1986). Contingent payment procedures for smoking reduction and cessation. *Journal of Applied Behavioral Analysis, 19*, 197–202.

Substance Abuse and Mental Health Services Administration. (2005). *Results from the 2004 National Survey on Drug Use and Health: National findings* (NSDUH Series H-28, DHHS Publication No. SMA 05-4062). Rockville, MD: Office of Applied Studies.

Tidey, J. W., O'Neill, S. C., & Higgins, S. T. (2002). Contingent monetary reinforcement of smoking reductions, with and without transdermal nicotine, in outpatients with schizophrenia. *Experimental and Clinical Psychopharmacology, 10*, 241–247.

U.S. Department of Health and Human Services. (2000). *Smoking cessation: Clinical practice guideline*. Washington, DC: Public Health Service, Centers for Disease Control and Prevention.

U.S. Department of Health and Human Services. (2001). *Women and smoking: A report of the Surgeon General*. Rockville, MD: Public Health Service, Centers for Disease Control and Prevention, Office of Smoking and Health.

Volpp, K. G., Levy, A. G., Asch, D. A., Berlin, J. A., Murphy, J. J., Gomez. A., et al. (2006). A randomized controlled trial of financial incentives for smoking cessation. *Cancer Epidemiology Biomarkers and Prevention, 15*, 12–18.

Winett, R. A. (1973). Parameters of deposit contracts in the modification of smoking. *The Psychological Record, 23*, 49–60.

Woodruff, S. I., Edwards, C. C., Conway, T. L., & Elliot, S. P. (2001). Pilot test of an Internet virtual world chat room for rural teen smokers. *Journal of Adolescent Health, 29*, 239–243.

Yudkin, P. L., Jones, L., Lancaster, T., & Fowler, G. H. (1996). Which smokers are helped to give up smoking using transdermal nicotine patches? Results from a randomized, double-blind, placebo-controlled trial. *British Journal of General Practice, 46*, 145–148.

CHAPTER 7

ALCOHOL

Conrad J. Wong, Kenneth Silverman,
and George E. Bigelow

Alcohol abuse and dependence represent major public health problems in the United States and most other industrialized countries. In the 2004 U.S. National Survey on Drug Use and Health, for example, 18.6 million (7.8%) of those ages 12 years or older met criteria for alcohol abuse or dependence (Substance Abuse and Mental Health Services Administration, 2005). This chapter reviews the research on the efficacy of behavioral contingency management (CM) procedures for the treatment of alcohol abuse and dependence. The empirical basis for the application of CM procedures to treat alcohol abuse and dependence is derived from nonhuman and human laboratory studies demonstrating that alcohol self-administration is operant behavior controlled by its environmental context and consequences, that alcohol itself can serve as a powerful reinforcer, and that alcohol self-administration can be altered by manipulating environmental conditions, including the introduction and appropriate contingent scheduling of alternative reinforcers. This chapter summarizes research on the application of operant conditioning to the conceptualization and study of alcohol self-administration and to the treatment of alcohol problems.

CONCEPTUAL FRAMEWORK

CM interventions for alcohol abuse and dependence are based on extensive basic and applied research. The theoretical foundation of CM interventions for alcohol abuse and dependence is derived from fundamental principles of operant conditioning and behavioral pharmacology (see Higgins & Silverman, Chapter 1, this volume, for a more detailed discussion of these issues). Briefly, the primary tenets of operant conditioning are that many behaviors are learned, orderly, and controlled by their consequences. The fundamental operant principle of reinforcement exerts a powerful modulating influence on behavior, including alcohol use. Consequences that increase the likelihood of behavior occurring under similar circumstances in the future are considered reinforcing; those that decrease the likelihood of behavior occurring are considered punishing. Whether applied to alcohol self-administration itself or to other more adaptive behaviors, the fundamental principle of reinforcement is the root of CM interventions designed to increase and maintain therapeutically desired behaviors.

The field of behavioral pharmacology has demonstrated that alcohol and drug use are learned behaviors that are maintained in part through the reinforcing pharmacological actions of alcohol and drugs but also through other sources of reinforcement associated with alcohol and drug use (e.g., social reinforcement; Higgins & Katz, 1998). Behavioral pharmacology studies with animals and humans have demonstrated that alcohol functions as a reinforcer similar to primary reinforcers such as food, water, and sex (Schuster & Thompson, 1968; Samson, Pfeffer, & Tolliver, 1988; Spiga, Macenski, Meisch, & Roache, 1997). Moreover, studies have shown that alcohol use is amenable to change in the same way other behaviors are altered when alternative reinforcers are made contingent upon alternative behaviors (Carroll, 1987; Carroll, Rodefer, & Rawleigh, 1995; Foltin, 1998; Samson et al., 1988; Samson, Roehrs, & Tolliver, 1982; Spiga et al., 1997).

Operant behavioral approaches, including CM interventions and community reinforcement approach therapy for the treatment of alcoholism, have been developed with the goal of increasing the frequency and magnitude of reinforcement derived from healthier alternative activities, especially those that are incompatible with alcohol use.

Nonhuman Behavioral Pharmacology Alcohol Research

Several articles review the vast scientific literature with rodents and nonhuman primates demonstrating that operant responding can be initiated and maintained by the presentation of ethanol solutions (Grant & Bennett, 2003; Meisch, 2001; Samson & Czachowski, 2003; Samson et al., 1988). One of the early studies conducted in 1960 by Clark and Polish demonstrated that nonhuman primates would self-administer oral alcohol to avoid shock. Other early studies with monkeys and rats showed that lever-press response rates increased above baseline levels when intravenous (IV) ethanol administration was contingent upon lever pressing (Smith & Davis, 1974; Winger & Woods, 1973). Studies with rats and monkeys demonstrated that oral ethanol could serve as a reinforcer (Grant & Samson, 1985; Grant, Johanson, & Schuster, 1986), and that alcohol self-administration can be influenced by other factors including dose, schedule of reinforcement, and food restriction (Samson & Pfeffer, 1987).

The use of operant choice procedures, in which two or more potential reinforcers are concurrently available, has provided evidence that alcohol self-administration can be manipulated as a function of availability of alternative reinforcers in the organism's environment. Studies with nonhuman primates and rats have demonstrated that the availability of alternative reinforcers, such as sucrose and other drug reinforcers, could modulate alcohol self-administration (Carroll et al., 1995; Samson et al., 1982). For example, a study with rats showed that responding for ethanol could be decreased as a function of increased concentration of a sucrose alternative (Samson et al., 1982). Another study conducted by Carroll et al. (1995) in monkeys showed that ethanol consumption decreased as a function of increased response cost (fixed ratio) when concurrent saccharin solution was available. These experiments are just a few of the of studies in a vast scientific literature that provide the empirical basis that ethanol can serve as a reinforcer and that non-drug-alternative reinforcers can reduce ethanol self-administration.

Human Behavioral Pharmacology Alcohol Research

Consistent with studies with nonhumans, behavioral pharmacology studies with humans have shown that alcohol serves as a reinforcer and that alcohol self-administration can be manipulated as a function of operant contingencies, including the schedule of reinforcement and the availability of alternative reinforcers. In one of the earliest studies conducted by Mello and Mendelson (1965), two volunteers with long histories of alcoholism were given the opportunity to respond for alcohol or money on various fixed-ratio and fixed-interval schedules. The results from this seminal study showed that humans would respond for alcohol in preference to money for long periods of time in an operant conditioning paradigm (Mello & Mendelson, 1965).

Early laboratory studies with problem drinkers demonstrated that alcohol drinking could be controlled by systematically varying the consequences of alcohol drinking (Cohen, Liebson, Faillace, & Allen, 1971; Cohen, Liebson, & Faillace, 1972, 1973). This research group conducted a systematic series of human laboratory alcohol self-administration studies that were among the first, perhaps the very first, to demonstrate the ability of appropriately scheduled consequences of drinking to reduce alcoholics' drinking and to produce cessation of drinking even in the midst of an ongoing drinking episode. These were landmark studies, as scientific, clinical, and popular opinion at the time was that alcoholics' drinking was uncontrollable once initiated.

An early study conducted by Cohen, Liebson, Faillace, and Spears (1971) showed that alcohol consumption could be suppressed when money was offered as an alternative to drinking in a choice-procedure paradigm. In addition, that study showed that a larger-magnitude competing alternative was more effective than a lower-magnitude alternative in achieving abstinence, and that the efficacy of the alternative reinforcer was reduced when delays of reinforcement were introduced between the choice occasion and the reinforcer delivery.

In other studies (e.g., Cohen, Liebson, Faillace, & Allen, 1971) drinking excessively (more than five drinks in a day) determined whether the drinker lived in an "enriched" or "impoverished" residential laboratory environment. The enriched environment provided access to a variety of privileges, including social contacts, use of a recreation room, access to preferred regular hospital meals, opportunity to work in the hospital laundry for pay, and permission to receive visitors. In the impoverished environment subjects were restricted to their bedrooms, their opportunities for activities and socialization were severely restricted, and they received a pureed diet. A review of these studies by Bigelow et al. (1981) reported that alcoholic participants overwhelming chose to drink moderately and then stop when faced with the contingency that excessive drinking would result in immediate "impoverishment."

A subsequent study conducted by Bigelow and colleagues showed that the drinking of chronic problem drinkers could be suppressed by scheduling a brief period of isolation immediately contingent upon the receipt of each drink (Bigelow, Liebson, & Griffiths, 1974). The isolation contingency resulted in immediate, brief loss of availability of a broad range of reinforcers, including physical activities, social stimulation, and interaction. Further studies showed that contingent time out from social interactions alone was sufficient to reduce drinking in chronic problem drinkers (Griffiths, Bigelow, & Liebson, 1974, 1977).

A more recent study conducted by Spiga et al. (1997) evaluated the effects of work requirement on alcohol self-administration. Healthy volunteers self-administered 4%, 8%, or 16% ethanol solution contingent upon completion of a fixed-ratio response requirement. The response requirement was varied between 32, 64, and 128 responses. Results showed that alcohol consumption at lower doses decreased with an increase in response requirement. However, alcohol consumption at the highest dose was high across all ratio requirements and was unchanged by an increase in the ratio requirement. These data illustrate both the malleability of drinking behavior under certain conditions and its resistance to change under other conditions.

In another study conducted by Schmitz, Sayre, Hokanson, and Spiga (2003), an operant multiple-choice procedure was used to evaluate alcohol's reinforcing efficacy relative to other reinforcers (money and tobacco smoking) in concurrent alcohol and tobacco outpatient treatment seekers. Individuals were instructed to choose one of two potential reinforcers from a series of paired comparisons. In this procedure, participants chose alcohol less frequently as a function of increasing money amounts as the alternative. This study demonstrated the power of alternative reinforcers to reduce the behavioral control exerted by alcohol itself.

CM INTERVENTIONS FOR THE TREATMENT OF ALCOHOLISM

Controlled laboratory studies with problem drinkers showed that alcohol use could be modified by manipulating reinforcement contingencies for alcohol use and for abstinence. This research provides a firm scientific foundation for the application of CM interventions in the treatment for alcohol abuse and dependence. The primary objective of CM procedures for the treatment of alcoholism has been to arrange reinforcement for alcohol abstinence or other therapeutic behaviors, such as medication compliance or counseling attendance.

Abstinence-Reinforcement Procedures

Under alcohol-abstinence-reinforcement procedures, patients receive a desirable consequence or reinforcer contingent upon an objective measure of alcohol abstinence. Various types of consequences and abstinence-reinforcement procedures have been described to promote abstinence from alcohol in problem drinkers.

Miller (1972) described a case study in which a contingency contract was established between a wife and a husband to reduce the husband's excessive drinking. Under the contract, the husband agreed to restrict the amount, time, and location of drinking. Under the central feature of the contract, if the husband ever drank more than three drinks per day, he agreed to pay a $20 fine to the wife (to be spent on frivolous purchases) and the wife withdrew her attention to the husband. Daily recordings of drinking seemed to show that drinking decreased when the contract was arranged, although the study did not demonstrate clear experimental control of drinking.

In an early controlled study, Miller, Hersen, Eisler, and Watts (1974) applied and evaluated an alcohol-abstinence-reinforcement intervention in a 49-year-old male. This individual had a 20-year history of heavy drinking, at least 25 prior arrests for public drunkenness, and a recent history of drinking "from 1 pint to one-fifth of whiskey together with wine and beer on a daily basis" (p. 261). The patient provided breath samples on a quasi-random basis twice per week over 12 weeks. To collect breath samples, a research assistant called the patient at random times. Within an hour of the call, the research assistant went to the patient's home or place of employment to collect the sample. If the patient was not reached, the research assistant went into the community to find him. On occasion the patient was asked to come to the hospital to provide the sample.

After a 3-week baseline of simply collecting the samples, a contingency was arranged in which the patient could receive a $3 coupon booklet for every alcohol-negative breath sample. The coupons could be exchanged for items available at the hospital commissary. After 3 additional weeks, $3 coupons were provided for each breath sample independent of the results of the breath alcohol tests. After 3 weeks of noncontingent coupon delivery, coupons were again provided contingent upon alcohol-negative breath samples for 3 more weeks.

Breath alcohol levels (BALs) decreased when the contingency was imposed, increased when the coupons were provided on a noncontingent basis, and then decreased again when the contingency was reimposed. Visual display of the breath alcohol concentrations (BACs) across successive collections showed clearly that contingent delivery of the coupons decreased alcohol-positive breath samples.

In this brief early report, Miller demonstrated the effectiveness of abstinence reinforcement in reducing persistent alcohol use and made some thoughtful observations that provide useful guidance today:

> Relatively basic reinforcers, such as those used in the present study may have most influence on low income or Skid Row alcoholics. With more varied alcoholic populations in which longer term periods of sobriety are desired, a more comprehensive approach utilizing both a wide selection of reinforcers for decreasing drinking and social punishing or loss of reinforcers for excessive drinking may be necessary. In this regard, activities that occur in the natural environment at a high frequency (e.g., working or socializing) may be made contingent upon decreased alcohol consumption. (pp. 262–263)

In a subsequent study, Miller (1975) evaluated a novel and comprehensive abstinence-reinforcement intervention, similar to the one envisioned in his report described earlier, in 20 men who were described as "skid row alcoholics." Participants were included in the study if they reported at least a 5-year history of abusive drinking; a sporadic work history; residence in downtown "rooming houses, hotels, or missions"; and repeated arrests for public drunkenness. Those men were randomly assigned to a control or a CM group. At the time of the study, local social service agencies were providing this population of "skid row alcoholics" with a range of goods and services including food, clothing, housing, and employment. Thus, control participants received these standard goods and services, which were being provided to this population routinely. CM participants could receive the same goods and services; however, if they were observed using alcohol, they lost access to those goods and services for 5 days. Alcohol use was assessed in CM participants through random breath alcohol tests or by direct observation of gross intoxication.

Breath samples were not collected from both groups, so the study could not examine the effects on the CM intervention on a direct measure of drinking. However, the study showed that the CM intervention significantly decreased arrests for public drunkenness and increased the days of employment, relative to the control group.

Brigham et al. (1981) described the use of an abstinence-reinforcement intervention in three adolescents who had histories of excessive alcohol drinking. Under the abstinence-reinforcement interventions, each adolescent could earn 5 points and $1 every day he or she abstained from alcohol. The points could be "exchanged for either special privileges (movies, camping trips, athletic events), or to avoid aversive tasks (lawn cutting, washing dishing)" (p. 78). Alcohol use was assessed primarily through self-reports by the adolescents themselves, although there was some effort to corroborate those self-reports through the use of breath alcohol tests administered by the parents and the parental reports of drinking. The study did not provide clear experimental evidence that the abstinence-reinforcement intervention decreased drinking in these individuals, although it provided an early example of a potentially useful abstinence-reinforcement intervention.

Peniston (1988) examined the use of a CM intervention to reduce drinking in 15 male veterans diagnosed with schizophrenia while they resided on an inpatient psychiatric ward. Although drinking was not a problem while these individuals were on the inpatient ward, patients did drink while in the community on day passes. The CM intervention focused on four target behaviors: reducing verbally abusive behaviors, increasing attendance at therapeutic activities, improving personal grooming, and reducing alcohol drinking while on day passes in the community. To measure instances of drinking, two independent observers recorded whether or not a patient returned intoxicated to the ward from an outing. Under the CM intervention, the patients could earn $35 every week and a day pass every 2 weeks if they maintained 60 consecutive days without exhibiting the target behaviors. If a patient exhibited a targeted behavior, the weekly $35 payments were discontinued and patients were switched to a program in which they could earn $5 canteen books daily, which could be used to purchase personal items twice daily. If a patient exhibited one of the target behaviors, a $1 fine was imposed immediately, which reduced the amount earned in canteen books the following day. A multiple-baseline across-behaviors design was used to show that the CM intervention reduced verbal abusive behavior, decreased nonattendance, improved personal grooming, and reduced drinking. The study provided reasonably good evidence of the effectiveness of this CM intervention in improving the target behaviors, although the evidence of the effectiveness of the intervention on drinking was weaker than for the other target behaviors.

Petry, Martin, Conney, and Kranzler (2000) evaluated the effectiveness of a CM intervention for alcohol-dependent veterans during an 8-week outpatient treatment. Those individuals were randomly assigned to receive standard outpatient treatment or to receive the standard treatment plus a prize CM intervention. Under the CM intervention, participants could earn the opportunity to draw, in a lottery-like procedure, for prizes worth between $1 and $100 for providing alcohol-negative breath samples and for performing treatment-related activities (see Petry & Alessi, Chapter 14, this volume, for a more detailed description of the prize reinforcement system). Breath samples were collected once per day every weekday that the participant reported to the treatment clinic. Participants in the CM group earn $200 in prizes, on average. The study provided clear evidence that the CM intervention increased retention in treatment. The study also provided limited evidence that the CM intervention may have increased abstinence from alcohol. However, the effects of the CM intervention on alcohol use was confounded by differential rates of retention and differential rates of breath sample collection in the two groups, which precluded comparable measurement of rates of alcohol use in the control and CM groups.

Employment-based abstinence reinforcement, using access to paid employment to reinforce abstinence, has been shown effective in promoting drug abstinence in cocaine-abusing methadone patients (see Donlin, Knealing, & Silverman, Chapter 17, this volume). A recent study (Wong, Kolodner, Fingerhood, Bigelow, & Silverman, 2005) was completed that sought to replicate the effectiveness of employment-based abstinence reinforcement in a population of homeless alcohol-dependent individuals. Individuals who were homeless, unemployed, and alcohol dependent were randomly assigned to a work only (WO; $n = 42$), abstinence and work (AW; $n = 43$) or no voucher (NV; $n = 39$) group. All participants were invited to work in a workplace for 4 hours per day for 26 weeks. Breath samples were collected and tested for alcohol prior to start of each workday and at random times throughout each week (including weekends). Participants in the WO and AW groups could earn up to $5 per hour in base pay and additional earnings for performance on training programs. WO participants could work and earn wages independent of their daily or random breath results. AW participants could work and earn wages only when their daily and random breath samples demonstrated alcohol abstinence; positive samples also resulted in a temporary reset of base pay to a low amount. NV participants could work in the workplace independent of daily and random breath sample results but did not receive vouchers. Preliminary results show that mean rates of attendance for the WO and AW groups were similar but were significantly higher than for the NV group. Breath sample collection rates were similar for the AW and WO groups, but the NV group's rate was significantly lower than the WO group's. Preliminary analyses showed that AW participants had lower rates of alcohol-positive samples (BAL > 0.003 g/100ml) and samples with a BAL $\geq$ 0.05 g/100 ml compared to the WO group. The preliminary results from this study suggest that reinforcement can increase work attendance and alcohol abstinence in a population of homeless alcohol-dependent individuals.

Reinforcement of Disulfiram Use

Disulfiram is a medication that has considerable potential in the treatment of alcohol addiction. Disulfiram has little or no effects when taken alone; however, when an individual is taking therapeutic doses of disulfiram regularly, drinking even small amounts of alcohol promptly causes an extremely unpleasant reaction that can include headache, nausea, vomiting, sweating, chest pains, and so on. Because of the prompt and unpleasant nature of the disulfiram–alcohol reaction, individuals who are maintained on disulfiram treatment avoid drinking alcohol. Therapeutic disulfiram blood levels can typically be achieved by daily ingestion of 250 mg disulfiram or by ingestion of higher doses 3 days per week. Disulfiram can be a highly effective medication; however, it has one critical limitation: Patients frequently refuse to take it. Beginning in the 1970s, several studies have shown that CM interventions can be used to promote disulfiram ingestion.

Disulfiram in Methadone Patients

Liebson, Bigelow, and Flamer (1973) reported on a CM intervention to reinforce disulfiram in an adult enrolled in a methadone treatment program for heroin addiction. Methadone is an opioid medication that is extremely effective in reducing heroin use. Taken in adequate doses, methadone can block the stimulus effects of heroin and can reduce or eliminate opiate withdrawal signs and symptoms commonly associated with stopping heroin use. In addition to its effects on heroin use, Liebson et al. (1973) observed that methadone is also very attractive to methadone patients and could possibly be used as a reinforcer to increase therapeutic behavior change. In this early case study, Liebson and colleagues arranged a contingency to promote disulfiram use in a 36-year-old man who was drinking alcohol excessively and persistently while enrolled in a community methadone treatment program. Under the contingency, this man was required to take disulfiram to continue in methadone treatment. Each day when he arrived at the methadone treatment program to take his daily dose of methadone, he was first required to drink a solution that contained his daily dose of disulfiram. He then would receive his daily methadone dose. Under this program, the man continued to take disulfiram and appeared to have stopped drinking. This study did not experimentally evaluate the methadone reinforcement contingency but illustrated the potential utility of this approach.

In a subsequent study, Liebson, Tommasello, and Bigelow (1978) experimentally evaluated a similar CM intervention to promote disulfiram use in 25 adults who had been discharged from methadone treatment or were at risk of being discharged because of their persistent alcohol use. Using a CM intervention similar to that described by Liebson et al. (1973) in which participants were required to take their daily dose of disulfiram under observation before receiving their daily dose of methadone, these men were all inducted onto disulfiram treatment and randomly assigned to a CM or control group. CM participants were required to continue taking disulfiram to receive each daily dose of methadone and to continue in methadone treatment. If a participant ever refused to take disulfiram, a 21-day methadone-dose taper was initiated in which the participant's methadone dose was gradually reduced. If the participant agreed to resume disulfiram treatment, the methadone doses would be increased and standard methadone treatment resumed. Control participants were given disulfiram to take on their own at home. Participants were randomized to their respective conditions for 6 months. Participants in the CM group had significantly fewer days of drinking (2% of days) than did participants in the control group (21% of days).

A within-subjects reversal design experiment conducted by Bickel et al. (1989) assessed whether the threat of a transfer to another methadone maintenance clinic could be used to manage alcohol use among alcoholic methadone patients. During the intervention period, three alcoholic methadone patients were provided continued methadone maintenance treatment contingent upon disulfiram ingestion. Failure to take disulfiram resulted in the transfer of the patient to another methadone program in the community. Subjects showed decreased alcohol use and improved clinic attendance during the intervention period, suggesting that a less severe consequence could be used to manage alcohol use in this population (Bickel et al., 1989).

Disulfiram in Hospital Employees

Two early studies were conducted on hospital employees in Baltimore and used employment as a reinforcer to promote disulfiram use. Cohen, Bigelow, Hargett, Allen, and Halsted (1973) described uncontrolled case studies in four hospital employees who were at risk for being terminated due to their drinking. The report described individualized treatment programs in which three of the participants were required to take daily doses of disulfiram under a nurse's observation to work. All four participants were required to provide routine breath samples that were tested for alcohol. If a participant failed to take a dose of disulfiram or provided a sample that was positive for alcohol, he was suspended from work for 1 day without pay. Although this study did not demonstrate the effectiveness of this intervention, the study provided an early description of potential contingencies that could be arranged in a workplace to promote disulfiram ingestion and abstinence from alcohol.

Robichaud, Strickler, Bigelow, and Liebson (1979) evaluated an employment-based intervention to promote disulfiram ingestion in 21 industrial employees who were referred to treatment due to drinking-related problems on the job. Participants in this program were required to ingest disulfiram under a nurse's observation daily for 14 days and every other day thereafter. Every 2 weeks, the treatment program sent a letter to the each participant's employer indicating whether or not the participant had attended treatment. Treatment durations varied across participants and lasted between 3 and 30.3 months. During the treatment period, participants were absent from work on significantly fewer days (2%) than before (10% of days) or after (7% of days) treatment. The study did not prove the direct effects of the intervention on alcohol use; however, it provided an early controlled demonstration of the use of employment-based contingencies to promote disulfiram use.

Deposit Contracting to Promote Disulfiram Use

Bigelow, Stickler, Liebson, and Griffiths (1976) applied a deposit contracting intervention to promote disulfiram ingestions in 20 male adults who had histories of drinking problems. All participants were seeking treatment, their ages ranged from 28 to 54, 60% were married, and 80% were employed full time. Under the outpatient treatment contract, patients were required to take disulfiram under a nurse's observation for a minimum of 3 months. Patients could visit the treatment unit anytime between 7:30 A.M. and 11:00 P.M. to take a dose of disulfiram under the nurse's observation. Patients were required to report to the treatment unit every day for the first 14 days and every other day thereafter. To promote disulfiram use, all patients were required to leave an initial monetary security deposit, which they could lose if they failed to take scheduled disulfiram doses. The amount of initial security deposit was negotiated with the patient, although patients were encouraged to leave between $100 and $150. A patient could lose $5 or $10 of the deposit for failing to take a scheduled dose. Although the study did not experimentally evaluate the procedure, it did show that patients were willing to leave a deposit and to attend clinic frequently to take doses of disulfiram, and some patients were willing to re-enlist for extended periods of treatment. Participants left security deposits that averaged $71.25, and only seven patients (35%) lost some portion of their security deposit. Participants in the study only missed taking 7.8% of the scheduled doses, and 14 of the participants (70%) re-enlisted for a second contract immediately upon completion of the initial contract period. Overall, the study demonstrated the acceptability and feasibility of employing deposit contracting to promote disulfiram use in adults with serious alcohol problems.

Court-Arranged Disulfiram Treatment

Haynes (1973) described a program adopted by the Municipal Court of Colorado Springs, Colorado, in which individuals who had frequent arrests for public drunkenness were offered a choice between disulfiram treatment or the typical 90-day jail sentence. Individuals who chose the disulfiram treatment were required to visit the probation office twice per week to take their court-provided disulfiram tablets. Participants were on probation for 1 year. Failure to take the scheduled disulfiram doses was considered a violation of probation and could result in immediate arrest, although participants were typically allowed one or two violations before incarceration. In the first year of the program, 141 individuals were offered disulfiram treatment as an alternative to incarceration and 138 chose to take the disulfiram treatment. Of the 138 individuals, 66 were receiving the disulfiram treatment at the end of a year. Although this was only a brief descriptive study, the experience suggests that disulfiram treatment can be maintained by avoidance of incarceration.

COMMUNITY REINFORCEMENT
APPROACH (CRA) THERAPY

In addition to the direct application of abstinence-reinforcement contingencies, a behavioral counseling intervention based on similar operant principles was developed in the 1970s, known as the Community Reinforcement Approach (CRA). CRA therapy is a therapist delivered multicomponent behavioral treatment that was originally developed for the treatment of severe alcoholics (Hunt & Azrin, 1973). CRA was designed to systematically facilitate changes in the client's daily environment to promote healthy behaviors and to arrange reinforcement for abstinence in the patient's naturalistic environment.

Under this intervention, CRA sessions are focused on several general issues. Patients are initially instructed in how to recognize the antecedents and consequences of their alcohol and drug use. During this process, therapists and patients learn about the conditions under which drinking occurs most frequently by the patient. The therapist attempts to help the patient make the connection between his or her involvement with the alcohol-using lifestyle and drinking. Patients are then counseled to restructure their daily activities to minimize contact with known antecedents of their alcohol use, to find healthy alternatives to alcohol use, and to make explicit the negative consequences for alcohol use.

The patient is also encouraged to develop a new social network of non-alcohol-using individuals and is counseled to increase spending time with non-alcohol-using people and discontinuing interactions with drinkers. Patients and their nonusing significant other are offered reciprocal relationship counseling, a validated intervention for helping couples negotiate positive changes in their relationship (Azrin, Naster, & Jones, 1973). The intervention is designed to teach couples positive communication skills and how to negotiate reciprocal contracts for desired changes in each other's behavior.

Unemployed patients are offered participation in a Job Club intervention, which is a method for assisting chronically unemployed individuals to obtain employment (Azrin & Besalel, 1980; Azrin, Flores, & Kaplan, 1975). During the Job Club intervention, the therapist assists the client in identifying jobs that match the client's interest and vocational abilities. Other Job Club activities include assistance in developing and sending a resume, finding potential job opportunities in the classified ads, and practicing interviewing skills.

Finally, alcohol-dependent patients might be offered disulfiram. To ensure medication compliance, CRA therapists assist the patients to identify individuals who may help monitor and reinforce medication compliance, including significant others or other family members.

Several randomized controlled evaluations have been conducted evaluating the CRA therapy with various alcohol-abusing populations. The following section briefly describes those studies.

The first matched control trial was conducted with alcohol abusers receiving inpatient treatment. In that study, 16 patients admitted for alcoholism were randomly assigned to receive either CRA therapy or standard hospital care based on the 12-Step program of Alcoholics Anonymous (AA) (Hunt & Azrin, 1973). In this initial study, CRA therapy included vocational, family, and social recreational counseling. CRA participants also received assistance with employment, with marital and family interactions, and with arranging non-alcohol-related social/recreational activities. At the 6-month follow-up, patients assigned to the CRA therapy reported drinking on 14% of the follow-up days, whereas patients who had received standard treatment reported drinking 79% of the follow-up days. Furthermore, compared to patients in the standard treatment group, CRA patients had lower rates of unemployment (5% vs. 62% of days unemployed) and were hospitalized fewer days (2% vs. 27%).

In the second controlled study, CRA was expanded to include disulfiram therapy with monitoring by a significant other for medication compliance, a "buddy" system for social support, and group rather than individual counseling (Azrin, 1976). Twenty men admitted for alcoholism in a state hospital were randomly assigned to a modified CRA group or standard treatment group. Follow-up data collected 6 months following discharge from the hospital showed that the CRA group showed significantly better outcomes compared to the standard treatment group with regard to reduced self-reported time spent drinking (2% vs. 55%), less time institutionalized (0% vs. 45%), and decreased rates of unemployment (20% vs. 56%).

A subsequent controlled trial with outpatient alcohol abusers dissociated the effects of monitored disulfiram therapy from other components of CRA (Arzrin, Sisson, Meyers, & Godley, 1982). In that study, 43 alcohol-dependent outpatients were randomized to receive standard treatment plus disulfiram monitoring without compliance support, standard treatment plus disulfiram therapy with significant other compliance support, or CRA with disulfiram therapy and significant other compliance support. Results showed that CRA plus disulfiram and significant other compliance support was most effective in reducing self-reported number of days drinking, number of days intoxicated, number of ounces of alcohol consumed per drinking episode, and time away from home or institutionalized. The disulfiram and significant other compliance group showed intermediate effects on those outcome measures.

The CRA therapy for alcoholism combined with abstinence-contingent access to housing has also been evaluated in homeless adults (Smith, Myers, & Delaney, 1998). In that study, 106 homeless alcohol-dependent adults were randomly assigned to either a CRA group or a usual-care group that received 12-Step AA counseling with employment counseling. All participants were housed in supported housing. Random breath samples were collected and tested for alcohol from CRA participants. A positive breath sample resulted in a temporary suspension from housing. CRA participants were allowed to return to housing once they had attended CRA groups and were abstinent for 1 week. Random breath samples were not collected from usual-care participants, but they were suspended from housing if disruptive behavior was reported. Assessments were conducted at 2, 4, 6, 9, and 12 months after enrollment into the study. Compared to the usual-care group, participants in the CRA group self-reported consuming significantly fewer total number of drinks per week at the 2-, 4-, 6-, and 12-month follow-up time points, but not at the 6-month follow-up. In addition, CRA participants reported significantly fewer drinking days per week compared to usual-care participants at the 4-, 6-, and 9-month follow-ups. Peak blood alcohol content, estimated from self-reported steady drinking pattern, was significantly lower in CRA participants compared to usual-care participants at all follow-up time points except at the 12-month follow-up. Blood samples were also collected and analyzed for blood chemistry profiles at intake, 6-, and 12-month follow-up. At the 6-month follow-up, blood chemistry profiles showed significant decreases from abnormal to normal levels in the CRA group. In contrast, blood chemistry levels in the standard group remained elevated from intake levels. This controlled evaluation showed promising results regarding the overall effectiveness of CRA to promote alcohol abstinence in a population of difficult to treat homeless alcoholics. However, the study has some limitations with regard to the experimental design. Specifically, abstinence was required for all participants while living in supported housing, but routine breathalyzer tests were conducted only on CRA participants as part of their behavioral contingency. Thus, it is not clear from this study whether the observed effects in the CRA group resulted from the CRA treatment, the abstinence-contingent access to housing, or a combination of the two treatment elements.

In summary, the research to date suggests that the CRA therapy may reduce drinking in alcohol-dependent adults. However, the available evidence of CRA's effectiveness is based on self-reports of alcohol use. Future studies are needed that utilize direct, biological measures of alcohol use. Without the systematic collection of objective biological measures of alcohol use, we cannot be fully confident in the contribution of CRA therapy in promoting alcohol abstinence.

BARRIERS TO ABSTINENCE-REINFORCEMENT PROCEDURES FOR THE TREATMENT OF ALCOHOLISM

A major challenge in arranging reinforcement contingencies for alcohol abstinence has been identifying a reliable and valid biological marker for monitoring recent alcohol use. The absence of an biological marker with an appropriate detection duration makes it difficult to reinforce or punish alcohol use. For example, BAC is an objective measure of alcohol use that is relatively unobtrusive and easily collected. However, BAC only provides evidence of recent alcohol use because alcohol has a relatively short half-life in the body. Specifically, oral ingestion of alcohol results in an initial rise in BAC that represents absorption from the intestine, peaking usually within 1 hour. Then there follows an approximately linear decline in BAC with time. (For a review, see Lands, 1998).

Due the relatively quick elimination rate of alcohol from the body, frequent collection of breath samples for the purpose of monitoring and detecting alcohol use is necessary. As a result, the BAC may be an impractical objective measure for monitoring and reinforcing when an individual is or is not using alcohol.

Collecting breath samples on a random and unpredictable schedule may be a more effective method for monitoring and reinforcing alcohol use. To test such a procedure, a recent study conducted by Wong et al. (2004) evaluated a random breath sample collection procedure to monitor alcohol use among 92 homeless alcohol-dependent individuals participating in a clinical trial evaluating an employment-based abstinence-reinforcement intervention. Under this procedure, breath samples were collected on a random schedule on average two times per week, 7 days per week, between 900 and 1,700 hours. At the start of the study, participants were assigned a pager or cell phone, and were paid $35 in vouchers if they answered a randomly scheduled page or phone call and allowed research staff to collect a breath sample. Breath samples were tested for alcohol using an Alco-Sensor III device. Overall, 96% of participants provided at least one random breath sample over a 26-week period, 64% of all random breath samples were collected, and 29% of collected samples tested positive (BAL 0.003 g/ 100 ml) for alcohol. While this procedure needs further improvements, these preliminary data suggest that a procedure to collect breath sample on a random and unpredictable schedule may provide a valid outcome measure and monitoring procedure for alcohol use in treatment, especially for CM interventions.

CONCLUDING COMMENTS

Extensive animal and human laboratory research has shown that alcohol use can be conceptualized as operant behavior and can be modified by manipulation of its consequences. That research provides an empirical basis for the application of operant principles to the treatment of alcohol abuse and dependence. These principles have been applied in CM interventions that arrange reinforcement contingencies for abstinence and for treatment adherence (most notably medication compliance), and in CRA counseling. The number of clinical studies that have evaluated CM interventions and CRA to control alcohol use in problem drinkers is limited and many of the studies have serious methodological shortcomings. Many of the studies have not employed adequate experimental designs and many have relied on self-report measures of alcohol use. Given these limitations, it is difficult to make definitive statements about the effectiveness of CM interventions or CRA in treating alcohol abuse and dependence. Nevertheless, the case studies and controlled evaluations provide promising evidence that CM interventions and CRA are feasible and appear effective in promoting therapeutic behavior change, including disulfiram ingestion and alcohol abstinence.

Based on our review of the literature, further rigorous research employing sound experimental designs and objective measures of alcohol are needed to fully determine the effectiveness of CM interventions and CRA to treat alcohol abuse and dependence. Perhaps most critically, research is needed to develop innovative methodology to monitor and reinforce alcohol abstinence. Recent research integrating the use of technology and the Internet has led to new procedures to monitor smoking and to arrange reinforcement for smoking abstinence (Dallery, Glenn, & Raiff, 2007), which may also hold promise for the treatment of alcohol problems. Under this procedure, a smoker records a video clip on a computer while providing a breath sample into a device that measures and displays the smoker's carbon monoxide level. Carbon monoxide levels below a specified cutoff can provide evidence of recent smoking abstinence. The video clip is transmitted through the Internet to a central location where a clinician or technician can verify the individual's smoking status. If the carbon monoxide reading displayed in the video clip verifies that the individual is abstinent from smoking, reinforcement is provided immediately via e-mail to the participant (Dallery, Glenn, & Raiff, 2007). Similar procedures could be easily adapted and implemented for the monitoring and reinforcing of alcohol abstinence in treatment-seeking problem drinkers.

In summary, studies conducted in both the laboratory and in clinical treatment setting suggest that operant interventions, particularly CM procedures, could be extremely effective in the treatment of alcohol abuse and dependence. However, additional treatment research utilizing rigorous experimental designs and adequate outcome measures are needed before definitive judgments can be made on the effectiveness and utility of this approach. Until further rigorous research is conducted to evaluate the effectiveness of CM interventions and CRA to promote alcohol abstinence, it will be difficult to encourage the alcohol treatment field to apply these procedures for the treatment of alcohol abuse and dependence.

ACKNOWLEDGMENTS

Preparation of the chapter was supported by Grant No. R01 AA012154 from the National Institute on Alcohol Abuse and Alcoholism and Grant No. R21 DA017885 from the National Institute on Drug Abuse.

REFERENCES

Azrin, N. H. (1976). Improvements in the community reinforcement approach to alcoholism. *Behaviour Research and Therapy, 14*, 339–348.

Azrin, N. H., & Besalel, V. A. (1980). *Job Club counselor's manual*. Baltimore: University Park Press.

Azrin, N. H., Flores, T., & Kaplan, S. J. (1975). Job-finding club: A group-assisted program for obtaining employment. *Behaviour Research and Therapy, 13*, 17–27.

Azrin, N. H., Naster, B. J., & Jones, R. (1973). Reciprocity counseling: A rapid learning-based procedure for marital counseling. *Behaviour Research and Therapy, 11*, 365–382.

Azrin, N. H., Sisson, R. W., Meyers, R. J., & Godley, M. (1982). Alcoholism treatment by disulfiram and community reinforcement therapy. *Journal of Behavior Therapy and Experimental Psychiatry, 13,* 105–112.

Bickel, W. K., Rizzuto, P., Zielony, R. D., Klobas, J., Pangiosonlis, P., Mernit, R., et al. (1989). Combined behavioral and pharmacological treatment of alcoholic methadone patients. *Journal of Substance Abuse, 1,* 161–171.

Bigelow, G., Liebson, I., & Griffiths, R. (1974). Alcoholic drinking: Suppression by a brief time-out procedure. *Behaviour Research and Therapy, 12,* 107–115.

Bigelow, G. E., Stitzer, M. L., Griffiths, R. R., & Liebson, I. A. (1981). Contingency management approaches to drug self-administration and drug abuse: Efficacy and limitations. *Addictive Behaviors, 6,* 241–252.

Bigelow, G., Strickler, D., Liebson, I., & Griffiths, R. (1976). Maintaining disulfiram ingestion among outpatient alcoholics: A security deposit contingency contracting procedure. *Behaviour Research and Therapy, 14,* 378–381.

Brigham, S. L., Brekers, G. A., Rosen, A. C., Swihart, J. J., Pfrimmer, G., & Ferguson, L. N. (1981). Contingency management in the treatment of adolescent alcohol drinking problems. *Journal of Psychology, 109,* 73–85.

Carroll, M. E. (1987). Self-administration of orally-delivered phencyclidine and ethanol under concurrent fixed-ratio schedules in rhesus monkeys. *Psychopharmacology, 93,* 1–7.

Carroll, M. E., Rodefer, J. S., & Rawleigh, J. M. (1995). Concurrent self-administration of ethanol and an alternative nondrug reinforcer in monkeys: Effects of income (session length) on demand for drug. *Psychopharmacology, 120,* 1–9.

Clark, R., & Polish, E. (1960). Avoidance conditioning and alcohol consumption in rhesus monkeys. *Science, 132,* 223–224.

Cohen, M., Bigelow, G., Hargett, A., Allen, R., & Halsted, C. (1973). The use of contingency management procedures for the treatment of alcoholism in a work setting. *Alcoholism, 9,* 97–104.

Cohen, M., Liebson, I. A., & Faillace, L. A. (1972). A technique for establishing controlled drinking in chronic alcoholics. *Diseases of the Nervous System, 33,* 46–49.

Cohen, M., Liebson, I. A., & Faillace, L. A. (1973). Controlled drinking by chronic alcoholics over extended periods of free access. *Psychological Reports, 32,* 1107–1110.

Cohen, M., Liebson, I. A., Faillace, L. A., & Allen, R. P. (1971). Moderate drinking by chronic alcoholics: A schedule-dependent phenomenon. *Journal of Nervous and Mental Disorders, 153,* 434–444.

Cohen, M., Liebson, I. A., Faillace, L. A., & Speers, W. (1971). Alcoholism: Controlled drinking and incentives for abstinence. *Psychological Reports, 28,* 575–580.

Dallery, J., Glenn, I. M., & Raiff, B. R. (2007). An Internet-based abstinence reinforcement treatment for cigarette smoking. *Drug and Alcohol Dependence, 86,* 230–238.

Foltin, R. W. (1998). Ethanol and food pellet self-administration by baboons. *Alcohol, 16,* 183–188.

Grant, K. A., & Bennett, A. J. (2003). Advances in nonhuman primate alcohol abuse and alcoholism research. *Pharmacology and Therapeutics, 100,* 235–255.

Grant, K. A., Johanson, C. E., & Schuster, C. R. (1986). Effect of increased access to ethanol on oral ethanol self-administration by Rhesus monkeys. *Alcohol Clinical Experimental Research, 10,* 113.

Grant, K. A., & Samson, H. H. (1985). Oral self-administration of ethanol in free-feeding rats. *Alcohol, 2,* 317–322.

Griffiths, R. R., Bigelow, G. E., & Liebson, I. A. (1974). Suppression of ethanol self-administration in alcoholics by contingent time-out from social interactions in alcoholics. *Behaviour Research and Therapy, 12*, 327–334.

Griffiths, R. R., Bigelow, G. E., & Liebson, I. A. (1977). Comparison of social time-out and activity time-out procedures in suppressing ethanol self-administration in alcoholics. *Behaviour Research and Therapy, 15*, 329–336.

Haynes, S. N. (1973). Contingency management in a municipally-administered Antabuse program for alcoholics. *Journal of Behavior Therapy and Experimental Psychiatry, 4*, 31–32.

Higgins, S. T., & Katz, J. L. (1998). *Cocaine abuse: Behavior, pharmacology, and clinical applications.* San Diego: Academic Press.

Hunt, G. M., & Azrin, N. H. (1973). A community reinforcement approach to alcoholism. *Behaviour Research and Therapy, 11*, 91–104.

Lands, W. E. M. (1998). A review of alcohol clearance in humans. *Alcohol, 15*, 147–160.

Liebson, I., Bigelow, G., & Flamer, R. (1973). Alcoholism among methadone patients: A specific treatment method. *American Journal of Psychiatry, 130*, 483–485.

Liebson, I. A., Tommasello, A., & Bigelow, G. E. (1978). A behavioral treatment of alcoholic methadone patients. *Annals of Internal Medicine, 89*, 342–344.

Meisch, R. A. (2001). Oral drug self-administration: an overview of laboratory animal studies. *Alcohol, 24*, 117–128.

Mello, N. K., & Mendelson, J. H. (1965). Operant analysis of drinking patterns of chronic alcoholics. *Nature, 206*, 43–46.

Miller, P. M. (1972). The use of behavioral contracting in the treatment of alcoholism: A case report. *Behavior Therapy, 3*, 593–596.

Miller, P. M. (1975). A behavioral intervention program for chronic public drunkenness offenders. *Archives of General Psychiatry, 32*, 915–918.

Miller, P. M., Hersen, M., Eisler, R. M., & Watts, J. G. (1974). Contingent reinforcement of lowered blood-alcohol levels in an outpatient chronic alcoholic. *Behaviour Research and Therapy, 12*, 261–263.

Peniston, E. G. (1988). Evaluation of long-term therapeutic efficacy of behavior modification program with chronic male psychiatric inpatients. *Journal of Behavior Therapy and Experimental Psychiatry, 19*, 95–101.

Petry, N. M., Martin, B., Cooney, J. L., & Kranzler, H. R. (2000). Give them prizes, and they will come: Contingency management for treatment of alcohol dependence. *Journal of Consulting and Clinical Psychology, 68*, 250–257.

Robichaud, C., Strickler, D., Bigelow, G., & Liebson, I. (1979). Disulfiram maintenance employee alcoholism treatment: A three-phase evaluation. *Behaviour Research and Therapy, 17*, 618–621.

Samson, H. H., & Czachowski, C. L. (2003). Behavioral measures of alcohol self-administration and intake control: Rodent models. *International Review of Neurobiology, 54*, 107–143.

Samson, H. H., & Pfeffer, A. O. (1987). Initiation of ethanol-maintained responding using a schedule-induction procedure in free feeding rats. *Alcohol Drug Research, 7*, 461–469.

Samson, H. H., Pfeffer, A. O., & Tolliver, G. A. (1988). Oral ethanol self-administration in rats: Models of alcohol-seeking behavior. *Alcoholism: Clinical and Experimental Research, 12*, 591–598.

Samson, H. H., Roehrs, T. A., & Tolliver, G. A. (1982). Ethanol reinforced responding in the rat: A concurrent analysis using sucrose as the alternate choice. *Pharmacology, Biochemistry and Behavior, 17*, 333–339.

Schmitz, J. M., Sayre, S. L., Hokanson, P. S., & Spiga, R. (2003). Assessment of the relative reinforcement value of smoking and drinking using a multiple-choice measurement strategy. *Nicotine and Tobacco Research, 5,* 729–734.

Schuster, C. R., & Thomspon, T. (1969). Self administration of and behavioral dependence on drugs. *Annual Review of Pharmacology, 9,* 483–502.

Smith, J. E., Meyers, R. J., & Delaney, H. D. (1998). The community reinforcement approach with homeless alcohol-dependent individuals. *Journal of Consulting and Clinical Psychology, 66,* 541–548.

Smith, S. G., & Davis, W. M. (1974). Intravenous alcohol self-administration in the rat. *Pharmacology Research Communications, 6,* 394–402.

Spiga, R., Macenski, M. J., Meisch, R. A., & Roache, J. D. (1997). Human ethanol self-administration I: The interaction between response requirement and ethanol dose. *Behavioural Pharmacology, 8,* 91–100.

Substance Abuse and Mental Health Services Administration. (2005). *Results from the 2004 National Survey on Drug Use and Health: National Findings* (NSDUH Series H-28, DHHS Publication No. SMA 05-406). Rockville, MD: Office of Applied Studies.

Winger, G. D., & Woods, J. H. (1973). The reinforcing property of ethanol: I. Initiation, maintenance and termination of ethanol-reinforced responding. *Annals of the New York Academy of Sciences, 215,* 162–175.

Wong, C. J., Diemer, K., Webb, L., Taylor, C., Knealing, T., Fingerhood, M., et al. (2004). *Random breath sample collection to detect alcohol use in homeless alcoholics.* Paper presented at the College on Problems of Drug Dependence, San Juan, Puerto Rico.

Wong, C. J., Kolodner, K., Fingerhood, M., Bigelow, G. E., & Silverman, K. (2005). *A therapeutic workplace for homeless alcohol-dependent individuals.* Paper presented at the College on Problems of Drug Dependence, Orlando, FL.

CHAPTER 8

MEDICATION COMPLIANCE

Bruce J. Rounsaville, Marc Rosen,
and Kathleen M. Carroll

The great strength of contingency management (CM) as a treatment for addictions is its power to bring about changes in a wide range of sharply defined target behaviors. Nearly any given behavior can be changed by providing contingent incentives. Given the comparatively circumscribed nature of medication consumption behaviors, medication compliance would seem to be an ideal target for CM. High rates of noncompliance with prescribed medications are typical in treatment of patient groups in general (Haynes, McDonald, Garg, & Montague, 2000; Haynes, Taylor, & Sackett, 1979; Horwitz & Horwitz, 1993) and substance-abusing populations specifically (Drake & Brunette, 1998; Weiss, 2004).

In addition to CM, a broad array of remedies have been devised and subjected to efficacy testing, including educational strategies, family interventions, the use of devices to prompt pill taking, directly observed administration, skills training, and motivational enhancement (Haynes, McDonald, & Garg, 2002; Meichenbaum & Turk, 1987). Systematic reviews of the general medication compliance enhancement literature have documented effects favoring experimental conditions in only around half of published reports (Sackett & Snow, 1979) and CM approaches have been used in only a small fraction of reviewed studies (Roter et al., 1998). Notably, our literature review in preparation for this chapter identified few studies of CM for medication compliance enhancement in addicts, with the majority focusing on reinforcing compliance with naltrexone treatment for opioid dependence (Carroll et al., 2001; Carroll, Sinha, Nich, Babuscio, & Rounsaville, 2002; Grabowski et al., 1979; Preston et al., 1999) or family contracts for medication taking (Anton, Hogan, Jalali, Riordan, & Kleber, 1981; Chick et al., 1992; Fals-Stewart & O'Farrell, 2003; O'Farrell, Cutter, Choquette, & Floyd, 1992). In this chapter, we attempt to identify ways to build on the comparatively sparse literature on CM for medication compliance for addictions by (1) identifying promising targets for CM, (2) reviewing the challenges to applying CM for medication compliance enhancement, and (3) suggesting directions for refinements of CM that combat these challenges.

MEDICATIONS TO TARGET WITH CM

Individuals with substance abuse or dependence are not protected from illnesses that may be treated with medications, and hence substance abusers are presumably included as an unidentified subgroup in general studies of medication compliance (Wadland & Ferenchick, 2004). Nonetheless, within homogenous groups of treated substance abusers, medications of special interest include (1) drugs to reduce substance use, including agonists (e.g., methadone for opioids), antagonists (e.g., naltrexone for opioids), aversive agents (e.g., disulfiram for alcohol), and anticraving agents (e.g., naltrexone for alcohol and buproprion for nicotine); (2) HIV (human immunodeficiency virus) treatments (e.g., highly active antiretroviral therapy for HIV-positive patients); (3) antibiotics (e.g., antituberculosis regimens); and (4) medications to treat comorbid mental disorders (e.g., antipsychotics and antidepressants).

Compliance enhancement is particularly salient for substance-abusing populations because of generally low or mixed motivations to curtail substance use in the majority of treatment-seeking patients (Miller, 1985), high rates of HIV and other infections in substance abusers (Klinkenberg, Sacks, & HIV/AIDS Treatment Adherence Health Outcomes and Cost Study Group, 2004; O'Connor, Selwyn, & Schottenfeld, 1994), and high rates and negative prognostic significance of comorbid psychopathology in substance-abusing patients (Brady & Sinha, 2005; Compton, Thomas, Conway, & Colliver, 2005; Kessler et al., 1997). Factors underlying poor compliance among substance-using patients include (1) lack of immediate benefit from taking the medication, (2) ambivalence about giving up drugs, (3) adverse reactions, (4) need for protracted treatment, (5) complexity of dosing schedules, and (6) logistic difficulties in filling prescriptions.

The most salient limitation of most of these types of medications is the lack of immediate rewarding effects. Medications that physicians prescribe for drug abusers generally represent the converse of abused substances in terms of the immediacy of positive reinforcement. Abused drugs tend to have immediate positive effects followed by delayed adverse effects. With few exceptions, prescribed medications either provide no immediate reward or cause initial side effects and generate positive reinforcements that are delayed and/or subtle. For medicines prescribed with the aim of curtailing or reducing drug use, the immediate effect on the addict is to take away a valued reinforcer.

One exception to the tendency to provide delayed benefits is the group of agonist treatments, in which a longer-acting agent is substituted for an abused substance that has greater short-term effects. Agonist agents are well accepted by substance abusers and no studies have evaluated CM to enhance medication taking for agonist treatments, although CM has frequently been combined with methadone maintenance in order to reduce the use of illicit opiates (e.g., Stitzer, Bickel, Bigelow, & Liebson, 1986; Stitzer, Iguchi, & Felch, 1992). Other medications that provide relatively rapid reinforcing benefits are painkillers and quick-acting antibiotics.

CM may usefully be adapted to address the short-term disincentives to take many nonagonist medications. In the remainder of this section, we review how CM has been applied to agents for drug reduction, HIV treatment, antibiotic treatment, and treatment for comorbid psychopathology.

Medications to Reduce Drug Use

As noted previously, it takes some time for an addict to obtain noticeable benefit from stopping drug use. Restoration of health, improved social functioning, and cultivation of rewarding alternative behaviors all tend to take place gradually, while withdrawal effects, intense drug craving, medication side effects, and the threat of permanent loss of drug rewards are experienced with little or no delay after stopping use. After a period of protracted abstinence, the intrinsic benefits of taking the prescribed medication may become apparent and reduce the need for compliance enhancement efforts, but CM may be particularly important during initial phases of treatment.

The reinforcement power of antidrug agents is mitigated by the fact that the addict may receive far less immediate benefit than members of his or her social network while the addict alone suffers the negative aspects of giving up substance use. This dynamic underlies the enlistment of family members and significant others in some of the most successful CM strategies to improve addicts' compliance with antidrug medications (Chick et al., 1992; Fals-Stewart & O'Farrell, 2003; Higgins, Budney, Bickel, Hughes, & Foerg, 1993).

The need for CM to reinforce medication compliance is hence most marked for those agents that are highly effective in producing abstinence, like naltrexone for opioid dependence and disulfiram for alcoholism. Both of these agents require detoxification prior to use and both more or less preclude continued substance use as long as the medication is taken as directed. Hence, compliance with these agents is nearly equivalent to treatment success (Fuller et al., 1986; Volpicelli et al., 1997). Not surprisingly, these two agents figure prominently in the CM literature on medication compliance. Interestingly enough, medication compliance represents less of a problem for antidrug agents that have more subtle and partial effects on drug use, such as naltrexone for alcoholism and buproprion for tobacco dependence, and there are no studies targeting them with CM.

Nevertheless, systematic evaluations of the effect of CM on naltrexone compliance and outcome have consistently demonstrated positive results. As early as the 1970s, several investigators (Grabowski et al., 1979; Meyer, Mirin, Altman, & McNamee, 1976) reported success using comparatively small contingency payments as reinforcements for naltrexone consumption. More recently, some of the most promising data regarding strategies to enhance retention and outcome in naltrexone treatment have come from investigators evaluating CM approaches. Preston et al. (1999) evaluated voucher-based reinforcement of compliance with thrice-weekly naltrexone versus noncontingent vouchers and no vouchers in 58 outpatients. They reported that contingent vouchers were associated with significant improvements in retention and compliance with naltrexone compared with the other two conditions; however, marked differences in rates of drug use were not seen.

To evaluate whether outcomes could be improved by also reinforcing drug-free urine tests, two studies by our group provided voucher-based reinforcement both for verified compliance with thrice-weekly naltrexone treatment and for submission of drug-free urine specimens. In the first study (Carroll et al., 2001), 127 recently detoxified opioid-dependent individuals were randomly assigned to one of three conditions: (1) naltrexone + weekly cognitive-behavioral therapy (CBT), (2) naltrexone and CBT + CM with delivery of vouchers contingent upon naltrexone compliance and drug-free urine specimens, or (3) naltrexone, CBT, CM + significant other (SO) involvement, where a family member was invited to participate in up to six family counseling sessions. CM was associated with significant improvements in both retention and reduction in opioid use. Although the additional SO involvement did not significantly improve retention, compliance, or substance-abuse outcomes compared with CM overall, significant benefits were seen for the subgroup that attended at least one family session.

In a parallel second study designed to evaluate the effect of magnitude of reinforcement on compliance and outcome in this population (Carroll et al., 2002), 55 detoxified opioid-dependent individuals were randomly assigned to either standard naltrexone maintenance; standard naltrexone + lower-value CM (maximum value $561); or standard naltrexone + higher-value CM (maximum value $1,152). Assignment to either CM condition was associated with significant reductions in opioid use over time compared with standard naltrexone treatment. However, contrasts of higher- versus lower-value reinforcement magnitude were not significant, suggesting no relative value of higher- over lower-value incentives in this population.

In contrast with these studies that focus naltrexone CM contracts on positive incentives, naltrexone has been most successful in patient groups for which there are powerful negative contingencies if medication is missed and/or drug use is resumed, including probation populations who face returning to incarceration and medical practitioners who face loss of license (e.g., Cornish et al., 1997).

For disulfiram treatment of alcoholism, the most important factor in treatment success is medication compliance and patients must accept a treatment goal of complete abstinence from alcohol as long as medication is taken. Notably, despite the intrinsically powerful effects of disulfiram to curtail alcohol use, in clinical settings it has been found to be no more powerful than placebo because of high rates of noncompliance when no extrinsic contingencies for pill taking are provided (Fuller et al., 1986). In contrast, a number of CM strategies have been shown to increase compliance with disulfiram with robust effects on reduced alcohol use and other alcohol-related outcomes. First, disulfiram for alcoholism has been shown to be highly powerful when prescribed within the context of behavioral family treatments that include a contract for spouse-administered treatment (Chick et al., 1992; O'Farrell et al., 1992; O'Farrell & Litten, 1992). In addition to reinforcing medication compliance, per se, family behavioral contracts can target the problem of delayed benefits from stopping drinking by including agreements by family members to provide rewards for continued abstinence. Second, in patients with concurrent opioid dependence and alcoholism, making provision of methadone contingent upon disulfiram ingestion has been reported to increase compliance in an uncontrolled case series (Bickel et al., 1988) and a randomized clinical trial (Liebson, Tomasello, & Bigelow, 1978). Third, disulfiram compliance has been enhanced in an uncontrolled trial of alcoholic volunteers using a security-deposit box contingency contracting approach (Bigelow, Strickler, Liebson, & Griffiths, 1976). Therapists deposit an agreed-on amount of the patient's own money into a safe-deposit box with return of the full sum contingent upon disulfiram compliance and achievement of specified treatment goals. Failure to take disulfiram or to achieve specified treatment goals results in specified sums of money to be removed from the deposit box and donated to charity. In addition to its efficacy, this strategy has the advantage of defraying the costs of incentives by using the patient's own funds. Fourth, linking disulfiram compliance with directly observed administration in a workplace setting was shown to reduce absenteeism in an uncontrolled trial of volunteer industrial workers who had a history of alcohol-related workplace incidents (Robichaud, Strickler, Bigelow, & Liebson, 1979). In all these strategies, disulfiram compliance is enhanced by providing comparatively strong social (marital, job), pharmacological (contingent methadone), or financial (safe-deposit box) incentives that antedate and supplement intrinsic rewards from being abstinent from alcohol.

Antiretroviral Treatments for HIV-Positive Substance Abusers

While untreated HIV is associated with severe illness and high death rates within 6 years of infection, increasingly powerful highly active antiretroviral therapy (HAART) regimens greatly reduce the morbidity and mortality associated with HIV infection (Baker, 1997; Palella et al., 1998). Indeed, many adequately treated patients experience few symptoms and appear to have nearly normal life expectancy. Intuitively, the literally live-saving and life-enhancing effects of HAART would seem to provide more than sufficient motivation for HIV-positive patients to comply with treatment. Nonetheless, HIV-infected drug abusers have been reported to display high rates of medication noncompliance (Udall, Palmer, Whetten, Mellins, & HIV/AIDS Treatment Adherence Health Outcomes and Cost Study Group, 2004). Factors working against medication compliance include unpleasant medication side effects, complexity of many HIV medication regimens, slow progression of HIV symptoms, cognitive deficits in many HIV-positive drug abusers, the irregular schedules kept by many drug abusers, stigma associated with HIV-positive status, and strong motivation for denial of this life-threatening infection (Ammassari et al., 2002; Bouhnik et al., 2002; Ickovics & Meade, 2002). On the other side, optimal adherence is required for an optimal response to HAART. In one widely cited study, 78% of patients taking 95% of prescribed doses had detectable viral loads but only 39% of patients with slightly lower adherence between 80% and 95% had undetectable viral loads (Paterson et al., 2000). The interrelated phenomena of nonadherence and drug resistance are thought to be the most important reasons for failed treatment (Perno et al., 2002). Patients who intermittently adhere to HAART may temporarily select for partially resistant virus and then allow the virus to multiply unchecked (Vanhove, Schapiro, Winters, Merigan, & Blaschke, 1996). Economic factors also underscore the value of antiretroviral medication compliance as the average costs of HAART, including associated monitoring, have been estimated to exceed $10,000 per year for each treated patient (Bozzette et al., 2001) but are lower than the cumulative costs of treating advanced HIV disease (Schackman et al., 2001).

The use of CM to enhance antiretroviral medication compliance supports the general strategy of providing short-latency, tangible incentives to make up for the delayed benefits and immediate negative aspects of adherence with treatment. Applying CM for this indication entails numerous challenges because HAART involves multiple medications, complex medication schedules, and the need for compliance with other aspects of treatment such as blood draws. Our group has applied CM to this problem by linking monetary incentives to evidence of timely medication use of a single agent monitored by an electronic sensor embedded in the cap of the medication dispenser (MEMS [Medicatiom Event Monitoring System] cap) (Rigsby et al., 2000). The MEMS (developed by Aprex Corporation, Fremont, California) cap data are then downloaded to a computer to provide a printout listing the date and time of each bottle opening over the preceding months. In addition to providing incentives for MEMS-verified medication taking, this CM approach is combined with training in which the counselor helps the client identify environmental cues to prompt medication taking (Rosen, Ryan, & Rigsby, 2002).

In an initial trial of this approach, 4 weeks of CM resulted in an average of 92% of doses taken on time in comparison with 70% in the non-CM controls. Notably, reinforcement of a single component of the HAART regimen was associated with increased compliance with other nonreinforced medications in the regimen. Also, compliance with antiretroviral medications was not contingent upon maintaining drug abstinence as there was no association between antiretroviral medication compliance and number of days of substance abuse (Rosen, personal communication, 2005). More recently, Sorensen and colleagues (Sorensen, 2004) and our group (M. Rosen, September 15, 2005) have replicated these findings in a larger sample and using a longer duration of CM treatment. Unfortunately, in all three trials of CM to enhance antiretroviral compliance, increased medication compliance associated with CM rapidly reverted back to control levels after incentives had been withdrawn.

Antibiotic Treatments

While the link between intravenous substance abuse and needle-borne infections is clear, an important but less recognized problem is the recent resurgence of medication-resistant tuberculosis (TB), especially in treated substance abuse populations (Batki, Gruber, Bradley, Bradley, & Delucchi, 2002; O'Connor & Samet, 2002; Perlman et al., 1995). Like HIV infection, TB can be life threatening, but mortality rates are comparatively low and there is typically a long latency between infection and noticeable symptoms. Hence, most cases are discovered when the patient is asymptomatic and the benefits of complying with antitubercular regimens are comparatively distant or abstract from the patient's perspective. From the perspective of treatment providers the need for treatment is urgent in order to protect the safety of other patients and of society at large. As with antiretroviral therapy, TB antibiotic treatments require long-term compliance and induce unpleasant side effects, and its subjective benefits are minimal. CM can address these factors by providing immediate and tangible rewards for medication compliance. Several studies have demonstrated significant effects of the provision of small contingent payments ($10 or less) on compliance with isoniazid therapy (Chaisson et al., 2001) or rates of return for TB skin test readings (Malotte, Hollingshead, & Rhodes, 1999) among drug users. Elk et al. (1993) also demonstrated marked increases in adherence with isoniazid among methadone-maintained opioid-dependent individuals when methadone was dispensed contingent upon isoniazid ingestion.

Medications for Comorbid Psychopathology

Community surveys and reports from substance abuse clinical settings have repeatedly documented excess rates of comorbid mental illness in treated substance abusers (Anthony, Warner, & Kessler, 1994; Kessler et al., 1997) and the poorer prognosis conveyed by psychiatric comorbidity (Rounsaville, Dolinsky, Babor, & Meyer, 1987; Rounsaville, Kosten, Weissman, & Kleber, 1986). Many of these comorbid mental illnesses are readily treated with medications, most notably antidepressant, antimanic, and antipsychotic agents (O'Brien, 1997). Medication noncompliance in substance abusers with psychiatric comorbidity has been shown to be prevalent and associated with relapse to both types of disorders (Drake et al., 2001). For example, rehospitalization in schizophrenic patients is frequently precipitated by an episode of substance abuse combined with discontinuation of antipsychotic medications (Dixon, Haas, Weiden, Sweeney, & Frances, 1991). For example, Nunes et al.'s (1998) study of the efficacy of the tricyclic antidepressant imipramine for reducing depression and illicit drug use among depressed methadone-maintained patients reported a 38.7% rate of completion of an "adequate trial" of 6 weeks of imipramine, as measured by self-report and directly observed ingestion (direct observation was for approximately half of the doses). This rate of adherence is similar to other rates of adherence in other pharmacological studies of depressed cocaine- or opioid-dependent patients (Goldstein et al., cited in Woody, O'Brien, McLellan, Marcovici, & Evans, 1982; Kleber et al., 1983; Titievsky, Seco, Barranco, & Kyle, 1982; Woody, O'Brien, & Rickels, 1975; Woody et al., 1982), except for studies, in which patients received directly observed therapy, in which adherence rates were substantially higher (e.g., Petrakis et al., 1998).

Currently, our group is conducting a randomized controlled trial of enhancing compliance with medication for psychiatric conditions among outpatients with severe mental illness and co-occurring substance abuse (M. V. Pantalon, personal communication, October 17, 2005) Specifically, the study requires that the eligible patient demonstrates < 75% compliance with the use of a MEMS during a 2-week baseline. Once this requirement is established the patient is randomly assigned to one of the following, medication compliance enhancement conditions: (1) adherence feedback (AF;

Cramer & Rosenheck, 1998), in which patients receive computerized feedback on medication and counseling adherence, based on MEMS data and attendance records, (2) AF + CM (i.e., $200 for perfect compliance throughout; Budney & Higgins, 1998), or (3) AF + motivational enhancement therapy (MET) (Miller & Rollnick, 2002; D'Onofrio, Pantalon, Degutis, Fiellin, & O'Connor, 2005). Each intervention is brief (5–10 minutes for AF + CM; 20 minutes for AF + MET).

LIMITATIONS/DRAWBACKS FOR CM
TO ENHANCE MEDICATION COMPLIANCE

From this brief review, all controlled trials have supported the efficacy of CM to enhance compliance with the targeted medication type. As noted earlier, CM is most applicable to shape behaviors that are discrete and clearly identified, like complying with medication instructions. Nonetheless, CM is seldom used in practice and even CM research has focused only on a small number of medication compliance issues. If CM is to be more widely used, the barriers to its use need to be identified and dealt with.

Despite its strengths, CM has a number of weaknesses as a tool to enhance medication compliance. First, the costs of providing material incentives are not provided for in budgets of typical substance abuse or primary-care medical settings. Given the novelty of CM treatments for these applications, there are no ready ways for program administrators to recover these costs using third-party payment procedure codes. Second, the skills needed to apply CM are generally unfamiliar to medically trained personnel. In addition, the types of recordkeeping required to keep track of anything but the simplest reinforcement schedules are likely to be burdensome in a busy primary-care clinic. Third, the provision of tangible incentives can be seen as enhancing only extrinsic motivation to perform the desired behavior while failing to address intrinsic motivations to comply with prescribed treatments (Deci, Koestner, & Ryan, 1999). This criticism of current CM approaches has been validated by those studies that have documented substantial reductions in targeted behaviors when incentives are removed (e.g., Rigsby et al., 2000).

STRATEGIES TO COUNTER CM DRAWBACKS

Offset Costs: Select Applications with Large Potential CM Benefits

Given the costs and other barriers to widespread use of CM for medication compliance, it is important to pick applications in which the potential benefits far outweigh these costs. As a primary consideration, CM should be reserved for those applications when the medication is crucial to reach treatment goals and the consequences of noncompliance are severe. Notably, these conditions prevail for all of the applications reviewed previously, including (1) naltrexone for opioid dependence and disulfiram for alcoholism, where compliance is synonymous with abstinence; (2) antiretroviral treatment for HIV infection, for which high rates of compliance are needed not only to achieve benefits but also to prevent emergence of new medication resistant strains of HIV; (3) anti-TB antibiotics that are needed to prevent disease progression and to protect society from recurrence of a TB epidemic; and (4) medications to treat severe comorbid psychopathology (e.g., antipsychotic and antimanic agents) that can prevent the need for costly rehospitalizations.

Vaccines aimed at inactivating abused drugs are costly but potentially powerful, and they might benefit from the reinforcement of taking injections. At present, the type of vaccine with the most promise targets cocaine dependence (Kosten & Biegel, 2002). While the anticocaine antigen titers are potentially long lasting and promise to convey sustained benefit, repeated vaccine injections over an 8-week period are needed to achieve clinically significant antigen titers (Kosten et al., 2002). During that time, both compliance with vaccine injection schedules and maintenance of abstinence are vitally important to ensure success. If patients continue to use cocaine when anticocaine titers are low, they are likely to perceive the treatment as completely ineffective and to drop out prematurely or to simply raise the dose of abused cocaine to compensate for the vaccine's effect. This initial 10-week treatment induction period is an ideal time to use powerful, voucher-based CM conditions with escalating rewards (Higgins et al., 1991) that have been repeatedly demonstrated to foster sustained periods of abstinence as long as incentives are provided. Adequate anticocaine antigen titers can then potentially prevent the reemergence of cocaine use that often accompanies the withdrawal of the comparatively expensive incentives used in this approach.

Several secondary factors should be considered when choosing medications to target with CM. First, CM should be reserved for medications in which other, less intensive compliance enhancements are not available or ineffective. For example, because patients prescribed daily antipsychotic medications can simply be switched to long-acting depot formulations, adding CM to improve antipsychotic pill compliance may not be the most cost-effective course of action. Second, CM is likely to be necessary only for medications with characteristics that reduce the likelihood of compliance such as low or highly delayed perceived benefit, aversive side effects, need for sustained use, and complex dosing schedules. As noted previously, these characteristics apply to all the types of medications that have been targeted for clinical trials of CM with substance abusers and generally do not apply with other types of medications prescribed for drug abusers. Hence, the major solution to the problem of CM costs is the choice of applications in which these costs can be readily offset.

Reduce Training Burdens: Simplify/Enhance Efficiency of CM

Even though compliance with prescribed medications can make the difference between treatment success and treatment failure, behavioral aspects of medical treatment are seldom emphasized in medical/nursing education and the time allotted for each patient contact is highly limited, particularly in managed care settings. Hence, the likelihood that a CM compliance enhancement scheme will be adopted is directly proportional to the brevity and simplicity of administering this intervention. The need for enhancing compliance over extended time periods adds further to the need for quick and simple strategies. Unfortunately, some of the strategies that have been found to be most efficacious for treating abusers are somewhat complex, including the voucher-based, escalating-dose strategy devised by Higgins and colleagues (Budney & Higgins, 1998) and the variable-ratio, prize-incentive method pioneered by Petry, Martin, Cooney, and Kranzler (2000). Simple, fixed-ratio reinforcement schedules have tended to be less effective when applied in substance abuse populations (Petry, 2000).

Simple or easily applied reinforcement schedules may be more feasible than the comparatively complex and/or intensive CM interventions applied over a comparatively brief time period that are typical of published clinical trials. In practice settings, even simple CM interventions still require considerable staff training, and more intensive short-term efforts might have to be performed by specially trained behavioral therapy consultants. Ideally, the simpler strategies could be used throughout the course of medication treatment.

An example of a simple and treatment-compatible CM intervention piloted by our group involves providing participants with a cell phone contingent upon their also using the phone to participate in phone-based counseling around medication compliance. Among the eight participants, average compliance was approximately 10% higher after beginning the counseling. The benefits of the counseling were also suggested by numerically higher adherence on days counselors called than on comparison, noncounseled days.

The use of computer technology shows great promise for facilitating the general strategy of developing simple, user-friendly compliance en hancement methods. One computer-delivered CM intervention that showed preliminary evidence of efficacy involved reinforcing smokers for daily abstinence. Abstinence was verified by carbon monoxide readings that were e-mailed to a web server (Dallery et al., 2004). Even complex reinforcement schedules can be programmed to calculate the amount of rewards for target behaviors and to even provide automatic feedback to patients when the behavior is performed (Marsch & Bickel, 2004).

Our use of cellular telephones to foster compliance with the antiretroviral treatment described earlier might be less expensive if automated prompts were provided to each patient and delivered remotely through pagers or telephones. While the initial costs of developing automated CM programs are likely to be high, substantial savings will accrue from greater consistency in treatment delivery and time savings for ongoing treatment delivery.

Enhance Durability of Effect: Strategies to Increase Intrinsic Motivation for Treatment

Long-term compliance with prescribed treatments requires either continued application of incentives or the development of intrinsic motivation to continue medication taking. In substance-abusing samples, posttreatment CM effects on abstinence have generally been shown to drop off substantially in the small number of studies in which treatment durability has been addressed (Higgins, Wong, Badger, Haug-Ogden, & Dantona, 2000; Rawson et al., 2002) and a lack of sustained benefits was also seen when CM was applied to antiretroviral adherence (Rosen, 2005; Sorensen et al., 2004). Given the need for extended medication compliance for applications we have reviewed, this is the most important weakness for future research to address. Next, we briefly outline several general approaches.

First, we must increase attention to the beneficial effects of medication compliance. All the medications targeted for compliance enhancement are intended to benefit the patient, although the effects tend to be delayed, subtle, or mixed. A comparatively simple strategy to enhance the salience of these benefits would utilize clear feedback on progress toward treatment goals. For example, charting of successive test results (e.g., Hamilton Depression Inventory scores [Hamilton, 1960] and viral loads) may provide tangible reminders that treatment is helping. For medications that eliminate illicit drug use such as naltrexone for opioids, gradually increasing benefits of sustained abstinence are often apparent with each successive week. Providing formal ratings of these changes to the patient and/or significant others may increase the motivation to sustain recovery.

Second, we must manage the transition away from CM. The most straightforward approach to manage the cessation of incentive delivery is to develop a tapering scheme that utilizes basic behavior strategies that foster sustained behavior. These include transitioning from fixed-ratio schedules to intermittent or variable-ratio reinforcement schedules (Crowley, 1999). A second general approach entails attempting to shift the type of incentive for medication compliance away from artificial and costly extrinsic rewards provided by the treater (e.g., prizes) to incentives that can be delivered outside the treatment setting, such as receiving praise or support from family members. A third general strategy entails broadening the types of target behaviors that will result in delivering contingent rewards. Clearly, medication compliance is a single behavior in the complex repertoire of behaviors that foster recovery, including the use of skills to avoid drug exposure and the development of rewarding behaviors that substitute for incentives provided by drug use. Hence, in addition to or as a substitute for providing incentives for pill taking, clinicians may incentivize other behaviors that may have a more enduring impact on substance use such as attendance at substance abuse treatment, providing negative urine specimens, completing homework assignments in CBT (Carroll, Nich, & Ball, 2005), meeting short-term treatment goals (Iguchi, Belding, Morral, Lamb, & Husband, 1997), or engaging in rewarding social activities (Petry et al., 2006). Timing of interventions is a key issue in bringing about the shift from therapist-delivered tangible incentives for narrowly targeted medication compliance to naturally occurring rewards for a broad range of recovery behaviors. Such a transition entails moving from a discrete, easily identified target behavior with comparatively simple rewards to complex behaviors and less tangible rewards. Hence, a period of combined reinforcement schedules is likely to be needed to facilitate a smooth withdrawal of tangible incentives for medication compliance. This combined treatment may be provided from the start of treatment or in conjunction with the process of tapering away from more narrowly defined CM for medication compliance enhancement.

CONCLUDING COMMENTS

In substance abusers, medication compliance enhancement would appear to be an ideal application for CM treatments. Despite this, the literature on CM to enhance medication compliance in substance abusers is rather sparse. The existing literature demonstrates CM's short-term efficacy in enhancing compliance with medications that reduce drug use, medications for HIV treatment and anti-TB antibiotics. More widespread application of CM with drug abusers is impeded by costs, the need for extensive training, and limited evidence for enduring effects. Future treatment development of CM for medication compliance needs to counter these issues by focusing on CM applications with large potential benefit, developing simple or automated methods for CM delivery, and placing greater emphasis on the process of transitioning away from formal CM treatment.

ACKNOWLEDGMENTS

This work was supported by National Institute on Drug Abuse Grant Nos. P50-DA09241, K05-DA00089 (to Bruce J. Rounsaville), K05-DA00457 (to Kathleen M. Carroll) and K02-DA017277 (to Marc Rosen) and by the U.S. Veterans Health Administration New England Mental Illness Research, Education and Clinical Center.

REFERENCES

Ammassari, A., Antinori, A., Cozzi-Lepri, A., Trotta, M.P., Nasti, G., Ridolfo, A. L., et al. (2002). Relationship between HAART adherence and adipose tissue alterations. *Journal of Acquired Immune Deficiency Syndromes, 31*(Suppl. 3), S140–S144.

Anthony, J. C., Warner, L. A., & Kessler, R. C. (1994). Comparative epidemiology of dependence on tobacco, alcohol, controlled substances and inhalants. Basic findings from the National Comorbidity Study. *Experimental and Clinical Psychopharmacology, 2,* 244–268.

Anton, R. F., Hogan, I., Jalali, B., Riordan, C. E., & Kleber, H. D. (1981). Multiple family therapy and naltrexone in the treatment of opioid dependence. *Drug and Alcohol Dependence, 8,* 157–168.

Batki, S. L., Gruber, V. A., Bradley, J. M., Bradley, M., & Delucchi, K. L. (2002). A controlled trial of methadone treatment combined with directly observed isoniazid for tuberculosis prevention in injection drug users. *Drug and Alcohol Dependence, 66*(3), 283–293.

Bickel, W. K., Ruzzuto, P., Zielony, R. D., Klobas, J., Pangiosonlis, P., Mernit, R., et al. (1988). Combined behavioral and pharmacological treatment of alcoholic methadone patients. *Journal of Substance Abuse, 1*(2), 161–171.

Bigelow, G., Strickler, D., Liebson, I., & Griffiths, R. (1976). Maintaining disulfiram ingestion among outpatient alcoholics: A security-deposit contingency contracting procedure. *Behavior Research Therapy, 14,* 378–381.

Bouhnik, A. D., Chesney, M., Carrieri, P., Gallais, H., Moreau, J., Moatti, J. P., et al. (2002). Nonadherence among HIV-infected injecting drug users: The impact of social instability. *Journal of Acquired Immune Deficiency Syndromes, 31*(Suppl. 3), S149–S153.

Bozzette, S. A., Joyce, G., McCaffrey, D. F., Leibowitz, A. A., Morton, S. C., Berry, S. H., et al. (2001). Expenditures for the care of HIV-infected patients in the era of highly active antiretroviral therapy [see comment]. *New England Journal of Medicine, 344*(11), 817–823.

Brady, K. T., & Sinha, R. (2005). Co-occuring mental and substance use disorders: The neurobiological effects of chronic stress. *American Journal of Psychiatry, 162*(8), 1483–1493.

Budney, A. J., & Higgins, S. T. (1998). A community reinforcement plus vouchers approach: Treating cocaine addiction. *NIDA Therapy Manuals for Drug Addiction* (NIH Publication No. 98-4309).

Carroll, K. M., Ball, S. A., Nich, C., O'Connor, P. G., Eagan, D., Frankforter, T. L., et al. (2001). Targeting behavioral therapies to enhance naltrexone treatment of opioid dependence: Efficacy of contingency management and significant other involvement. *Archives of General Psychiatry, 58,* 755–761.

Carroll, K. M., Nich, C., & Ball, S. A. (2005). Practice makes progress: Homework completion as a mediator of skills acquisition and outcome of cognitive behavioral therapy for cocaine dependence. *Journal of Consulting and Clinical Psychology, 73*(4), 749–755.

Carroll, K. M., Sinha, R., Nich, C., Babuscio, T., & Rounsaville, B. J. (2002). Contingency management to enhance naltrexone treatment of opioid dependence: A randomized clinical trial of reinforcement magnitude. *Experimental and Clinical Psychopharmacology, 10,* 54–63.

Chaisson, R. E., Barnes, G. L., Hackman, J., Watkinson, L., Kimbrough, L., Metha, S., et al. (2001). A randomized controlled trial of interventions to improve adherence to isoniazid therapy to prevent tuberculosis in injection drug users. *American Journal of Medicine, 110*(8), 610–615.

Chick, J., Gough, K., Falkowski, W., Kershaw, P., Hore, B., Mehta, B., et al. (1992). Disulfiram treatment of alcoholism. *British Journal of Psychiatry, 161*, 84–89.

Compton, W. M., Thomas, Y. F., Conway, K. P., & Colliver, J. D. (2005). Developments in the epidemiology of drug use and drug use disorders. *American Journal of Psychiatry, 162*(8), 1494–1502.

Cornish, J. W., Metzger, D., Woody, G. E., Wilson, D., McLellan, A. T., Vandergrift, B., et al. (1997). Naltrexone pharmacotherapy for opioid dependent federal probationers. *Journal of Substance Abuse Treatment, 14*, 529–534.

Cramer, J. A., & Rosenheck, R. (1998). Compliance with medication regimens for mental and physical disorders [see comment]. *Psychiatric Services, 49*(2), 196–201.

Crowley, T. J. (1999). Research on contingency management treatment of drug dependence: Clinical implications and future directions. In S. T. Higgins & K. Silverman (Eds.), *Motivating behavior change among illicit drug abusers* (pp. 345–370). Washington, DC: American Psychological Association.

Dallery, J., Manders, I. G. T., Silverman, K., Branch, M., Locey, M., Raiff, B. (2004). *An Internet-based voucher program for smoking abstinence.* Paper presented at the College on the Problems of Drug Dependence, San Juan, Puerto Rico.

Deci, F. L., Koestner, R., & Ryan, R. M. (1999). A meta-analytic review of experiments examining the effects of extrinsic rewards on intrinsic motivation. *Psychological Bulletin, 128*, 627–668.

Dixon, L., Haas, G., Weiden, P. J., Sweeney, J., & Frances, A. K. (1991). Drug abuse in schizophrenic patients: Clinical correlates and reasons for use. *American Journal of Psychiatry, 148*, 224–230.

D'Onofrio, G., Pantalon, M. V., Degutis, L. C., Fiellin, D. A., & O'Connor, P. G. (2005). Development and implementation of an emergency practitioner-performed brief intervention for harmful and hazardous drinkers in the emergency department. *Academic Emergency Medicine, 12*(3), 249–256.

Drake, R. E., & Brunette, M. F. (1998). Complications of severe mental illness related to alcohol and drug use disorders. *Recent Developments in Alcoholism, 14*, 285–299.

Drake, R. E., Essock, S. M., Shaner, A., Carey, K. B., Minkoff, K., Kola, L., et al. (2001). Implementing dual diagnosis services for clients with severe mental illness. *Psychiatric Services, 52*, 469–476.

Elk, R., Grabowski, J., Rhoades, H. M., Spiga, R., Schmitz, J. M., & Jennings, W. (1993). Compliance with tuberculosis treatment in methadone-maintained patients: Behavioral interventions. *Journal of Substance Abuse Treatment, 10*(4), 371–382.

Fals-Stewart, W., & O'Farrell, T. J. (2003). Behavioral family counseling and naltrexone for male opioid-dependent patients. *Journal of Consulting and Clinical Psychology, 71*, 432–442.

Fuller, R. K., Branchey, L., Brightwell, D. R., Derman, R. M., Emrick, C. D., Iber, F. L., et al. (1986). Disulfiram treatment of alcoholism: A Veterans Administration cooperative study. *Journal of the American Medical Association, 256*, 1449–1455.

Grabowski, J., O'Brien, C. P., Greenstein, R. A., Long, M., Steinberg-Donato, S., & Ternes, J. (1979). Effects of contingent payments on compliance with a naltrexone regimen. *American Journal of Drug and Alcohol Abuse, 6*, 355–365.

Hamilton, M. (1960). A rating scale for depression. *Journal of Neurology, Neurosurgery and Psychiatry, 23*, 56–62.

Haynes, R. B., McDonald, H. P., & Garg, A. X. (2002). Helping patients follow prescribed treatment: Clinical applications. *Journal of the American Medical Association, 288*(22), 2880–2883.

Haynes, R. B., McDonald, H. P., Garg, A. X., & Montague, P. (2000). Interventions for helping patients to follow prescriptions for medications. *Cochrane Database Systematic Review, 2,* CD000011.

Haynes, R. B., Taylor, D. W., & Sackett, D. L. (1979). *Compliance in health care.* Baltimore: Johns Hopkins University Press.

Higgins, S. T., Budney, A. J., Bickel, W. K., Hughes, J. R., & Foerg, F. (1993). Disulfiram therapy in patients abusing cocaine and alcohol. *American Journal of Psychiatry, 150,* 675–676.

Higgins, S. T., Delany, D. D., Budney, A. J., Bickel, W. K., Hughes, J. R., Foerg, F., et al. (1991). A behavioral approach to achieving initial cocaine abstinence. *American Journal of Psychiatry, 148,* 1218–1224.

Higgins, S. T., Wong, C. J., Badger, G. J., Haug-Ogden, D. E., & Dantona, R. L. (2000). Contingent reinforcement increases cocaine abstinence during outpatient treatment and one year follow-up. *Journal of Consulting and Clinical Psychology, 68,* 64–72.

Horwitz, R. I., & Horwitz, S. M. (1993). Adherence to treatment and health outcomes. *Archives of Internal Medicine, 153,* 1863–1869.

Ickovics, J. R., & Meade, C. S. (2002). Adherence to antiretroviral therapy among patients with HIV: A critical link between behavioral and biomedical sciences. *Journal of Acquired Immune Deficiency Syndromes, 31*(Suppl. 3), S98–S102.

Iguchi, M. Y., Belding, M. A., Morral, A. R., Lamb, R. J., & Husband, S. D. (1997). Reinforcing operants other than abstinence in drug abuse treatment: An effective alternative for reducing drug use. *Journal of Consulting and Clinical Psychology, 65,* 421–428.

Kessler, R. C., Crum, R. M., Warner, L. A., Nelson, C. B., Schulenberg, J., & Anthony, J. C. (1997). Lifetime co-occurrence of DSM-III-R alcohol abuse and dependence with other psychiatric disorders in the National Comorbidity Study. *Archives of General Psychiatry, 54,* 313–321.

Kleber, H. D., Weissman, M. M., Rounsaville, B. J., Wilber, C. H., Prusoff, B. A., & Riordan, C. E. (1983). Imipramine as treatment for depression in addicts. *Archives of General Psychiatry, 40*(6), 649–653.

Klinkenberg, W. D., Sacks, S., & HIV/AIDS Treatment Adherence Health Outcomes and Cost Study Group. (2004). Mental disorders and drug abuse in persons living with HIV/AIDS. *AIDS Care, 16*(Suppl. 1), S22–S42.

Kosten, T. R., Rosen, M. I., Bond, I., Settles, M., Roberts, J. S., Shields, J., et al. (2002). Human therapeutic cocaine vaccine: Safety and immunogenicity. *Vaccine, 20,* 1196–1204.

Liebson, I. A., Tommasello, A., & Bigelow, G. E. (1978). A behavioral treatment of alcoholic methadone patients. *Annals of Internal Medicine, 89,* 342–344.

Malotte, C. K., Hollingshead, J. R., & Rhodes, F. (1999). Monetary versus nonmonetary incentives for TB skin test reading among drug users. *American Journal of Preventive Medicine, 16*(3), 182–188.

Marsch, L. A., & Bickel, W. K. (2004). Efficacy of computer-based HIV/AIDS education for injection drug users. *American Journal of Health Behaviors, 28*(4), 316–327.

Meichenbaum, D. H., & Turk, D. C. (Eds.). (1987). *Facilitating treatment adherence.* New York: Plenum Press.

Meyer, R. E., Mirin, S. M., Altman, J. L., & McNamee, H. B. (1976). A behavioral paradigm for the evaluation of narcotic antagonists. *Archives of General Psychiatry, 33,* 371–377.

Miller, W. R. (1985). Motivation for treatment: A review with special emphasis on alcoholism. *Psychological Bulletin, 98*(1), 84–107.

Miller, W. R., & Rollnick, S. (2002). *Motivational interviewing: Preparing people for change* (2nd ed.). New York: Guilford Press.

Nunes, E. V., Quitkin, F. M., Donovan, S. J., Deliyannides, D., Ocepek-Welikson, K., Koenig, T., et al. (1998). Imipramine treatment of opiate-dependent patients with depressive disorders: A placebo-controlled trial. *Archives of General Psychiatry, 55*, 153–160.

O'Brien, C. P. (1997). A range of research-based pharmacotherapies for addiction. *Science, 278*, 66–70.

O'Connor, P. G., & Samet, J. H. (2002). Substance abuse: The expanding role of general internal medicine. *Journal of General Internal Medicine, 17*, 398–399.

O'Connor, P. G., Selwyn, P. A., & Schottenfeld, R. S. (1994). Medical care for injection-drug users with human immunodeficiency virus infection. *New England Journal of Medicine, 331*(7), 450–459.

O'Farrell, T. J., Cutter, H. S., Choquette, K. A., & Floyd, F. J. (1992). Behavioral marital therapy for male alcoholics: Marital and drinking adjustment during two years after treatment. *Behavior Therapy, 23*, 529–549.

O'Farrell, T. J., & Litten, R. Z. (1992). Techniques to enhance compliance with disulfiram. *Alcohol: Clinical and Experimental Research, 16*, 1035–1041.

Palella, F. J., Jr., Delaney, K. M., Moorman, A. C., Loveless, M. O., Fuhrer, J., Satten, G. A., et al. (1998). Declining morbidity and mortality among patients with advanced human immunodeficiency virus infection. *New England Journal of Medicine, 338*(13), 853–860.

Paterson, D. L., Swindells, S., Mohr, J., Brester, M., Vergis, E. N., Squier, C., et al. (2000). Adherence to protease inhibitor therapy and outcomes in patients with HIV infection. *Annals of Internal Medicine, 133*(1), 21–30.

Perlman, D. C., Salomon, N., Perkins, M. P., Yancovitz, S., Paone, D., & DesJarlais, D. C. (1995). Tuberculosis in drug users. *Clinics in Infectious Disease, 21*(5), 1253–1264.

Perno, C. F., Ceccherini-Silberstein, F., De Luca, A., Cozzi-Lepri, A., Gori, C., Cingolani, A., et al. (2002). Virologic correlates of adherence to antiretroviral medications and therapeutic failure. *Journal of Acquired Immune Deficiency Syndromes, 31*(Suppl. 3), S118–S122.

Petrakis, I., Carroll, K. M., Nich, C., Gordon, L., Kosten, T., & Rounsaville, B. (1998). Fluoxetine treatment of depressive disorders in methadone-maintained opioid addicts. *Drug and Alcohol Dependence, 50*(3), 221–226.

Petry, N. M. (2000). A comprehensive guide to the application of contigency management procedures in clinical settings. *Drug and Alcohol Dependence, 58*, 9–25.

Petry, N. M., Alessi, S. M., Carroll, K. M., Hanson, T., MacKinnon, S., Rounsaville, B., et al. (2006). Contingency management treatments: Reinforcing abstinence versus adherence with goal-related activities. *Journal of Consulting and Clinical Psychology, 74*, 592–601.

Petry, N. M., Martin, B., Cooney, J. L., & Kranzler, H. R. (2000). Give them prizes and they will come: Contingency management treatment of alcohol dependence. *Journal of Consulting and Clinical Psychology, 68*, 250–257.

Preston, K. L., Silverman, K., Umbricht, A., DeJesus, A., Montoya, I. D., & Schuster, C. R. (1999). Improvement in naltrexone treatment compliance with contingency management. *Drug and Alcohol Dependence, 54*, 127–135.

Rawson, R. A., Huber, A., McCann, M. J., Shoptaw, S., Farabee, D., Reiber, C., et al. (2002). A comparison of contingency management and cognitive-behavioral approaches during methadone maintenance for cocaine dependence. *Archives of General Psychiatry, 59*, 817–824.

Rigsby, M. O., Rosen, M. I., Beauvais, J., Cramer, J. A., Rainey, P. M., O'Malley, S. S., et al. (2000). Cue dose training with monetary reinforcement: Pilot study of an antiretroviral adherence intervention. *Journal of General Internal Medicine, 15*, 841–847.

Robichaud, C., Strickler, D., Bigelow, G., & Liebson, I. (1979). Disulfiram maintenance employee alcoholism treatment: A three-phase evaluation. *Behaviour Research Therapy, 17*, 618–621.

Rosen, M. I. (2005). *Use of electronic monitoring to improve adherence to prescribed medications among drug-using patients.* Paper presented at the College on the Problems of Drug Dependence, Orlando, FL.

Rosen, M. I., Ryan, C., & Rigsby, M. (2002). Motivational enhancement and MEMS review to improve medication adherence. *Behaviour Change, 19*(4), 183–190.

Roter, D. L., Hall, J. A., Merisca, R., Nordstrom, B., Cretin, D., & Svarstad, B. (1998). Effectiveness of interventions to improve patient compliance: A meta-analysis. *Medical Care, 36*(8), 1138–1161.

Rounsaville, B. J., Dolinsky, Z. S., Babor, T. F., & Meyer, R. E. (1987). Psychopathology as a predictor of treatment outcome in alcoholics. *Archives of General Psychiatry, 44*, 505–513.

Rounsaville, B. J., Kosten, T. R., Weissman, M. M., & Kleber, H. D. (1986). Prognostic significance of psychopathology in treated opiate addicts. *Archives of General Psychiatry, 43*, 739–745.

Sackett, D. L., & Snow, J. C. (1979). The magnitude of compliance and noncompliance. In R. B. Haynes, D. W. Taylor, & D. L. Sackett (Eds.), *Compliance in health care* (pp. 423–435). Baltimore: Johns Hopkins University Press.

Schackman, B. R., Goldie, S. J., Weinstein, M. C., Losina, E., Zhang, H., & Freedberg, K. A. (2001). Cost-effectiveness of earlier initiation of antiretroviral therapy for uninsured HIV-infected adults. *American Journal of Public Health, 91*(9), 1456–1463.

Sorensen, J. L., Haug, N., Delucchi, K., Gruber, V., Tulsky, J., & Hall, S. M. (2004). *Voucher reinforcement trial to improve methadone treatment for injection drug users with HIV infection.* Paper presented at the College on the Problems of Drug Dependence, San Juan, Puerto Rico.

Stitzer, M. L., Bickel, W. K., Bigelow, G. E., & Liebson, I. A. (1986). Effect of methadone dose contingencies on urinalysis test results of polydrug abusing methadone maintenance patients. *Drug and Alcohol Dependence, 18*, 341–348.

Stitzer, M. L., Iguchi, M. Y., & Felch, L. J. (1992). Contingent take-home incentives: Effects on drug use of methadone maintenance patients. *Journal of Consulting and Clinical Psychology, 60*, 927–934.

Titievsky, J., Seco, G., Barranco, M., & Kyle, E. M. (1982). Doxepin as adjunctive therapy for depressed methadone maintenance patients: A double-blind study. *Journal of Clinical Psychiatry, 43*(11), 454–456.

Udall, K. K., Palmer, N. B., Whetten, K., Mellins, C., & HIV/AIDS Treatment Adherence Health Outcomes and Cost Study Group. (2004). Adherence in people living with HIV/AIDS, mental illness, and chemical dependency: A review of the literature. *AIDS Care, 16*(Suppl. 1), S71–S96.

Vanhove, G. F., Schapiro, J. M., Winters, M. A., Merigan, T. C., & Blaschke, T. F. (1996). Patient compliance and drug failure in protease inhibitor monotherapy. *Journal of the American Medical Association, 276*(24), 1955–1956.

Volpicelli, J. R., Rhines, K. C., Rhines, J. S., Volpicelli, L. A., Alterman, A. I., & O'Brien, C. P. (1997). Naltrexone and alcohol dependence: Role of subject compliance. *Archives of General Psychiatry, 54*(8), 737–742.

Wadland, W. C., & Ferenchick, G. S. (2004). Medical comorbidity in addictive disorders. *Psychiatric Clinics of North America, 27*(4), 675–687.

Weiss, R. D. (2004). Adherence to pharmacotherapy in patients with alcohol and opioid dependence. *Addiction, 99*(11), 1382–1392.

Woody, G. E., O'Brien, C. P., McLellan, A. T., Marcovici, M., & Evans, B. D. (1982). The use of antidepressants with methadone in depressed maintenance patients. *Annals of the New York Academy of Sciences, 398*, 120–127.

Woody, G. E., O'Brien, C. P., & Rickels, K. (1975). Depression and anxiety in heroin addicts: A placebo-controlled study of doxepin in combination with methadone. *American Journal of Psychiatry, 132*(4), 447–450.

PART II

SPECIAL POPULATIONS

CHAPTER 9

HOMELESS POPULATIONS

Jesse B. Milby *and* Joseph Schumacher

This chapter uses a research-supported intervention for cocaine-dependent homeless persons to illustrate how to use contingency management (CM) effectively to treat this population. A review of clinical trials on which the intervention is based provides evidence for its effectiveness and identifies components that yield robust effects on reduced drug use, improved homelessness, and employment. The chapter also describes typical services for this vulnerable population. The changing nature of U.S. homelessness and comparisons with world homelessness provide a global view of homelessness. The salient role of substance abuse in homelessness is described in the context of research elucidating its unique morbidity and mortality. Limitations of the recommended intervention are discussed and challenges for future research are identified. Finally, we address ethical concerns for the use of contingency-managed housing (CMH) and the sensitivity of providers who serve the homeless.

HOMELESSNESS IN PERSPECTIVE

Before the rise in homelessness in the United States starting in the 1980s, substance abuse has always been prevalent among marginally housed persons who lived on the skid rows and flophouses of our cities. But, the homeless in previous decades usually had stable shelter arrangements in skid row hotels. Few spent nights on the streets. However, since the 1980s many homeless are literally without shelter (Burt, 1992). Since then, shelter and health care providers reported higher levels of substance abuse, and more literal homelessness. But, estimating the prevalence of homelessness from service providers' data is fraught with difficulties. Case identification, co-occurrence with mental disorders, lack of scientific sampling, and the overall rigor of scientific methodology vary greatly (Fischer & Breakey, 1991). Assuming these concerns are valid, findings generally show that homeless people usually live in extreme poverty, with poor access to health care. They tend to underutilize public entitlements and benefits, and single persons, especially males, are found to be isolated from existing family, friends, or other social supports.

HOMELESSNESS PREVALENCE IN THE UNITED STATES

A population-based survey of homeless prevalence in the United States, using the 1990 census, suggests there were about 500,000–650,000 homeless persons at any time in the United States during the early 1990s (Link et al., 1994). Another census-based study estimates homelessness affected 3.5–6% of Americans during their lifetime, with prevalence estimated at 1% of the general population, and about 6.3% of those living in poverty (Burt & Aron, 2001; Burt et al., 1999). In 1998, the U.S. Conference of Mayors reported that in 1994 there were between 4.95 and 9.32 million persons homeless in the United States (Martens, 2001–2002). Families with children comprised 37%, the fastest-growing segment.

HOMELESS PREVALENCE IN THE UNITED STATES COMPARED TO WESTERN EUROPE

Lack of general agreement on international prevalence also stems from the absence of a unified definition of homelessness and dissimilar estimating methods (Fischer & Breakey, 1991; Martens, 2001–2002). However, homelessness is pervasive across the world. Expected in developing countries and those torn by political strife, ethnic conflicts, famine, earthquakes, and floods, homelessness is still surprisingly prevalent in richer countries. A relatively recent population-based survey suggests that prevalence in the United States may be several times greater than in Germany (Tompsett et al., 2003). Singer (2003) alleges current U.S. homelessness is two to five times greater than in Western Europe. But in the United States and Western Europe, homelessness may have more to do with poor employment skills, lack of available low-cost housing for the poor, and social disaffiliation from family and other social support.

ETIOLOGY OF HOMELESSNESS: RISK FACTORS

In our reading of the literature on the causes of homelessness several factors emerge repeatedly. They include serious mental illness, unavailability of low-cost housing, reduction of public benefits, a declining local economy with increased unemployment, lack of social affiliation and social support, and substance abuse (Burt, 1992; Folsom et al., 2005; Koegel, Burnam, & Farr, 1988a, 1988b; O'Flaherty, 1996; Reardon, Burns, Preist, Sachs-Ericsson, & Lang, 2003; Rosenheck & Koegel, 1993). A recent study of risk factors for homelessness in a cohort of 10,340 being treated for schizophrenia, bipolar disorder, or major depression in San Diego County's public mental health services in 1999–2000, showed that 15% were homeless. Homelessness was associated with male gender, African American ethnicity, lack of Medicaid, and substance use disorder (Folsom et al., 2005). Rosenheck (1994) and colleagues studied a large cohort of homeless veterans in multiple programs. Many factors contributed to homelessness, but the presence of a substance abuse disorder was one of the common paths to homelessness and accounted for a large proportion of the variance in predicted homelessness (Rosenheck, 1994). For a different view which eschews causal roles of serious mental illness and substance abuse and looks to economic factors to explain the recent increase of homelessness, see O'Flaherty (1996). He attributes its sharp rise since the 1980s to economic changes, especially the decline of available low-cost housing in America's urban areas.

CHANGING DEMOGRAPHICS AMONG THE HOMELESS

Characteristics of the homeless population have been changing (Burt, 1992; Burt & Aron, 2001; U.S. Conference of Mayors, 1998). In Birmingham, between 1986 and the early 1990s, the prevalence of homelessness, and who was affected, dramatically shifted. In the late 1980s, homelessness was most prominent among Caucasian men with alcohol dependence. In less than 5 years it shifted to greater prevalence among crack-cocaine-dependent African Americans, with a substantial increase in homeless women and children (Raczynski et al., 1993; Ritchey, La Gory, Fitzpatrick, & Mullis, 1990). Prevalence studies across three decades in St. Louis show similar shifts. Mood and substance use disorders dramatically increased, as did the frequency of minority homelessness (North, Eyrich, Pollio, & Spitznagel, 2004).

HEALTH RISKS AMONG THE HOMELESS

Risks to general health among the homeless are associated with some uniquely high health vulnerabilities with increasing morbidity and mortality. In spite of the increased prevalence of multiple diseases, most of them are eminently treatable and should not be fatal. However, homeless persons experience restricted access to health care. One study described shelter staffs trying to gain access to care for clients within a system designed to keep them out (Hatton, Kleffel, Bennett, & Gaffrey, 2001). Many morbidities and substantial mortality among homeless persons are due to increased risks associated with substance abuse and dependence. Along with substance use disorders, homeless persons are more likely to have a history of incarceration which adds to their social isolation and exposure to infectious disease (Haddad, Wilson, Ijaz, Marks, & Moore, 2005; Kushel, Hahn, Evans, Bangsberg, & Moss, 2005).

Respiratory diseases, especially bronchitis, asthma and tuberculosis (TB), are prominent among the homeless (Plumb, 1997). Of 185,870 cases of TB reported in the National TB Surveillance System from all states and the District of Columbia in 1994–2003, 11,369 were among homeless persons. Compared to the nonhomeless, homeless persons with TB had a higher prevalence of substance abuse. In addition, TB among homeless persons was more likely to be infectious, and 34% had co-infection with HIV (human immunodeficiency virus) (Haddad et al., 2005). TB is also prominent, especially among those incarcerated (Zolopa et al., 1994). Sexually transmitted disease rates are elevated among homeless persons but are even higher among those who are incarcerated, as are rates of HIV/AIDS and hepatitis A and C (Riley, Bangsberg, Guzman, Perry, & Moss, 2005). A recent study of homeless, seriously mentally ill with co-occurring substance abuse, used serological testing to assess prevalence of HIV and hepatitis B and C. Pretreatment, 11 of 172 participants were HIV positive, 37 of 114 who volunteered for hepatitis testing evidenced prior exposure to hepatitis B, and 34 evidenced exposure to hepatitis C. Those with reactive tests to hepatitis B or C (44%) were much more likely to be substance abusers, especially those with a history of injection use (Klinkenberg et al., 2003). However, those who are HIV infected but able to sustain antiretroviral therapy may have a lower risk of death than those whose instability does not allow sustained antiretroviral therapy (Riley et al., 2005).

A significant proportion of homeless persons have serious mental illness (SMI). In spite of their eligibility for housing, medical, social and mental health services, they tend to move from one shelter or marginal housing situation to another, swelling the ranks of the chronically homeless (Acosta & Toro, 2000; Folsom et al., 2005; Reardon et al., 2003). Homeless persons with SMI and alcohol abuse or dependence appear to have increased at least 500% between 1980 and 1987. Access to social security income and social security disability income was cut during this period, and the value of these benefits and federal general assistance decreased for those who qualified for them (Burt, 1992).

SUBSTANCE ABUSE RISK AMONG THE HOMELESS

Estimates for the prevalence of substance abuse disorders among the home-less range widely. A recent review found estimates ranging between 20 and 75% (Martens, 2001–2002). Estimates vary depending on the source of case identification and epoch. However, most reports range between 30 and 65%, and they tend to be higher if the study's focus is alcohol dependence and lower if it is dependence on other illicit drugs (Corrigan & Anderson, 1984; Gelberg, Linn, & Leake, 1988; Koegel et al., 1988a, 1988b). The prevalence of substance abuse disorders among men exceeds that for women. For example, Geissler, Borman, Kwiatkowski, Brancht, and Reichardt (1995) studied 323 homeless persons and found 71% of the men and 33% of the women reported problems with drugs, with crack cocaine the pri-mary abused drug.

Though more homelessness is found among those living in poverty, presence of a substance use disorder adds additional risk for becoming homeless. Toro et al. (1995) randomly sampled currently homeless, previously homeless, and never homeless poor. They found the currently homeless almost twice as likely to have a lifetime substance abuse disorder as the never homeless. When lower-income women were compared for the prevalence of drug dependence and other mental disorders, Bassuk and Weinreb (1996) found more of both among homeless women than among housed women.

INTERVENTIONS FOR HOMELESS SUBSTANCE ABUSERS

Health services for the homeless vary greatly across states. Many homeless services are publicly supported; thus local benefits and entitlements add variation to federal and state support. States or cities with a larger commit-ment to homeless persons tend to have more comprehensive and expensive services available. But coordination is a challenge for service providers. The most common intervention for substance-abusing homeless is intensive case management. One case manager, usually trained in social work, coordi-nates and seeks access to services for a small number of homeless persons. Where managers have small caseloads, coordinated interventions vary widely and can include health promotion and prevention; medical, dental, and surgical consultation; and treatment. Substance abuse services typically include inpatient detoxification, day treatment, and substance abuse medi-cations. Assistance with job finding, vocational evaluation and retraining, and remedial education and access to GED (general equivalency diploma) testing can be important. Referrals for legal aid, intervention with proba-tion and parole officers, and child and family services for women can be strategic in recovery. The needs of individual homeless persons can be daunting, especially for managers with large caseloads and poor access to services. It would seem that interventions that combine services would be most effective, like residential care and therapeutic communities. However, there are very few controlled intervention studies for homeless substance abusers, and those that have been conducted are not very encouraging. Conrad, Hultman, and Lyons (1993) reviewed 14 controlled studies which shared the same outcome assessment battery. Several interventions were studied in randomized controlled trials which compared an enhanced intervention with extant usual case (UC). Less rigorous studies assessed residential therapeutic community, intensive case management, day treatment, and shelter-based case management. Only the early version of contingency-managed behavioral day treatment (CMBDT) showed robust 6-month abstinence outcomes for drug and alcohol use (Milby et al., 1996). For 2 months CMBDT provided daily transport to and from treatment and a noon meal each day, and it utilized a combination of individual and group counseling and multiple psychoeducation groups in the context of random urine testing. Four months of aftercare provided vocational training, paid work experiences, CMH, transportation, and noon meals. At 6 months, abstinence for cocaine- and alcohol-dependent subjects averaged over 50% (Milby et al., 1996). This intervention led to a series of enhancement and dismantling studies that improved retention and abstinence and is reviewed in the following section.

CMBDT INTERVENTIONS

Adapted from the Birmingham VAMC Day Hospital, Milby et al. (199 developed a behavioral intervention which combined interventions for substance abuse and homelessness (Raczynski et al., 1993). It included transportation, noon meals, work, and housing. This CMBDT used three phases of treatment. Phase I (months 1–2) provided behavioral day treatment (BDT) + CMH; Phase II (months 3–6) provided aftercare, contingency-managed work therapy (CMWT), and CMH for modest rent; and Phase 3 (months 7–12) provided continued aftercare. As research evolved, BDT was enhanced by the use of therapeutic goals management (TGM). Computer training and Job Club were added to CMWT in our current study. CMBDT interventions were continuously developed, including practical details on implementation of interest to clinicians or policymakers who might wish to adopt them. They are described below. Manuals can be obtained from the authors.

BDT with TGM

BDT is a Phase I multidimensional psychosocial intervention targeting drug and alcohol abuse and dependency. It utilizes group and individual counseling and didactic approaches to recovery skills learning. BDT lasts 2 months, 5 days a week, and approximately 5 hours per day. In Phase II, less intensive aftercare sessions are provided weekly for 4 months. Structured programs, some evidenced based, are offered in relapse prevention, a 12-Step model, cocaine education, cognitive-behavioral therapy components, recreational therapy, and HIV prevention. Treatment is delivered by master's-degree-trained counselors. Transportation and lunch are provided. Throughout both phases, via individual goal formulation, review and treatment goal attainment reinforced with vouchers, and regularly scheduled recreational activities, the intervention emphasizes continuous exposure to, and reinforcement provided by, wholesome non-drug-related social/recreational activities. These activities are used to counter the reinforcing effects of cocaine use and to establish multiple competing sources of non-drug-related social/recreational activities.

TGM is the development, monitoring, and reinforcement of objectively defined individualized goals during BDT. TGM is designed to reduce hazardous alcohol and other drug use and negative consequences associated with such use and to enhance functioning in major life areas. TGM elicits and negotiates, rather than assigns, individualized measurable goals, typically in five life areas: substance abuse, housing, employment, non-drug-related social/recreation activities, and mental health and behavioral problems. Where needed, physical health goals, including HIV/AIDS treatment compliance, are added. Initial goal development is based on a behavioral assessment and conducted by a trained psychologist. The initial TGM plan tends to jump-start treatment by helping clients take small steps toward goals that previously were perceived as overwhelming and unattainable. The TGM plan is reviewed weekly by counselors and peers in a goal-review group to assess goal progress and provide reinforcement. Goal attainment is based on observable, verifiable evidence (e.g., drug-testing logs, canceled event tickets, letters to family members, etc.) and reinforced. Social reinforcement (congratulations, clapping, high-fives, etc.) and tangible reinforcers (scheduled or variable reinforcement of monetary vouchers for recreational goods, personal hygiene items, or paying bills) are delivered contingent on goal attainment. As short-term goals are accomplished, new goals are added in each of the life areas in a weekly goal-development group to maintain a trajectory toward accomplishing long-term goals. Many clients maintain up to 20 active short-term goals and most clients achieve 80–100% weekly verifiable goal accomplishment.

Abstinence-Contingent Housing

Abstinence-contingent housing (ACH) is a Phase I and II behavioral intervention for substance abuse. It simultaneously reinforces drug abstinence and provides safe housing during participation in BDT and aftercare.

Housing is a furnished apartment with a roommate or a group house with approximately five other clients. The apartment or group house is equipped with bedding, flatware, a week's worth of food, and a key. ACH is free during Phase I, but requires a modest rent during Phase II, deducted from work therapy earned stipends or paid from private-sector wages. Random weekly urine-toxicology testing is used to regulate housing access. Initial entry to housing can require a period of abstinence (1 week or two consecutive drug-free drug tests) or can be accessed without abstinence contingency (e.g., for 1 week to serve as an exposure to the reinforcement). Continued housing reinforcement is contingent upon weekly drug-free toxicology testing. One study, however, investigated the effect of housing with and without abstinence contingencies. In ACH, a positive drug test results in the immediate removal from program-provided housing by the housing manager and transportation to a safe shelter. Participation in and transportation to BDT and a noon meal are continuously provided during the removal of housing period. Two consecutive drug-free tests result in the immediate return to housing while continuing in BDT or aftercare.

CMWT and Job Club

CMWT is a Phase II behavioral treatment for drug abuse which simultaneously provides work training and experiences during aftercare. Upon completion of Phase I BDT, clients have access to basic construction, landscaping/maintenance, food service, or computer training experiences. CMWT is contingent upon drug abstinence in the same way CMH is delivered. If a positive urine test is obtained, clients do not participate in work therapy and lose earnings until abstinence is re-attained as evidenced by consecutive drug-free urine tests. On the morning of a positive test, clients are transported to a shelter or other housing until abstinence is re-established. Construction work consists of refurbishing/repair of housing or working in kitchen and lawn care jobs. Construction work is supervised by "Bad Boy Builders," a team of recovering construction workers serving as on-the-job trainers. Computer training is held in a computer lab with 12 networked computers. It includes typing; word processing; Internet navigation; and the use of telephone, fax machine, and printer, supervised by a vocational rehabilitation specialist. On-the-job behaviors and vocational goals are monitored and reinforced by stipends to assist in the rent payments for CMH. Work ethic and on-the-job goals consist of on-time attendance, professional behavior, completion of assigned tasks, appropriate dress, and other behaviors. CMWT is supplemented with Job Club. Job Club is modeled after Azin, Flores, and Kaplan's (1975) original concept of vocational rehabilitation, and it offers training in completing job applications and conducting job interviews. Guidance by a vocational rehabilitation specialist in identifying job opportunities through the newspaper, submitting applications, conducting job interviews, and so on is provided.

RESEARCH ON TREATMENT OF COCAINE DISORDERS AMONG THE HOMELESS BY THE INVESTIGATIVE TEAM

An early effort by O'Brien, Alterman, Walter, Childress, and McLellan (1989) showed that day treatment reduced cocaine use, but none of the homeless cocaine-dependent patients were retained in treatment. Soon after, in a series of studies starting with Homeless I (H-I), Milby et al. (1996) demonstrated that homeless persons with primary crack cocaine addictions can be effectively retained and treated using innovative BDT and CM interventions designed to reinforce drug abstinence with safe and drug-free housing and paid work experiences. Throughout this series of studies, ACH has been a core component of this multimodal intervention. Also, ACH has been manualized and its procedures progressively refined so that ACH can be therapeutically managed by a caring but kind and firm nonprofessional. A summary of the findings from this 15-year research program is presented below.

Enhanced Day Treatment and ACH Improved Outcomes (Homeless I)

Milby et al. (1996) designed an intervention addressing both substance abuse and homelessness in a group of homeless persons with substance use disorders. Enhanced care (EC) consisted of BDT, including TGM for substance use disorders, and, to address homelessness, provided transportation, meals, paid contingency-managed work experiences, and low-cost ACH. After 2 months of day treatment, EC clients experienced 4 months of ACH, utilizing TGM for housing goals to foster housing independence, and work therapy, with aftercare group sessions available two afternoons per week. This intervention was compared to UC. UC utilized once-per-week individual and group counseling following the Alcoholics Anonymous (AA) model. Individual counseling was scheduled once per week or more, and clients were referred for housing and vocational services available in the community. For EC, ACH and work therapy both reinforced drug abstinence and provided safe, drug-free housing and work experiences. A total of 131 subjects were treated and followed. Intention-to-treat analyses revealed that the proportion of participants abstinent at scheduled follow-up urine tests for UC versus EC, respectively, was 62% versus 56% abstinent at baseline, 51% versus 76% at 2 months, 48% versus 54% at 6 months, and 40% versus 50% at 12 months. The average follow-up rates across all time points were 67.9%. There were no follow-up rate differences between follow-up points or treatment groups. Longitudinal Wei-Lachin analyses of proportions for point cocaine urine-toxicology tests revealed a significant group difference across 12 months ($p = .008$) favoring EC. Differences favoring EC were found for reduced homelessness at 6 and 12 months, and within-group differences for employment over 12 months. The largest between-group differences and effect sizes were found for alcohol use and homelessness (Milby et al., 1996).

ACH Improved Outcomes Beyond Intensive Day Treatment (Homeless II)

Because H-I could not disentangle the differential impact of the day-treatment and CM interventions, Homeless II (H-II) utilized a systematic replication of the intensive day treatment as the new UC (BDT) and compared it to BDT + ACH and work interventions (BDT+). H-II also controlled for confounding variables that were present in H-I. Cocaine-dependent homeless persons with nonpsychotic dual diagnoses were randomly assigned to the two groups and treated by the same counselors at the same times and in the same places. Treatment phases were the same as H-I. Comparison of weekly abstinence rates during the first 8 weeks (i.e., Phase I of day treatment [left panel in Figure 9.1]) exemplifies the therapeutic power of ACH. During Phase I all other treatment conditions were held constant and there was no confounding effect of abstinence-contingent work therapy that began as Phase II in week 9. At the end of Phase I the abstinence rates after 2 months were 72% for BDT+ vs. 30% for BDT, yielding an effect size of 0.85.

Throughout both phases, BDT+ clients were always more abstinent than BDT clients at any week. Generalized linear model analyses suggest that abstinence varied as a function of treatment group and phase with no evidence of a treatment by phase interaction. Best estimates of abstinence prevalence during Phase I were 0.42 for BDT and 0.69 for BDT+. For Phase II, the estimates were 0.18 for BDT and 0.54 for BDT+. At 12 months, both groups showed improvement at all time points from baseline. Both housing and employment outcomes showed within-group, but not between-group, differences at 6- and 12-month follow-ups. More details on this study are found in Milby (2000).

Housing with or without an Abstinence Contingency Was Better Than Day Treatment without Housing (Homeless III)

While H-I and H-II revealed superior drug abstinence outcomes up to 6 months utilizing CM with program-provided ACH and abstinence-contingent work therapy as reinforcement, neither study examined the possibility that provision of housing without an abstinence contingency, along with the effective day treatment, may have been sufficient for improved outcomes. To address the role and importance of whether and how housing is managed for homeless substance abusers, Homeless III (H-III) examined the role of provided versus abstinence-contingent-provided housing. Both housing groups were compared to a UC control of no housing (NH), which in-

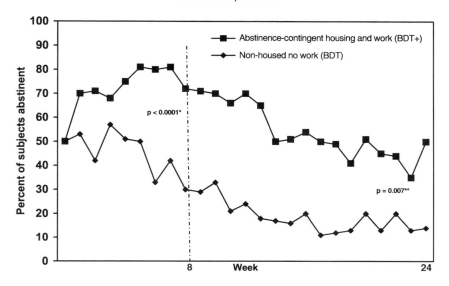

FIGURE 9.1. Weekly percent of abstinent participants during treatment and aftercare (Homeless II). From Milby et al. (2000). Copyright 2000 by Elsevier. Reprinted by permission.

cluded all other elements of the day treatment. As in H-II, cocaine-dependent homeless persons with nonpsychotic dual diagnoses were randomly assigned to these groups. All groups were treated by the same counselors, in the same rooms, at the same times. At midstudy, the apartment complexes housing the two housed groups were switched on a declared moving day, to control for any effects of housing structure and social effects of neighborhoods. Figure 9.2 shows results from this study. Intention-to-treat analyses suggest that ACH increased abstinence, relative to provided but non-abstinent-contingent housing (NACH), and even greater abstinence than for NH. Because the NACH clients had maximum incentive for attendance with no negative consequences for drug-positive urine tests, their attendance was higher than that of ACH and NH groups. When the contribution of attendance to abstinence was controlled, only ACH showed greater abstinence than NH (Milby, Schumacher, Wallace, Freedman, & Vuchinich, 2005).

TGM Effects in Long-Term Homeless IV Study Outcomes

Our current study, Homeless IV (H-IV), suggests that high levels of abstinence may be achieved with ACH in conjunction with CMWT (i.e., without BDT). One group, CM, received *only* ACH and abstinence-contingent work training. The second, CM+, received these same CM interventions

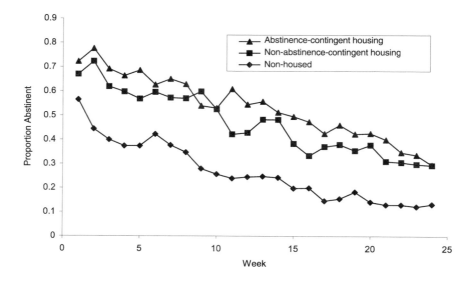

FIGURE 9.2. Weekly proportion of abstinent participants during treatment and after-care (Homeless III). From Milby, Schumacher, Wallace, Freedman, and Vuchinich (2005). Copyright 2005 by the American Public Health Association. Reprinted by permission.

plus the BDT. Interventions lasted 6 months. Abstinence was measured by urine surveillance during active treatment three times per week and following active treatment, randomly one per week in months 7–12, and once per 2 months in months 13–18. Preliminary results to date reveal that the CM+ group showed small but consistently greater abstinence in each of the 24 weeks of active treatment but much greater abstinence above 55% at 12 and 18 months. Figure 9.3 illustrates these results. It should be noted that though there is only one subject difference in numbers of subjects retained in each group at 12 and 18 months, data are still being gathered and results are preliminary (Milby, Schumacher, Wallace, Freedman, Kertesz, et al., 2005). There are two notable aspects of these preliminary findings. First, high levels of abstinence were achieved by the CM group. It averaged 75% abstinent after 2 months and was not significantly different from the 80% abstinence observed for CM+. These high abstinence rates were observed in response to ACH and abstinence-contingent vocational training combined. Though investigators cannot parse out the unique contribution of ACH, the findings suggest a potentially robust therapeutic impact with a much less complex, abstinence-contingent intervention. Second, the impact of BDT, as measured in the CM+ group that received the same abstinence-contingent work intervention as CM, may be delayed and only observed as

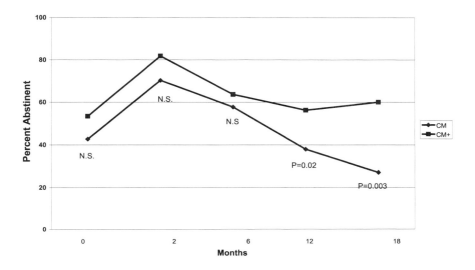

FIGURE 9.3. Preliminary abstinence outcomes at follow-ups (Homeless IV).

more sustained abstinence at long-term follow-up. Another aspect of this study needs emphasis. We used a more assertive urine surveillance procedure which obtained urine specimens in the community when subjects could not get to the clinic for urine testing. This greatly reduced missing data and added to the validity of our abstinence measures by reducing the number of missed urine tests we attributed to drug use.

Houston Technology Transfer Study: CMH plus BDT Can Be Transported with Beneficial Short-Term Abstinence Results

Another indication of the effectiveness of CMBDT combined with ACH is found in our systematic replication of the H-II intervention. This was implemented in a new city with new investigators and new community service resources for housing, work therapy, and UC as a control comparison. Our H-II manualized BDT with ACH was compared to UC in Houston for cocaine-addicted homeless persons. Houston's UC was an inpatient intervention for 1 month (an inpatient intervention not received by the BDT) followed by intensive day treatment for 5+ months. For months 2–6, UC subjects received comparable outpatient intervention like the BDT but *not* ACH. Follow-up data are still being collected at this writing. However, the pilot study is completed (Norwood et al., 2004). Homeless cocaine-dependent subjects (*n* = 55) with nonpsychotic psychiatric symptoms, were randomly assigned to receive 1 month UC with weekly aftercare, job development, and housing assistance (n = 23) or to BDT + ACH. This 2-month outpatient BDT was combined with abstinence-contingent program-provided housing, and 4 months ACH and job development (n = 32). Groups did not differ at baseline on demographics or measures of homelessness, employment, substance abuse, or psychiatric distress. Significant differences in current use at 1- and 2-month follow-up were found as evidenced by urine toxicology assessed within 1 week following the 1-month time point or 2 weeks following the 2-month time point. At 1 month, 72% (23/32) of all clients randomized to the BDT + ACH condition tested negative for cocaine, marijuana, alcohol, amphetamines, sedatives, and opiates, compared to 39% (9/23) of all clients randomized to UC. At 2 months, 66% (21/32) of BDT + ACH clients tested negative for all drugs, compared to 35% (8/23) of UC clients. These results provide evidence that CMH + BDT can be successfully transferred to new providers with beneficial results.

(Transporting Treatment) Housing Contingency Reduces Homelessness

From the same pilot study, information about housing was collected at 1-month, 2-month, and 6-month follow-up. Average percentage of days homeless since last assessment was computed for each group at each time point. At 1 month, BDT + ACH clients averaged 19% of days homeless versus 5% of days homeless for UC. At 2 months: BDT + ACH had 8% days homeless versus UC 24%, and at six-months, BDT + ACH had 15% days homeless vs. UC 23%. Univariate repeated measures analyses indicate a significant group by time interaction. These results provide preliminary evidence that BDT in combination with CM ACH may initially increase days homeless during treatment (as the contingency is applied) but reduce homelessness over time (Llewellyn et al., 2005).

LIMITATIONS, CHALLENGES, AND POLICY IMPLICATIONS OF RESEARCH ON CMBDT FOR HOMELESS DRUG ABUSERS

There are several limitations to this research which present challenges for further research. All studies used a UC comparison control. Thus, though enhancements of CMBDT were always superior to UC, we cannot logically conclude that they were superior to no treatment. However, H-I through H-IV studies were conducted in the same city, using the same referral mechanisms and study entry criteria with indistinguishable demographic characteristics. In all but one study, the comparison intervention (UC) was the enhanced intervention from the previous study. Thus, though experimental methods were limited, it is likely these interventions would have been superior to both the comparison intervention and a no-treatment control had that comparison also been utilized.

Though all these studies have shown reduced drug use at 6 months, we have not been able to gather sufficient random urine tests to observe credible drug use data from 6 to 12 months, and 12 to 18 months. Our point-prevalence measures of drug use at follow-up have always been able to be rescheduled, thus allowing the possibility that, although clients were using at follow-up, after rescheduling they could test drug negative. Our current study has greatly reduced missed urine test data, but it is unknown whether these procedures have yielded credible random urine test results that are not potentially biased by missing data.

The labor-intensive complexity and cost of CMBDT is another limitation. Integrated CMBDT, including work, training, and housing components, is expensive, and in spite of its effectiveness, it may not be financially feasible for many communities to adopt (Schumacher, Mennemeyer, Milby, Wallace, & Nolan, 2002). However, preliminary results from our current stepped-care study suggest that a CMH and work-training component alone may be effective as a less costly and complex initial intervention that more communities could utilize (Milby, Schumacher, Wallace, Freedman, Kertesz, et al., 2005). It is also possible that urban communities, where core components of CMBDT already exist, could implement this intervention with substantial savings, as in the replication of CMBDT at Houston, Texas (Norwood et al., 2004).

Because all of our studies have been conducted with participants who presented for substance abuse treatment, it is unknown whether this type of intervention would be effective with substance-abusing homeless who were not interested in treatment. Could ACH alone, without BDT, be effective for those who were only interested in access to housing? This is an important empirical question that could be answered by policy-relevant research. National surveys show that only a small percentage of those who need treatment actually receive it. Offering ACH without substance abuse treatment may be a way to engage this large group to help improve their housing, health, and illicit drug use, so that those who choose may benefit from other service options available to them.

Though this research was conducted with seriously impaired homeless persons who had nonpsychotic Axis I disorders in addition to their substance use disorder, it excluded homeless persons with serious psychotic mental illness. Thus, we do not know whether this intervention would be effective with an SMI cohort. However, we do know that the presence of one or more nonpsychotic Axis I disorders, in addition to cocaine dependence, did not make a difference in abstinence, housing, and employment outcomes, relative to patients who did not have additional Axis I disorders (McNamara, Schumacher, Milby, Wallace, & Usdan, 2001).

Our CMBDT, with ACH and work, is philosophically and procedurally different from the housing-first approach (without an abstinence contingency) that has been shown by Tsemberis and colleagues to improve housing stability for SMI homeless persons (Tsemberis, Gulcur, & Nakae, 2004). However, their randomized controlled trial comparing housing first showed no difference in substance abuse outcomes compared to UC which utilized housing contingent upon treatment participation and sobriety. The UC intervention did not offer the array of integrated services included in the CMBDT, and it had no previous history of treatment effectiveness. Housing first is designed to help stabilize SMI homeless persons so that they can participate in mental health and substance abuse treatment. Though this may be a viable treatment approach to improve housing stability, it is unknown whether our CMBDT could be more effective, especially for reducing illicit drug use along with improved housing and employment stability. The two interventions have never been compared for homeless substance abusers with SMI. It is quite possible that CMBDT, especially if supplemented with a consultant or liaison psychiatry expertise, could yield better and more sustained housing and reduced illicit drug use. This is not so much a limitation of our research but a challenge for future policy-relevant research.

Another challenge occurs where shelters are not available as backup for ACH when clients are removed from program housing. This situation may be a limitation to implementing ACH. ACH, as we use it, should provide a safety net of secure shelter backup if the abstinence contingency is violated. Equally important is implementation so that termination from provided housing is only temporary until abstinence is re-established. Procedures should allow multiple terminations and returns to ACH so that the contingency has a chance to impact drug-seeking behavior. For public-supported substance abuse programs serving nonpsychotic homeless persons, ACH as described here, is recommended as a research-based effective intervention.

Where objection to the use of strict ACH is a challenge to implementation, providers could utilize quality levels of housing via an abstinence contingency while still providing basic secure shelter housing for all participants regardless of substance use. Evidence of continued use could be the occasion for providing secure but spartan housing, where personal space, storage, and accoutrements are restricted. As control over drug use is being sustained, homeless clients could become eligible for an increment in housing quality (i.e., more secure space, better furniture, and decorations), with access to a variety of recreational and leisure options, and so on.

Another possible limitation to implementation is transportation. Provision of transport to and from housing to treatment is not required for ethical implementation of ACH. However, depending on transportation resources in particular areas, availability of transport may impact program effectiveness. Providing transport or transport tokens may greatly facilitate program effectiveness by increasing the likelihood that clients will continue in daily treatment sessions and noon meals.

Housing providers may not resist or object to using an abstinence contingency. However, few housing providers have resources for urine testing to maintain the contingency. This may be a limitation to implementation. Though such testing is usually seen as a service provided by substance abuse treatment, available urine screening tests are relatively inexpensive and can be conducted at the housing units as demonstrated by Norwood et al. (2004).

ETHICAL ISSUES TO BE CONSIDERED IN IMPLEMENTING ACH INTERVENTIONS

Control over the provision of housing for homeless persons can be controversial. In America's urban areas multiple sources of housing are provided by charitable and government organizations. Each housing provider has rules for eligibility, length of stay, eviction, and so forth, which strongly impact the lives of very vulnerable people. This mix of available housing sources inevitably results in housing availability disparities for low-priority groups. Some homeless persons are left to seek shelters or even to live on the streets or otherwise in ways and places not designed for human overnight habitation. Those seeking to integrate services with provided housing face a complexity of competing demands and ethical concerns for housing utilization sensitive to the needs of homeless persons. Contextual knowledge of housing resources is critical. For example, New York City considers safe housing a right of every citizen. To impose an abstinence contingency for public-provided housing, where evidence for active illicit drug use would involve termination of housing, may be impossible given local law and policies.

The ethical principle on which ACH is implemented is reflected in procedures we use to address the basic needs of homeless persons. These procedures respect individual rights to disengage from treatment that utilizes ACH. At any time our clients can obtain a referral for other treatment which does not utilize ACH or test as vigorously for illicit drug use. Those who participate in our ACH interventions are treatment seekers. As part of the treatment they request, they are informed of the program's abstinence contingencies for housing and the work intervention. They consent to participate after learning how it is implemented and that they have choices for other services where ACH is not utilized. They learn that though they will be removed from program-provided housing within 6 hours of a positive drug test, they are transported to secure shelter housing *and they are not* terminated from the program. Treatment continuation provides them with a noon meal and daily transport until they meet a 1-week abstinence contingency and are returned to their program-provided housing. Another important procedure in our ACH is the implementation of provided housing without an abstinence contingency during the first week of treatment. This facilitates both program participation and initiation of abstinence. Thus, via our van transport, provision of a noon meal, and daily participation in BDT, engagement continues until clients return to program housing as self-control over illicit use improves.

CONCLUDING COMMENTS

Taken together, all these studies show that behavioral intervention that included ACH always produced superior abstinence outcomes than did behavioral interventions that did not. Although our current study (H-IV) of BDT with ACH and our abstinent work intervention seems to produce the best, especially long-term abstinence results, these results must be considered preliminary. Also, the long-term impact of these two treatments on housing and employment are unknown. However, if considered from a public health perspective, the impact on abstinence of the less complex CMH and work intervention without day treatment is remarkable. We think a study of ACH as a stand-alone first-step intervention (i.e., without the abstinent-contingent work intervention used in H-IV) may be a viable intervention that could have important public policy implications for both substance abuse and housing interventions for homeless persons.

REFERENCES

Acosta, O., & Toro, P. A. (2000). Let's ask the homeless people themselves: A needs assessment based on a probability sample of adults. *American Journal of Community Psychology, 28*(3), 343–366.

Azin, N. H., Flores, T., & Kaplan, S. J. (1975). Job-finding club: A group assisted program for obtaining employment. *Behaviour Research and Therapy, 13*, 17–27.

Bassuk, E. L., & Weinreb, L. F. (1996). Substance abuse, mental disorders prevalent in homeless mothers. *Brown University Digest of Addiction Theory and Application, 15*, 1–3.

Burt, M. R. (1992). *Over the edge: The growth of homelessness in the 1980s*. New York: Russell Sage.

Burt, M. R., & Aron, L. Y. (2001). *Helping America's homeless*. Washington, DC: Urban Institute.

Burt, M. R., Aron, L. Y., Douglas, T., Valente, J., Lee, E., & Iwen, B. (1999). *Homelessness: Programs and the people they serve. Findings of the national survey of homeless assistance providers and clients*. Retrieved March 23, 2005, from *www.huduser.org/publications/homeless/homeless_tech.html*.

Conrad, K. J., Hultman, C. I., & Lyons, J. S. (1993). Treatment of the chemically dependent homeless: Theory and implementation in fourteen American projects. *Alcoholism Treatment Quarterly, 10*(3–4), 235–246.

Corrigan, E. M., & Anderson, S. C. (1984). Homeless alcoholic women on skid row. *American Journal of Drug and Alcohol Abuse, 10*, 535–549.

Fischer, P. J., & Breakey, W. R. (1991). The epidemiology of alcohol, drug, and mental disorders among homeless persons. *American Psychologist, 46*(11), 1115–1128.

Folsom, D. P., Hawthorne, W., Lindamer, L., Gilmer, T., Bailey, A., Golshan, S., et al. (2005). Prevalence and risk factors for homelessness and utilization of mental health services among 10,340 patients with serious mental illness in a large public mental health system. *American Journal of Psychiatry, 162*(2), 370–376.

Geissler, L. J., Borman, C. A., Kwiatkowski, C. F., Braucht, G. N., & Reichardt, C. S. (1995). Women, homelessness, and substance abuse. *Psychology of Women Quarterly, 19*, 65–83.

Gelberg, L., Linn, L. S., & Leake, B. D. (1988). Mental health, alcohol and drug use, and criminal history among homeless adults. *American Journal of Psychiatry, 145*(2), 191–196.

Haddad, M. B., Wilson, T. W., Ijaz, K., Marks, S. M., & Moore, M. (2005). Tuberculosis and homelessness in the United States, 1994–2003. *Journal of the American Medical Association, 293*(22), 2762–2766.

Hatton, D. C., Kleffel, D., Bennett, S., & Gaffrey, E. A. N. (2001). Homeless women and children's access to health care: A paradox. *Journal of Community Health Nursing, 18*(1), 25–34.

Klinkenberg, W. D., Caslyn, R. J., Morse, G. A., Yonker, R. D., McCudden, S., Ketema, F., et al. (2003). Prevalence of human immunodeficiency virus, hepatitis B, and hepatitis C among homeless persons with co-occurring severe mental illness and substance use disorders. *Comprehensive Psychiatry, 44*(4), 293–302.

Koegel, P., Burnam, M. A., & Farr, R. K. (1988a). Alcoholism among homeless adults in the inner city of Los Angeles. *Archives of General Psychiatry, 51*, 1011–1018.

Koegel, P., Burnam, M. A., & Farr, R. K. (1988b). The prevalence of specific psychiatric disorders among homeless individuals in the inner city of Los Angeles. *Archives of General Psychiatry, 45*, 1085–1092.

Kushel, M. B., Hahn, J. A., Evans, J. L., Bangsberg, D. R., & Moss, A. R. (2005). Revolving doors: Imprisonment among the homeless and marginally housed population. *American Journal of Public Health, 95*(10), 1747–1752.

Link, B. G., Susser, E., Stueve, A., Phelan, J., Moore R. E., & Stuening, E. (1994). Lifetime and five-year prevalence of homelessness in the United States. *American Journal of Public Health, 84*, 1907–1912.

Llewellyn, A., Norwood, W., Averill, P., Schumacher, J., Milby, J., & Rhoades, H. (2005). *Technology transfer of behavioral day treatment with contingency management for dually diagnosed homeless substance abusers: Homelessness at follow-up.* Paper presented at the 67th annual scientific meeting of the College on Problems of Drug Dependence, Orlando, FL.

Martens, W. H. (2001–2002). Homelessness and mental disorders: A comparative review of populations in various countries. *International Journal of Mental Health, 30*(4), 79–96.

McNamara, C., Schumacher, J. E., Milby, J. B., Wallace, D., & Usdan, S. (2001). Prevalence of nonpsychotic mental disorders does not affect treatment outcome in a homeless cocaine-dependent sample. *American Journal of Drug and Alcohol Abuse, 27*(1), 91–106.

Milby, J. B., Schumacher, J. E., McNamara, C., Wallace, D., Usdan, S., McGill, T., et al.

(2000). Initiating abstinence in cocaine abusing dually diagnosed homeless persons. *Drug and Alcohol Dependence, 60*(1), 55–67.

Milby, J. B., Schumacher, J. E., Raczynski, J. M., Caldwell, E., Engle, M., Michael, M., et al. (1996). Sufficient conditions for effective treatment of substance abusing homeless persons. *Drug and Alcohol Dependence, 43*(1–2), 39–47.

Milby, J. B., Schumacher, J. E., Wallace, D., Freedman, M. J., Kertesz, S., Viikinsalo, M., et al. (2005). *CM for housing and work performance are sufficient to establish sustained abstinence in homeless substance abusers.* Paper presented at the 67th annual scientific meeting of the College on Problems of Drug Dependence, Orlando, FL.

Milby, J. B., Schumacher, J. E., Wallace, D., Freedman, M. J., & Vuchinich, R. E. (2005). To house or not to house: The effects of providing housing to homeless substance abusers in treatment. *American Journal of Public Health, 95*(7), 1259–1265.

North, C. S., Eyrich, K. M., Pollio, D. E., & Spitznagel, E. L. (2004). Are rates of psychiatric disorders in the homeless population changing? *American Journal of Public Health, 94*(1), 103–108.

Norwood, W., Averill, P., Schumacher, J. E., Milby, J., Llewellyn, A., & Rhoades, H. (2004). *Technology transfer of behavioral day treatment with contingency management for dually diagnosed homeless substance abusers.* Paper presented at the 66th annual scientific meeting of the College on Problems of Drug Dependence, San Juan, Puerto Rico.

O'Brien, C. P., Alterman, A., Walter, D., Childress, A. R., & McLellan, A. T. (1989). Evaluation of treatment for cocaine dependence. *NIDA Research Monogram, 95*, 78–84.

O'Flaherty, B. (1996). *Making room: The economics of homelessness.* Cambridge, MA: Harvard University Press.

Plumb, J. D. (1997). Homelessness: Care, prevention and public policy. *Annual International Medicine, 126*(12), 973–975.

Raczynski, J. M., Schumacher, J. E., Milby, J. B., Michael, M., Engle, M., Lerner, M., et al. (1993). Comparing two substance abuse treatments for the homeless: The Birmingham project. *Alcoholism Treatment Quarterly, 10*(3–4), 217–233.

Reardon, M. L., Burns, A. B., Preist, R., Sachs-Ericsson, N., & Lang, A. R. (2003). Alcohol use and other psychiatric disorders in the formerly homeless and never homeless: Prevalence, age of onset, comorbidity, temporal sequencing, and service utilization. *Substance Use and Misuse, 38*(3–6), 601–644.

Riley, E. D., Bangsberg, D. R., Guzman, D., Perry, S., & Moss, A. R. (2005). Antiretroviral therapy, hepatitis C virus, and AIDS mortality among San Francisco's homeless and marginally housed. *Journal of Acquired Immunity Deficiency Syndrome, 38*(2), 191–195.

Ritchey, F. J., La Gory, M., Fitzpatrick, K. M., & Mullis, J. (1990). A comparison of homeless, community-wide, and selected distressed samples on the CES-depression scale. *American Journal of Public Health, 80*(11), 1384–1386.

Rosenheck, R. (1994). *Homelessness among veterans.* Paper presented at the Veterans Administration First National Conference on Homelessness, Washington, DC.

Rosenheck, R., & Koegel, P. (1993). Characteristics of veterans and nonveterans in three samples of homeless men. *Hospital and Community Psychiatry, 44*(9), 858–863.

Schumacher, J. E., Mennemeyer, S. T., Milby, J. B., Wallace, D., & Nolan, K. (2002). Costs and effectiveness of substance abuse treatments for homeless persons. *Journal of Mental Health Policy and Economics, 5*(1), 33–42.

Singer, J. (2003). Taking it to the streets: Homelessness, health, and health care in the United States. *Journal of General Internal Medicine, 18*(11), 964–965.

Tompsett, C. J., Toro, P. A., Guzicki, M., Schlienz, N., Blume, M., & Lombardo, S. (2003). Homelessness in the US and Germany: A cross-national analysis. *Journal of Community and Applied Social Psychology, 13*(3), 240–257.

Toro, P. A., Bellavia, C. W., Daeschler, C. V., Ownes, B. J., Wall, D. D., Passero, J. M., et al. (1995). Distinguishing homelessness from poverty: A comparative study. *Journal of Consulting and Clinical Psychology, 63,* 280–289.

Tsemberis, S., Gulcur, L., & Nakae, M. (2004). Housing first, consumer choice, and harm reduction for homeless individuals with a dual diagnosis. *American Journal of Public Health, 94*(4), 651–656.

U.S. Conference of Mayors. (1998). *A status report on hunger and homelessness in America's cities.* Washington, DC: U.S. Conference of Mayors.

Zolopa, A. R., Hahn, J. A., Gorter, R., Miranda, J., Wlodarczyk, D., Peterson, J., et al. (1994). HIV and tuberculosis infection in San Francisco's homeless adults. Prevalence and risk factors in a representative sample. *Journal of the American Medical Association, 272*(6), 455–461.

CHAPTER 10

PREGNANT AND POSTPARTUM WOMEN

Sarah H. Heil, Jin H. Yoon,
and Stephen T. Higgins

PREVALENCE, ADVERSE EFFECTS, AND COSTS
OF SUBSTANCE ABUSE DURING PREGNANCY

Nearly 1 of every 5 (18%) pregnant women in the United States reports smoking cigarettes in the past month, 1 of every 10 (10%) reports drinking alcohol and nearly 1 of every 20 (4.3%) reports using illicit drugs (Substance Abuse and Mental Health Services Administration, 2005). This translates into as many as 1.3 million substance-exposed babies being born in the U.S. each year. Of further concern is the likelihood that these figures are underestimations of the problem due to psychological, social and legal pressures to deny substance abuse during pregnancy (Bolnick & Rayburn, 2003; McCaul, Svikis, & Feng, 1991).

Substance abuse by pregnant women is a leading preventable cause of fetal and neonatal morbidity and mortality. Licit and illicit substance abuse during pregnancy increases the risk of miscarriage, stillbirth, premature birth, low birth weight, congenital defect, and neonatal death (Brady, Posner, Lang, & Rosati, 1994; Cnattingius, 2004; Richter & Richter, 2001; Young, 1997). Prenatal substance exposure may also manifest itself postpartum in the form of poor cognitive skills, mental retardation, and conduct disorders (Richter & Richter, 2001; Weinberg, 1997; Young, 1997).

Some of the adverse effects of substance use during pregnancy are direct physiological consequences of substance use. For example, smoking increases the flow of carbon monoxide to the fetus and decreases placental blood flow, increasing the likelihood of spontaneous abortion, intrauterine growth retardation, premature birth, and low birth weight (Cnattingius, 2004; Pollack, Lantz, & Frohna, 2000; Richter & Richter, 2001). Adverse effects may also result from or be compounded by environmental factors that often accompany substance abuse during pregnancy, such as poor prenatal care, poor nutrition, and poverty (Bolnick & Rayburn, 2003; Jansson et al., 1996).

The adverse consequences of substance abuse during pregnancy are also costly in direct economic terms. It has been estimated that the lifetime cost of caring for a child prenatally exposed to tobacco, alcohol, or drugs is between $750,000 and $1.4 million (National Center on Addiction and Substance Abuse at Columbia University, 2006). Most of that expense is a result of hospital costs at birth, including those related to complications during delivery and intensive care. Other costs are related to the treatment of physical, developmental, and psychological problems that may surface later in life. This sobering figure underscores the importance of treating substance abuse during pregnancy.

TREATMENT INTERVENTIONS FOR SUBSTANCE ABUSE DURING PREGNANCY AND POSTPARTUM

Becoming pregnant prompts some women to modify unhealthy behavior such as substance abuse, presumably in an effort to protect the health of the fetus (Daley, Argeriou, & McCarty, 1998; Woods, 1995). For example, women who smoke cigarettes are more likely to quit while pregnant than at any other time in their life and about 30% of pregnant smokers will quit with little or no intervention (Office of the Surgeon General, 2001; Solomon & Quinn, 2004). The vast majority of women, however, will continue to smoke during their pregnancy. Although we are unaware of any data on this topic, this trend is likely similar for other drugs of abuse and suggests that innovative and efficacious interventions are needed to treat pregnant women who continue to abuse drugs in order to avoid the serious and costly adverse consequences noted earlier.

Efficacious treatment interventions for substance abuse during pregnancy run the gamut, from brief (5–15 minutes) low-cost interventions delivered by prenatal care providers to relatively costly long-term residential treatment programs specially designed for pregnant substance abusers (Chang et al., 2005; Little et al., 2003; Melvin, Dolan-Mullen, Windsor, Whiteside, & Goldenberg, 2000; Worley, Conners, Crone, Williams, & Bokony, 2005). Contingency management (CM) interventions, most often delivered in intensive outpatient settings, have the potential to help fill the wide gap between these two ends of the intensity continuum. As suggested by results reviewed in this chapter, CM interventions may impact heavier users who typically do not respond to brief interventions (Chang, Wilkins-Haug, Berman, & Goetz, 1999; Melvin & Gaffney, 2004). CM interventions may also provide an efficacious treatment option for women who are unable to participate in residential treatment, due to childcare concerns for existing children and other barriers (Grella, 1997; Jansson et al., 1996).

CM involves systematic delivery of reinforcing or punishing consequences contingent upon the occurrence of a target response and the withholding of those consequences in the absence of the target response (Higgins & Silverman, 1999). The CM intervention that has garnered the most research attention is voucher-based reinforcement therapy wherein patients receive vouchers or related monetary-based incentives exchangeable for retail items contingent upon recent drug abstinence (Lussier, Heil, Mongeon, Badger, & Higgins, 2006). The aim of this chapter is to review the existing literature on CM interventions to promote drug abstinence and other behavior change in pregnant and postpartum women with substance abuse disorders.

CM INTERVENTIONS TARGETING DRUG ABSTINENCE IN PREGNANT AND POSTPARTUM WOMEN

A search of the literature identified 11 reports of studies published in peer-reviewed journals where the efficacy of CM interventions to promote drug abstinence in pregnant and postpartum women with substance abuse disorders was compared to that of an experimental comparison condition. These 11 reports were divided into studies in which the effects of the voucher intervention could (top of Table 10.1; $n = 8$) and could not (bottom of Table 10.1; $n = 3$) be experimentally isolated. In Table 10.1, we report basic characteristics of each study (the study n, setting, design, and the duration of the CM intervention) as well as four parameters of CM schedules that have been empirically demonstrated to impact efficacy. The first parameter is CM target, specifically whether abstinence from use of a single drug, two drugs, or multiple drugs, was reinforced. A recent meta-analysis by our group of 55 reports examining CM interventions with primarily nonpregnant substance abusers found that targeting abstinence from a single drug rather than multiple substances simultaneously is generally associated with larger effect sizes (Lussier et al., 2006). The second parameter is CM schedule type—that is, whether the magnitude of the reinforcer was fixed (e.g., $5 for every negative sample) or escalated in value over successive drug-negative specimens ($5 for the first negative sample, $6 for the second, etc.) with a reset contingency for drug use. Escalating schedules with reset con-

TABLE 10.1. Studies Targeting Abstinence in Pregnant Women

Study	n	Setting	Design	CM duration (weeks)	CM target	CM schedule type	Daily CM earnings (max.)	Voucher delivery	Positive outcome
Studies targeting abstinence in which the effects of CM could be experimentally isolated									
Elk et al. (1995)	7	DF	3	10	Cocaine	F	$7.29	D	Y
Ker et al. (1996)	22	DF	1[a]	8	Smoking	F	—	I	Y
Elk et al. (1998)	12	DF	1	16	Cocaine	F	$10.57	I	N
Jones et al. (2000)	93	MM	1	1	Cocaine and opiates	F	$12.14	I	N
Donatelle et al. (2000)	220	DF	1	32[b]	Smoking	F	$1.79	D	Y
Silverman et al. (2001)	40	MM	1	24	Cocaine and opiates	E	$16.85	I	Y
Silverman et al. (2002)	40	MM	1	72	Cocaine and opiates	E	$18.47	I	Y
Higgins et al. (2004)	58	DF	2[a]	38[c]	Smoking	E	$4.10	I	Y
Studies targeting abstinence in which the effects of CM could not be experimentally isolated									
Chang et al. (1992)	12	MM	1[a]	27	Polydrug	F	$2.14	—	N
Carroll et al. (1995)	14	MM	1	24	Polydrug	F	$2.14	—	N
Jones et al. (2004)	120	NTS	1[a]	4	Polydrug	F	$7.14	I	N

Note. n, sample size, all groups combined; Setting, setting in which study occurred: DF, drug-free clinic; MM, methadone maintenance clinic; NTS, nontreatment setting; Design, experimental design: 1, contingent vouchers versus no voucher control, parallel groups; 2, contingent vouchers versus noncontingent voucher control, parallel groups; 3, contingent vouchers versus no voucher control, within subject; CM duration, average weeks enrolled antepartum; CM schedule type: F, fixed magnitude; E, escalating magnitude with reset; Daily CM earnings, the maximum average amount that could be earned per day across the period that contingent vouchers were available; a dash (—) indicates insufficient information to determine; Voucher delivery: I, immediate (at the same visit the reinforcer was earned); D, delayed (at a visit after the reinforcer was earned); Positive outcome, whether or not a significant change was reported for the behavior targeted by the CM intervention: Y, yes; N, no.

[a]Not fully randomized.

[b]An average of 32 weeks antepartum and 8 weeks postpartum.

[c]An average of 26 weeks antepartum and 12 weeks postpartum.

185

tingencies have been shown to be more effective than fixed or escalating schedules without reset contingencies in sustaining drug abstinence (Roll & Higgins, 2000). The third parameter is daily CM earnings, which was the maximum amount that could be earned averaged across the period that contingent vouchers were available. The fourth parameter is the immediacy of voucher delivery, which was dichotomized into vouchers being delivered either immediately (i.e., presented at the same clinic visit in which the reinforcer was earned) or after a delay (i.e., presented at a clinic visit after the one in which reinforcement was earned). In the meta-analysis referenced previously, larger-magnitude incentives and more immediate delivery of earned incentives were both independently associated with larger effect sizes (Lussier et al., 2006). In the final column of Table 10.1, we report whether or not a significant change was reported for the behavior targeted by the CM intervention.

Studies Targeting Abstinence in Which the Effects of CM Could Be Experimentally Isolated

We begin with studies in which the effects of CM could be experimentally isolated because those represent the largest number of studies and the subset about which the greatest amount of systematic information could be obtained. Seventy-five percent (six of eight) of these reports noted positive outcomes for drug abstinence in pregnant and postpartum women.

Promoting Cocaine Abstinence

In the early 1990s, the need for cocaine treatment in the general population had increased sharply and there was particular concern about cocaine use by pregnant women and the fate of children who had been exposed to cocaine *in utero* (Pitts & Weinstein, 1990; Roland & Volpe, 1989; Rosenak, Diamant, Yaffe, & Hornstein, 1990). Our group demonstrated the efficacy of voucher-based incentives combined with psychosocial counseling for treating cocaine dependence in nonpregnant populations (Higgins et al., 1991, 1993, 1994). Following these reports, Elk et al. (1995) examined the use of incentives to promote cocaine abstinence in pregnant women using a multiple-baseline-across-participants design. During the baseline phase (average duration = 2 weeks), urine samples were collected thrice weekly and tested for cocaine and each participant was expected to attend weekly prenatal care visits. No explicit contingencies were placed on either behavior. During the intervention phase (average duration = 10 weeks), each participant received $10 each time her urine sample results indicated a significant decrease (15%) in cocaine metabolite levels relative to her prior sample or $12 for each sample that was cocaine negative. A participant could also earn a $15 bonus each week if (1) all three urine samples met the criteria above and (2) she attended her weekly prenatal care visit. Incentives earned at one visit were paid out at the participant's next visit. On average, participants submitted twice as many cocaine-negative urine samples during the intervention phase compared to the baseline phase (52% vs. 25%). Attendance at prenatal care visits was also increased during the intervention phase. These results provided the first evidence of the efficacy of CM in pregnant substance abusers.

Smoking Cessation

Three other reports with positive outcomes were studies examining the efficacy of CM to promote smoking cessation during pregnancy and postpartum. The initial report on the use of incentives with pregnant and postpartum smokers examined the efficacy of this approach among pregnant and postpartum women residing in a residential treatment program for other types of substance abuse (Ker, Leischow, Markowitz, & Merikle, 1996). Carbon monoxide (CO) levels were measured daily for approximately 8 weeks. Each day that a participant's CO level indicated smoking abstinence, she earned a credit that could be accumulated and redeemed for program privileges (e.g., extra phone or pass time) or prizes donated by community businesses (jewelry, children's toys, haircuts, etc.). Women who received incentives had lower mean daily CO levels compared to participants in another residential substance abuse treatment program for pregnant and postpartum women in the same area who simply provided daily CO samples but did not receive any incentives (3.07 vs. 12.42, respectively). This study provided compelling evidence that smoking is sensitive to CM interventions.

The seminal study was a more rigorous randomized trial involving low-income pregnant smokers (Donatelle, Prows, Champeau, & Hudson, 2000). Women were randomly assigned to CM or usual-care control conditions. In the CM condition, they received a monthly $50 voucher contingent upon biochemically verified smoking abstinence throughout pregnancy and for 2 months postpartum. In addition, women in the CM condition included a "social supporter" in treatment (i.e., a female non-smoker with whom the subject had a positive association) who also received vouchers when the subject was abstinent (i.e., a $50 voucher in the first and last months and a $25 voucher in each intervening month). Abstinence rates were significantly greater in the CM compared to the control condition at the end of pregnancy (34% vs. 9%, respectively) and the end of the voucher program at 2 months postpartum (22% vs. 6%, respectively). These results provided additional evidence that the low quit rates typically observed among low-income, pregnant smokers are not inevitable and that relapse rates postpartum are modifiable.

In our effort to further extend this approach, we conducted a pilot

study with low-income women who were still smoking upon entering prenatal care (Higgins et al., 2004). Participants were initially assigned to
either contingent or noncontingent voucher conditions as consecutive admissions and later randomly. Vouchers were available antepartum and
through 12 weeks postpartum and were earned for biochemically verified
smoking abstinence in the contingent condition and independent of smoking status in the noncontingent condition. Biochemically verified, 7-day
point-prevalence abstinence was significantly greater in the contingent than
the noncontingent conditions at the end-of-pregnancy (37% vs. 9%, respectively), 12-week postpartum (33% vs. 0%, respectively), and 24-week
postpartum (27% vs. 0%, respectively) assessments. Note that the 24-week
assessment occurred 12 weeks after vouchers were discontinued. Total
mean voucher earnings across antepartum and postpartum periods were
$397 ± 414 and $313 ± 142 in the contingent and noncontingent conditions, respectively. The magnitude of these treatment effects were consistent
with those reported by Donatelle et al. (2000) and exceeded levels typically
observed with low-income pregnant and recently postpartum smokers. In
addition, the maintenance of significant treatment effects through 24 weeks
postpartum extended the duration of treatment effects beyond any reported
previously in this population.

The Therapeutic Workplace

The remaining two reports of positive outcomes were by Silverman and
colleagues (Silverman, Svikis, Robles, Stitzer, & Bigelow, 2001; Silverman
et al., 2002). While the efficacy of CM interventions was relatively well established in nonpregnant populations by this time, there was concern that
practical funding mechanisms needed to be developed if the treatment was
going to have wide applicability. Silverman and colleagues designed and
evaluated a practical application of CM known as the Therapeutic Workplace. A more detailed discussion of the Therapeutic Workplace intervention can be found in Chapter 17 (Donlin, Knealing, & Silverman, this volume), but the first two studies evaluating the Therapeutic Workplace
are described is some detail here as the participants were methadone-
maintained pregnant women who continued to use heroin and cocaine.

In the Therapeutic Workplace, patients are hired and paid to work in a
model work program. Salary is linked to abstinence by requiring patients to
provide objective evidence of abstinence (i.e., a drug-free urine) to gain entrance to the workplace. Therefore, patients work and earn salary only
when abstinent. In addition, the daily salary increases as the patient's duration of sustained abstinence and workplace attendance increases. In the
workplace, patients participate in intensive job-skills training until they
meet strict criteria of sustained abstinence, workplace attendance, job
skills, and professional demeanor. Once these criteria are achieved, patients

can be hired as employees in an income-producing Therapeutic Workplace business, Hopkins Data Services (Silverman et al., 2005). Because employment can be sustained for years, this approach offers the possible advantage of maintaining high-magnitude salary-based abstinence reinforcement over extended periods of time.

In the first report (Silverman et al., 2001), 40 women were randomly assigned to either the Therapeutic Workplace group or to a usual-care control group. Urine samples were collected thrice weekly during the 24-week intervention in both groups and participants were compensated $3.50 for each sample. In the Therapeutic Workplace group, urine samples that were negative for both opiates and cocaine allowed the participant to enter the workplace that day. In the workplace, patients participated in basic skills education and job-skills training in 3-hour work shifts. On the first day a participant provided a negative urine sample and completed a 3-hour work shift, she earned a $7 voucher. Vouchers increased in value by $.50 for each consecutive successful day, to a maximum of $27. A drug-positive sample or failure to provide a sample reset the voucher value back to $7. After a reset, 9 consecutive days of abstinence and workplace attendance returned the voucher value back to the preset value. The majority of a participant's earning potential came from these contingencies promoting abstinence and attendance, but modest incentives were also available for productivity, punctuality, and professional behavior. These additional incentives are described in greater detail later in this chapter.

The results of the initial evaluation of the Therapeutic Workplace's effects on abstinence and attendance were quite promising. Over the course of the intervention, Therapeutic Workplace participants provided nearly twice as many cocaine- and opiate-negative urine samples compared to the usual-care control condition (59% vs. 33%, respectively). On average, 45% of the Therapeutic Workplace participants attended the workplace on a given day. In total, Therapeutic Workplace participants earned an average of $1,013 (range = $0 to $3,126) over the 6-month intervention period.

The Therapeutic Workplace participants were repeatedly offered re-enrollment in 6-month blocks to examine the long-term effects of the intervention. A second article by Silverman et al. (2002) reported abstinence outcomes based on urine samples collected at monthly assessments between months 18 and 36. Relative to the usual-care control group, cocaine and opiate abstinence was significantly higher in Therapeutic Workplace participants (28% vs. 54% and 37% vs. 60%, respectively). In addition, Therapeutic Workplace participants were six times more likely to show evidence of continuous cocaine and opiate abstinence over this extended assessment period than the usual-care group (30% vs. 5%, respectively). Across the entire 36-month intervention period, Therapeutic Workplace participants attended the workplace on 43% of the 780 workdays and had earned an average of $10.73 each workday in vouchers. Together, these two reports provide a unique demonstration of the ability of CM to produce long-term changes in drug use in an especially recalcitrant population.

Reports with Negative Outcomes

Only two articles in this category reported negative outcomes. In one, the reason appeared to be a ceiling effect resulting from high levels of abstinence at baseline. Elk, Mangus, Rhoades, Andres, and Grabowski (1998) used the same design as their 1995 report described earlier to examine the efficacy of CM to prevent relapse in cocaine-dependent women who reported using cocaine during the current pregnancy but had stopped use for at least 30 days prior to entering the study. Ninety-nine percent of all samples submitted were cocaine negative and there were no differences between the CM and control conditions. Prior results from this group suggested that pregnant women who were abstinent from cocaine at intake and received standard counseling generally maintained abstinence during the study (Elk et al., 1994), suggesting there was little room for improvement in this study with the addition of the CM intervention.

In the second report in this category, the reason for a negative outcome appeared to be an insufficient magnitude of reinforcement relative to the behavior change targeted (Jones, Haug, Stitzer, & Svikis, 2000). Pregnant women inducted onto methadone in Week 1 were offered $5/day in vouchers each day of Week 2 for providing cocaine- and opiate-negative samples. Participants also received bonus payments of $25 or $50 for attending the center 5–6 or 7 days, respectively. Given that the women were typically undergoing methadone dose stabilization during Week 2, continued drug use may have been an attempt to ward off withdrawal symptoms and the magnitude and fixed nature of the reinforcement offered may have been insufficient to compete.

Studies Targeting Abstinence in Which the Effects of CM Could Not Be Experimentally Isolated

We identified three additional studies in which CM interventions were included as one part of multicomponent treatment packages and the effects of the CM intervention could not be isolated from that of the other components of the intervention. None of these studies reported positive outcomes. Chang, Carroll, Behr, and Kosten (1992) and Carroll, Chang, Behr, Clinton, and Kosten (1995) provided sequential studies, the latter a randomized version of the former. In both studies, pregnant women in methadone-maintenance treatment continued in usual care (daily methadone dosing, counseling, and random urine screening) or participated in an enhanced treatment program that included monetary payments contingent upon thrice-weekly drug-negative urine screens (a fixed $15 weekly for three consecutive negative samples), as well as onsite prenatal care, weekly relapse prevention groups, and provision of therapeutic childcare during treatment visits for the duration of their pregnancy. In both studies, there were no differences in the percentage of urine drug screens positive for cocaine, illicit opiates, or other drugs. Unlike the study by Elk et al. (1998), no ceiling effect was apparent, with approximately 37% of all samples positive for at least one drug. With regard to the failure of the enhanced intervention to produce a treatment effect, the magnitude of the reinforcer in the CM component was relatively low in relation to the behavior targeted (a week of polydrug abstinence) and may have contributed to the negative findings.

A third study in which the effect of the CM intervention could not be isolated was reported by Jones, Svikis, Rosado, Tuten, and Kulstad (2004) and targeted non-treatment-seeking pregnant drug-abusing women attending prenatal care clinics. Women were offered the opportunity to participate in a CM intervention combined with motivational interviewing or both motivational interviewing and case management. The CM component averaged $6.67/day and was contingent upon providing samples negative for amphetamines, cocaine, marijuana, and morphine. Neither intervention was effective in increasing the number of drug-abstinent urine samples relative to a drug-free control condition. Once again, the lack of effect of the interventions that included a CM component may have been due to the amount of compensation, which did not appear commensurate with the behavior targeted, especially given that the participants were not seeking substance abuse treatment.

Monitoring Drug Use during Pregnancy

CM studies targeting drug abstinence require objective evidence of drug abstinence, typically in the form of a drug-negative urine, saliva, or breath sample, to deliver the incentive. While biochemical verification of abstinence is clearly necessary, there is relatively little systematic information available regarding appropriate tests and cutpoints for determining drug abstinence among pregnant and recently postpartum women. As one example, decreases in smoking rate and increases in nicotine and cotinine metabolism rates, among other changes during pregnancy, argue against adopting guidelines based on general populations of smokers (Dempsey, Jacob, & Benowitz, 2002; Rebagliato et al., 1998; SRNT Subcommittee on Biochemical Verification, 2002). We are also aware of data documenting the accelerated clearance of methadone in pregnancy (Pond, Kreek, Tong, Raghunath, & Benowitz, 1985; Wolff, Boys, Rostami-Hodjegan, Hay, & Raistrick, 2005). Accelerated clearance may be due in part to increases in the activity of the enzyme cytochrome P450 3A4 (Nekhayeva, Nanoovskaya, Deshmukh, & Zharikova, 2005). This enzyme is reported to be involved in the metabolism of more than 50% of all drugs (Wrighton & Stevens, 1992), suggesting that other opiates and other drug classes would likely be affected by this pregnancy-induced change as well. While some initial steps have been taken to investigate the ramifications of these differences in the area of smoking (Higgins et al., 2007), more systematic investigation of the use of different biomarkers, test types, and associated cutpoints across the range of abused substances is likely necessary to maximize the success of CM interventions in this population.

STUDIES TARGETING OUTCOME MEASURES OTHER THAN ABSTINENCE

In addition to the 10 studies using CM to target drug abstinence, our search of the literature also identified 6 studies targeting other outcomes. Three of the six were a series of studies targeting treatment attendance at the Center for Addiction and Pregnancy in Baltimore, Maryland (Jansson et al., 1996). Treatment attendance is related to positive treatment outcome and dropout is associated with relapse and adverse effects on the mother and the baby (Hubbard et al., 1989; McCaul & Svikis, 1996; Svikis, Golden, et al., 1997). Thus, improving treatment attendance is another mechanism by which maternal and fetal/neonatal outcomes may be enhanced. The remaining three studies targeting other outcomes all took place in the context of the Therapeutic Workplace intervention described earlier and were efforts to modify other types of behavior relevant to employment settings, such as on-time attendance. We provide more detail about both series of studies below.

The Center for Addiction and Pregnancy Studies

A series of three studies by Svikis, Jones, and colleagues examined the efficacy of CM for enhancing treatment attendance in opiate- and/or cocaine-dependent pregnant women. This series of studies began in response to observations of an alarming rate of treatment dropout after the transition from a 7-day inpatient stay to 30 days of intensive outpatient treatment in their comprehensive treatment program (Jansson et al., 1996). In the initial study (Svikis, Lee, Haug, & Stitzer, 1997), methadone-maintained (MM) and non-methadone-maintained (non-MM) pregnant women were randomly assigned to receive gift certificates of various magnitudes (i.e., $0, $1, $5, or $10) for attending at least 4 hours of treatment programming for the first seven days after transitioning from residential to outpatient care. The results indicated that voucher magnitude was efficacious only among non-MM pregnant women, with the larger $5 and $10 magnitudes producing significantly more attendance than the smaller $0 and $1 magnitudes (3.3 vs. 2.3 days, respectively). There was no magnitude effect among MM pregnant women, with all magnitude groups attending an average of 5.2 of the 7 days. The authors conclude that modest incentives can improve attendance in women who are not MM, but suggest that methadone itself reinforces attendance in MM women and the modest monetary incentives offered were not sufficient to provide additional benefit.

The second study in the series (Jones et al., 2000) attempted to replicate the foregoing finding in non-MM pregnant women, but shifted the targeted behavior in MM pregnant women from attendance to drug abstinence (results of this portion of the study were already described). Non-MM women received a $5 voucher for each day of attendance during the first 7 outpatient treatment days plus an additional $25 or $50 bonus for 5–6 or 7 days of attendance, respectively. The usual-care control condition did not receive vouchers. Contrary to the findings of Svikis, Lee, et al. (1997), there were no differences between conditions in the number of days attended. Both groups attending an average of 2.8 of the 7 days, compared to 2.3 and 3.3 days for the $0/$1 and $5/$10 conditions in the Svikis, Lee, et al. (1997) report. Although the authors suggest that some methodological differences in the way attendance data were collected in the two studies may account for differences across studies, it is also likely that the magnitude of the reinforcer was too low to reliably change attendance behavior.

The final study in this series focused solely on MM pregnant women and was designed to address both attendance and drug abstinence (Jones, Haug, Silverman, Stitzer, & Svikis, 2001). Participants were randomized to either usual-care or CM conditions. In the CM condition, participants earned incentives for treatment attendance during the first 7 days of treatment (i.e., the inpatient portion of treatment). For the second 7 days of treatment, when participants transitioned to intensive outpatient treatment, participants earned incentives for both (1) attending treatment and (2) providing a cocaine-negative urine sample. An escalating-voucher schedule was used whereby the initial voucher was worth $5 but escalated $5 in value for each consecutive day that the target behavior(s) were met. Results indicate that participants in the CM condition attended significantly more days of treatment compared to the usual-care condition (6.9 vs. 6.6 days, respectively). Attendance in the CM condition was also greater when compared over the entire 14-day study period (12.1 vs. 10.6 days, respectively). The effect on cocaine-positive samples during the second 7-day period was also significant, with half as many positive samples in the CM condition compared to the usual-care condition (12% vs. 24%, respectively). The rate of opiate-positive samples was also significant and of a similar magnitude (7% vs. 18%, respectively).

The Therapeutic Workplace Studies

A series of studies by Wong and colleagues as part of the Therapeutic Workplace intervention described earlier have used CM to modify other types of behavior pertinent to the job setting, including productivity, on-time attendance, and completed work shifts. All three studies used a within-subjects ABA reversal design. Briefly, the target behavior was first measured during a baseline period (A), then an intervention was introduced (B) and the target behavior measured again, and finally the intervention was removed (return to A) and the target behavior measured again. In all phases of all three studies, the primary contingencies to promote abstinence and attendance described earlier were held constant. These studies experimentally manipulated the other more modest contingencies available for productivity and punctuality.

Wong et al. (2003) examined data entry productivity in six Therapeutic Workplace participants who demonstrated relatively variable and low data-entry response rates. Data entry productivity was monitored during a 5-week baseline period during which the standard workplace productivity incentives were in place (i.e., $1 for each batch of approximately 3,600 characters of data entered minus $0.02 for every error). During the 5-week intervention period, the reinforcement magnitude increased tenfold (i.e., $10 for each batch of data entered minus $0.20 for each error). A 4-week return-to-baseline period followed in which the standard incentives were once again in place. Four of the six study participants showed clear increases in data-entry productivity during the intervention period followed by decreases once the intervention was removed.

After about 3 years of participation in the Therapeutic Workplace intervention, a number of the participants were hired as data entry operators in the Therapeutic Workplace data entry business, Hopkins Data Services (Silverman et al., 2005). After being hired to work in the business, operators frequently arrived at work late and also did not work complete shifts. Concerned that this pattern of behavior might jeopardize the business and decrease the income of the operators, Wong, Dillon, Sylvest, and Silverman (2004a) examined the effect of a CM intervention in which batch completion bonuses were temporarily reduced if operators arrived late or failed to work a complete work shift. The first four individuals hired as data entry operators in the business participated. The percentage of operators arriving to work on time (9 A.M.) and working complete work shifts (5.5 hr) was monitored during a 70-day baseline period during which the standard batch completion bonus was in place (i.e., $5 for each batch completed minus $0.08 for every error) and there were no explicit contingencies in place related to either arrival time or work shift completion. During the 50-day intervention period, if operators arrived at the workplace after 9 A.M., they were not allowed to work that day. In addition, if they arrived late or worked less than 5.5 hours that day, their batch completion bonus was reduced to $1 per batch minus $0.02 per error. Nine consecutive days of sustained abstinence, on-time arrivals, and completed work shifts returned the batch completion bonus to the prereset value. A 60-day return-to-baseline period followed in which the standard bonus was once again in place. On average, operators arrived at work on time significantly more often during the intervention phase compared to the baseline phases (95% vs. 18%). Likewise, operators completed significantly more work shifts (76% vs. 4%).

While these results were striking, participants complained about having to arrive exactly at 9 A.M. and research staff reported it was aversive to enforce the punctuality contingency. A subsequent study (Wong, Dillon, Sylvest, & Silverman, 2004b) examined the effect of a very similar CM intervention in which the batch completion bonus was temporarily reduced if work shifts were not completed, but there were no longer any explicit contingencies on arrival time. The modified intervention assumed that the business would thrive as long as participants consistently worked complete work shifts, regardless of whether or not they arrived at work exactly on time. Five operators participated, including the four operators from the prior study. An 80-day baseline was followed by a 72-day intervention period in which the batch completion bonus was reduced as described earlier only if the participant failed to work a complete work shift. This was followed by a 148-day return to baseline. On average, participants completed significantly more work shifts during the intervention phase compared to the baseline phases (63% vs. 6%). Although there was no longer an explicit contingency upon on-time arrival, the authors report that participants arrived to work on time significantly more often during the intervention phase compared to the baseline phase. Overall, the modified CM intervention generally maintained the impressive increase in completed work shifts observed in the prior study. Further, combining a contingency on completed work shifts with the limited operating hours of the workplace (09:00–12:00 and 13:00–16:00) likely helped keep arrival times flexible but within reasonable boundaries.

DISSEMINATING USE OF CM INTERVENTIONS DURING PREGNANCY AND POSTPARTUM

Overall, the results of studies to date on the use of CM in the treatment of pregnant and postpartum women with substance use disorders suggest that CM significantly improves treatment outcomes in this population. Replications and extensions of the studies reviewed here, including trials by other groups of investigators, are needed to further strengthen this literature. However, the data are sufficiently compelling and the consequences of continued substance abuse during pregnancy sufficiently dire that dissemination of CM interventions for pregnant substance abusers appears warranted at this time. Two potential challenges facing dissemination of CM interventions with this population outside of the research clinic are (1) the setting and (2) the cost.

Setting

One setting for dissemination may already be in place in the form of comprehensive treatment clinics like the aforementioned Center for Addiction and Pregnancy in Baltimore (Jansson et al., 1996), and others like it (e.g., Center for Addiction Research Education and Services in Little Rock, Arkansas, Worley et al., 2005; Milagro Program in Albuquerque, New Mexico, Curet & Hsi, 2002). These multidisciplinary treatment programs, which often provide "one-stop shopping" for mental health/substance abuse treatment, obstetric care, family planning, pediatric and other services, may be especially receptive to and benefit from inclusion of CM interventions. Among more traditional substance abuse treatment programs, nearly 20% already have specialized programs or groups for pregnant and postpartum women (Substance Abuse and Mental Health Services Administration, 2004). Given their recognition of the unique needs of substance-abusing pregnant and postpartum women, they may also be more open to the addition of CM interventions.

Cost

The cost of CM interventions is often cited as a barrier to their dissemination. However, pregnant women are likely a population where cost is less of an issue for at least two reasons. First, although most people find the idea of a pregnant woman using drugs disturbing and difficult to understand, they are also sympathetic to the fact that the fetus is potentially being harmed. As a result, communities may be more willing to support CM interventions targeting substance abuse by a pregnant woman to protect the health of the fetus. One form of support already documented in this literature is donation of goods and services to be used as incentives. In the reports by Ker et al. (1996) and Donatelle et al. (2000) described previously, incentives for their smoking-cessation interventions where provided by or purchased with funds donated by community agencies. Chapter 15 (Amass & Kamien, this volume) also describes successful donation solicitation programs to supply incentives for CM interventions for substance-abusing pregnant and parenting women.

A second reason that the cost of CM interventions may be less of an issue when those interventions are directed at substance-abusing pregnant women is that cost-benefit analyses are relatively easily calculated and compelling in this population. For example, the U.S. national costs of smoking during pregnancy have been estimated at $704 per maternal smoker (Centers for Disease Control and Prevention, 2004), or $1,570 in 2006 dollars (e.g., Bodenheimer, 2005). These are conservative cost estimates in that they are limited to only those costs associated with initial neonatal hospital stays following delivery. Children of women who smoke during pregnancy have a 1.5- to 2.0-fold higher risk of subsequent hospitalizations often related to the sequelae of intrauterine growth retardation (Cnattingius, 2004), suggesting that the true costs are significantly higher. Thus, the economic benefit of reducing or eliminating substance abuse by pregnant women using CM interventions would appear to be quite economical and justifiable.

CONCLUDING COMMENTS

This chapter merits several comments and conclusions regarding the use of CM interventions to promote drug abstinence and other behavior change in pregnant and postpartum women with substance abuse disorders. The overarching point to be noted is that the evidence to date suggests that CM significantly improves treatment outcomes in this population. Consistent with research in nonpregnant populations, studies with single drug targets, an escalating CM schedule, relatively larger-magnitude reinforcement, and/or immediate voucher delivery tended to have positive outcomes. As such, this review provides evidence supporting the efficacy of this approach and suggests that dissemination efforts are warranted. To that end, this review also highlights a number of the innovative settings and funding strategies that researchers in this area have examined, including models such as the Therapeutic Workplace and creative and practical demonstrations of how CM programs can be funded outside the research clinic. Future research replicating and extending these findings will provide additional evidence to further develop the use of this promising intervention in this truly special population.

ACKNOWLEDGMENTS

Preparation of this chapter was supported in part by National Institute on Drug Abuse Research Grant Nos. DA018410 and DA14028.

REFERENCES

Bodenheimer, T. (2005). High and rising health care costs. Part 1: Seeking an explanation. *Annals of Internal Medicine, 142,* 847–854.

Bolnick, J. M., & Rayburn, W. F. (2003). Substance use disorders in women: Special considerations during pregnancy. *Obstetrics and Gynecology Clinics of North America, 30,* 545–548.

Brady, J. P., Posner, M., Lang, C., & Rosati, M. J. (1994). *Risk and reality: The implications of prenatal exposure to alcohol and other drugs.* Washington, DC: U.S. Department of Education.

Carroll, K. M., Chang, G., Behr, H. M., Clinton, B., & Kosten, T. R. (1995). Improving treatment outcome in pregnant, methadone-maintained women: Results from a randomized clinical trial. *American Journal on Addictions, 4,* 56–59.

Centers for Disease Control and Prevention. (2004, October 8). State estimates of neonatal health-care costs associated with maternal smoking—United States, 1996. *Morbidity and Mortality Weekly Report, 53,* 915–917.

Chang, G., Carroll, K. M., Behr, H. M., & Kosten, T. R. (1992). Improving treatment outcome in pregnant opiate-dependent women. *Journal of Substance Abuse Treatment, 9,* 327–330.

Chang, G., McNamara, T. K., Orav, E. J., Koby, D., Lavigne, A., Ludman, B., et al. (2005). Brief intervention for prenatal alcohol use: A randomized trial. *Obstetrics and Gynecology, 105,* 991–998.

Chang, G., Wilkins-Haug, L., Berman, S., & Goetz, M. A. (1999). Brief intervention for alcohol use in pregnancy: A randomized trial. *Addiction, 94,* 1499–1508.

Cnattingius, S. (2004). The epidemiology of smoking during pregnancy: Smoking prevalence, maternal characteristics, and pregnancy outcomes. *Nicotine and Tobacco Research, 6,* S125–S140.

Curet, H. B., & Hsi, A. C. (2002). Drug abuse during pregnancy. *Clinical Obstetrics and Gynecology, 45,* 73–88.

Daley, M., Argeriou, M., & McCarty, D. (1998). Substance abuse treatment for pregnant women: A window of opportunity? *Addictive Behaviors, 23,* 239–249.

Dempsey, D., Jacob, P., III, & Benowitz, N. (2002). Accelerated metabolism of nicotine and cotinine in pregnant smokers. *Journal of Pharmacology and Experimental Therapeutics, 301,* 594–598.

Donatelle, R. J., Prows, S. L., Champeau, D., & Hudson, D. (2000). Randomized controlled trial using social support and financial incentives for high risk pregnant smokers: Significant other supporter (SOS) program. *Tobacco Control, 9*(Suppl. III), iii67–iii69.

Elk, R., Mangus, L., Rhoades, H., Andres, R., & Grabowski, J. (1998). Cessation of cocaine use during pregnancy: Effects of contingency management interventions on maintaining abstinence and complying with prenatal care. *Addictive Behaviors, 23,* 57–64.

Elk, R., Schmitz, J., Manfredi, L., Rhoades, H., Andres, R., & Grabowski, J. (1994). Cessation of cocaine use during pregnancy: A preliminary comparison. *Addictive Behaviors, 19,* 697–702.

Elk, R., Schmitz, J., Spiga, R., Rhoades, H., Andres, R., & Grabowski, J. (1995). Behavioral treatment of cocaine-dependent pregnant women and TB-exposed patients. *Addictive Behaviors, 20,* 533–542.

Grella, C. (1997). Services for perinatal women with substance abuse and mental health disorders: The unmet need. *Journal of Psychoactive Drugs, 29,* 67–78.

Higgins, S. T., Budney, A. J., Bickel, W. K., Foerg, F. E., Donham, R., & Badger, G. J. (1994). Incentives improve outcome in outpatient behavioral treatment of cocaine dependence. *Archives of General Psychiatry, 51,* 568–576.

Higgins, S. T., Budney, A. J., Bickel, W. K., Hughes, J. R., Foerg, F., & Badger, G. (1993). Achieving cocaine abstinence with a behavioral approach. *American Journal of Psychiatry, 150,* 763–769.

Higgins, S. T., Delaney, D. D., Budney, A. J., Bickel, W. K., Hughes, J. R., Foerg, F., et al. (1991). A behavioral approach to achieving initial cocaine abstinence. *American Journal of Psychiatry, 148,* 1218–1224.

Higgins, S. T., Heil, S. H., Badger, G. J., Mongeon, J. A., Solomon, L. J., McHale, L., et al.

(2007). Biochemical verification of smoking status in pregnant and recently post-partum women. *Experimental and Clinical Psychopharmacology, 15,* 58–66.

Higgins, S. T., Heil, S. H., Solomon, L. J., Bernstein, I. M., Lussier, J. P., Abel, R. L., et al. (2004). A pilot study on voucher-based incentives to promote abstinence from ciga-rette smoking during pregnancy and postpartum. *Nicotine and Tobacco Research, 6,* 1015–1020.

Higgins, S. T., & Silverman, K. (Eds.). (1999). *Motivating behavior change among illicit drug abusers.* Washington, DC: American Psychological Association.

Hubbard, R. L., Marsden, M. E., Rachal, J. V., Harwood, H. J., Cavanaugh, E. R., & Ginzburg, H. M. (1989). *Drug abuse treatment: A national study of effectiveness.* Chapel Hill: University of North Carolina Press.

Jansson, L. M., Svikis, D., Lee, J., Paluzzi, P., Rutigliano, P., & Hackerman, F. (1996). Preg-nancy and addiction. A comprehensive care model. *Journal of Substance Abuse Treatment, 13,* 321–329.

Jones, H. E., Haug, N., Silverman, K., Stitzer, M., & Svikis, D. (2001). The effectiveness of incentives in enhancing treatment attendance and drug abstinence in methadone-maintained pregnant women. *Drug and Alcohol Dependence, 61,* 297–306.

Jones, H. E., Haug, N., Stitzer, M. L., & Svikis, D. (2000). Improving treatment outcomes for pregnant drug-dependent women using low-magnitude voucher incentives. *Ad-dictive Behaviors, 25,* 263–267.

Jones, H. E., Svikis, D., Rosado, J., Tuten, M., & Kulstad, J. L. (2004). What if they do not want treatment?: Lessons learned from intervention studies of non-treatment-seeking, drug-using pregnant women. *American Journal on Addictions, 13,* 342–357.

Ker, M., Leischow, S., Markowitz, I. B., & Merikle, E. (1996). Involuntary smoking cessa-tion: A treatment option. *Journal of Psychoactive Drugs, 28,* 47–60.

Little, B. B., Snell, L. M., Van Beveren, T. T., Crowell, R. B., Trayler, S., & Johnston, W. L. (2003). Treatment of substance abuse during pregnancy and infant outcome. *Ameri-can Journal of Perinatology, 20,* 255–262.

Lussier, J. P., Heil, S. H., Mongeon, J. A., Badger, G. J., & Higgins, S. T. (2006). A meta-analysis of voucher-based reinforcement therapy for substance use disorders. *Addic-tion, 101,* 192–203.

McCaul, M. E., & Svikis, D. S. (1996). Measures of service utilization. *NIDA Research Monograph, 166,* 225–241.

McCaul, M. E., Svikis, D. S., & Feng, T. (1991). Pregnancy and addiction: Outcomes and interventions. *Maryland Medical Journal, 40,* 995–1001.

Melvin, C. L., Dolan-Mullen, P., Windsor, R. A., Whiteside, H. P. Jr., & Goldenberg, R. L. (2000). Recommended cessation counseling for pregnant women who smoke: A re-view of the evidence. *Tobacco Control, 9*(Suppl. 3), III80–III84.

Melvin, C. L., & Gaffney, C. A. (2004). Treating nicotine use and dependence of pregnant and parenting smokers: An update. *Nicotine and Tobacco Research, 6*(Suppl. 2), S107–S124.

National Center on Addiction and Substance Abuse at Columbia University. (2006). Preg-nancy and substance abuse. In *Women under the influence* (pp. 103–130). Baltimore: Johns Hopkins University Press.

Nekhayeva, I. A., Nanovskaya, T. N., Deshmukh, S. V., & Zharikova, O. L. (2005). Bidirectional transfer of methadone across human placenta. *Biochemical Pharmacol-ogy, 69,* 187–197.

Office of the Surgeon General. (2001). *Women and smoking: A report of the Surgeon Gen-eral.* Rockville, MD: Centers for Disease Control and Prevention.

Pitts, K. S., & Weinstein, L. (1990). Cocaine and pregnancy—A lethal combination. *Journal of Perinatology, 10,* 180–182.

Pollack, H., Lantz, P. M., & Frohna, J. G. (2000). Maternal smoking and adverse birth outcomes among singletons and twins. *American Journal of Public Health, 90,* 395–400.

Pond, S. M., Kreek, M. J., Tong, T. G., Raghunath, J., & Benowitz, N. L. (1985). Altered methadone pharmacokinetics in methadone-maintained pregnant women. *Journal of Pharmacology and Experimental Therapeutics, 233,* 1–6.

Rebagliato, M., Bolumar, F., Florey Cdu, V., Jarvis, M. J., Perez-Hoyos, S., Hernandez-Aguado, I., et al. (1998). Variations in cotinine levels in smokers during and after pregnancy. *American Journal of Obstetrics and Gynecology, 178,* 568–571.

Richter, L., & Richter, D. M. (2001). Exposure to parental tobacco and alcohol use: Effects on children's health and development. *American Journal of Orthopsychiatry, 71,* 182–203.

Roland, E. H., & Volpe, J. J. (1989). Effect of maternal cocaine use on the fetus and newborn: Review of the literature. *Pediatric Neuroscience, 15,* 88–94.

Roll, J. M., & Higgins, S. T. (2000). A within-subject comparison of three different schedules of reinforcement of drug abstinence using cigarette smoking as an exemplar. *Drug and Alcohol Dependence, 58,* 103–109.

Rosenak, D., Diamant, Y. Z., Yaffe, H., & Hornstein, E. (1990). Cocaine: Maternal use during pregnancy and its effects on the mother, fetus, and the infant. *Obstetrical and Gynecological Survey, 45,* 348–359.

Silverman, K., Svikis, D., Robles, E., Stitzer, M. L., & Bigelow, G. E. (2001). A reinforcement-based therapeutic workplace for the treatment of drug abuse: Six-month abstinence outcomes. *Experimental and Clinical Psychopharmacology, 9,* 14–23.

Silverman, K., Svikis, D., Wong, C. J., Hampton, J., Stitzer, M. L., & Bigelow, G. E. (2002). A reinforcement-based therapeutic workplace for the treatment of drug abuse: Three-year abstinence outcomes. *Experimental and Clinical Psychopharmacology, 10,* 228–240.

Silverman, K., Wong, C. J., Grabinski, M. J., Hampton, J., Sylvest, C. E., Dillon, E. M., et al. (2005). A web-based therapeutic workplace for the treatment of drug addiction and chronic unemployment. *Behavior Modification, 29,* 417–463.

Solomon, L. J., & Quinn, V. P. (2004). Spontaneous quitting: Self-initiated smoking cessation during early pregnancy. *Nicotine and Tobacco Research, 6*(Suppl. 2), S203–S216.

SRNT Subcommittee on Biochemical Verification. (2002). Biochemical verification of tobacco use and cessation. *Nicotine and Tobacco Research, 4,* 149–159.

Substance Abuse and Mental Health Services Administration. (2004). *National Survey of Substance Abuse Treatment Services (N-SSATS).* Rockville, MD: Author.

Substance Abuse and Mental Health Services Administration. (2005). *Substance use during pregnancy: 2002 and 2003 update.* Rockville, MD: Author.

Svikis, D. S., Golden, A. S., Huggins, G. R., Pickens, R. W., McCaul, M. E., Velez, M. L., et al. (1997). Cost-effectiveness of treatment for drug-abusing pregnant women. *Drug and Alcohol Dependence, 45,* 105–113.

Svikis, D. S., Lee, J. H., Haug, N. A., & Stitzer, M. L. (1997). Attendance incentives for outpatient treatment: Effects in methadone- and nonmethadone-maintained pregnant drug-dependent women. *Drug and Alcohol Dependence, 48,* 33–41.

Weinberg, N. Z. (1997). Cognitive and behavioral deficits associated with prenatal alcohol use. *Journal of the American Academy of Child and Adolescent Psychiatry, 36,* 1177–1186.

Wolff, K., Boys, A., Rostami-Hodjegan, A., Hay, A., & Raistrick, D. (2005). Changes to methadone clearance during pregnancy. *European Journal of Clinical Pharmacology, 61,* 763–768.

Wong, C. J., Dillon, E. M., Sylvest, C., & Silverman, K. (2004a). Contingency management of reliable attendance of chronically unemployed substance abusers in a therapeutic workplace. *Experimental and Clinical Psychopharmacology, 12,* 39–46.

Wong, C. J., Dillon, E. M., Sylvest, C., & Silverman, K. (2004b). Evaluation of a modified contingency management intervention for consistent attendance in therapeutic workplace participants. *Drug and Alcohol Dependence, 74,* 319–323.

Wong, C. J., Sheppard, J. M., Dallery, J., Bedient, G., Robles, E., Svikis, D., et al. (2003). Effects of reinforcer magnitude on data-entry productivity in chronically unemployed drug abusers participating in a therapeutic workplace. *Experimental and Clinical Psychopharmacology, 11,* 46–55.

Woods Jr., J. R. (1995). Clinical management of drug dependency in pregnancy. *NIDA Research Monograph, 149,* 39–57.

Worley, L. L., Conners, N. A., Crone, C. C., Williams, V. L., & Bokony, P. A. (2005). Building a residential treatment program for dually diagnosed women with their children. *Archives of Women's Mental Health, 8,* 105–111.

Wrighton, S. A., & Stevens, J. C. (1992). The human hepatic cytochrome P450 involved in drug metabolism. *Critical Reviews in Toxicology, 22,* 1–21.

Young, N. (1997). Alcohol and other drugs: The scope of the problem among pregnant and parenting women in California. *Journal of Psychoactive Drugs, 29,* 3–22.

CHAPTER 11

PEOPLE WITH MENTAL ILLNESS

Jennifer W. Tidey *and* Richard K. Ries

PREVALENCE AND IMPACT

Alcohol and other substance use disorders (SUDs) are highly prevalent among people with serious mental illness (SMI) in the United States. Epidemiological surveys have reported that 29% of people with any lifetime mental disorder also have a lifetime history of an addictive disorder, and this rate is higher (47%) for people with a SMI such as schizophrenia (Regier et al., 1990). Likewise, rates of cigarette smoking among people with SMI are approximately two to five times higher than in the general population (de Leon & Diaz, 2005; Lasser et al., 2000).

The co-occurrence of SMI and SUDs (SMI–SUDs) is a significant public health problem in the United States because of its association with a variety of negative outcomes. People with SMI–SUDs require longer and more intensive treatment and can have particularly poor medication and treatment compliance, leading to exacerbation of symptoms and increased utilization of health services (e.g., Rounsaville, Weissman, Kleber, & Wilber, 1982; Shaner et al., 1995). The list of negative outcomes from co-occurring disorders is long and includes homelessness, joblessness, incarceration, violence, and HIV (human immunodeficiency virus) and hepatitis C infection (Drake, Mueser, Brunette, & McHugo, 2004).

INTEGRATED TREATMENTS FOR PATIENTS WITH CO-OCCURRING DISORDERS

Since the early 1980s, there has been increasing recognition that the practice of addressing these patients' co-occurring disorders with separate SMI and SUDs treatments, whether delivered serially or in parallel, can lead to fragmentation and gaps in care (Drake et al., 2004; Center for Substance Abuse Treatment [CSAT], 1994). Currently, the most promising outpatient treatments are comprehensive programs with multidisciplinary teams that address engagement, motivation and retention through assertive outreach, motivational interventions, and cultural competence (Drake et al., 2004; CSAT, 2005; Ziedonis et al., 2005). Although some integrated treatment programs have produced good outcomes in terms of rehabilitation, decreased hospitalization, and other social variables (Drake et al., 2004), the Cochrane review of integrated treatment of SUDs–SMI disorders from 2000 concluded that "there is no clear advantage of any type of substance misuse programme for those with serious mental illness over the value of standard care" (Jeffrey, Ley, McLaren, & Siegfried, 2000). Thus, it remains unclear whether wraparound integrated treatment for SUDs–SMI, as described above, is particularly effective for substance abuse.

Fully integrated models are complex and costly, involving co-trained staff, and integrated facilities, policies, and even funding streams (CSAT, 2005). Others have commented that although some treatment centers are engaged in the provision of fully integrated substance abuse and mental health rehabilitation treatment, most are not overly successful in changing substance use, though they may have other positive outcomes. Several other strategies have been investigated for targeting SUD in the context of mental health provision. The most effective of these to date have been motivational interviewing combined with cognitive-behavioral therapy and family education (Barrowclough et al., 2001) and an eclectic approach combining aspects of motivational interviewing, contingency management, social-skills training, coping-skills training, and relapse prevention (Bennett, Bellack, & Gearon, 2001). However, these models also require extensive staff training and integration and likely will also face the same barriers to adoption that the other more complex models face. Finally, as found in a national survey (Watkins, Burnam, Kung, & Paddock, 2001), fully integrated substance abuse treatment for patients with SMI rarely occurs. Thus, providers of service to those with severe mental disorders who want to target substance abuse in their patients face two large initial barriers in using the fully integrated models: (1) the data are not highly compelling regarding changes to substance abuse; and (2) high costs, integration of staff, and regulatory issues hinder wide adoption, as found in Watkins et al. (2001). Clearly, more feasible and effective models are needed.

In the following sections we propose some methods of contingency management (CM) focusing solely on substance abuse delivered in the context of ongoing mental health care. The goal would be to provide efficacious service with a model which could easily be added to most mental health treatment systems with little effort or expense relative to other substance abuse treatment strategies that have been tried. Although it is likely that other, more complicated and wraparound services may be needed for ongoing vocational rehabilitation and substance and mental illness recovery of this population (U.S. Department of Health and Human Services [USDHHS], 2005), a practical method of initial engagement and treatment of substance abuse, especially stimulant abuse, in this population needs to be developed and documented. The following section begins by reviewing results from Phase 1 (efficacy) studies of CM's effects in SMI populations.

CM INTERVENTIONS FOR POPULATIONS WITH SMI

CM techniques have a long history of use in the treatment of persons with SMI (Ullman & Krasner, 1965). These types of interventions have been used to reinstate verbal behavior (Isaacs, Thomas, & Goldiamond, 1960), modify eating behavior (Ayllon & Michael, 1959), increase appropriate activity levels (Haughton & Ayllon, 1965; King, Armitage, & Tilton, 1960), and increase prosocial activity (Hingtgen, Sanders, & DeMeyer, 1965). CM has also been demonstrated, in a number of Phase 1 studies, to be successful at reducing the drug use of persons suffering from SMI (reviewed below). In a recent article, Carroll (2004) suggested that on the basis of this preliminary work and the large body of evidence supporting CM for treating drug abuse, CM would likely be an effective treatment component for addressing the substance use of individuals with a comorbid SMI.

Psychotic Disorders

Approximately 20% of patients with schizophrenia use cocaine (Regier et al., 1990; Swartz et al., 2006). Cocaine use in these patients can lead to poor medication compliance, worsening of psychotic symptoms, and high utilization of emergency services (Shaner et al., 1995). In an influential study, Shaner et al. (1995) examined how cocaine use, psychiatric symptoms, and psychiatric hospitalizations were influenced by the availability of disability income. These data were collected over a 15-week period, collapsed into 10 3-day bins, and then averaged to produce a prototypical month. The results of this analysis showed the influence of time of month on cocaine use and psychiatric admissions: cocaine use, psychiatric symptoms and hospitalizations are shown to sharply increase at the beginning of the month, after the delivery of disability payments (Shaner et al., 1995; although see Ries, Short, Dyck, & Srebnik, 2004).

The findings from the Shaner et al. (1995) study suggested that the availability of disability benefits can strongly influence cocaine use among people with schizophrenia. A logical extension of this work was to test whether introducing an abstinence contingency on these benefits could reduce cocaine use in these patients. In a preliminary study, a within-subjects reversal design was used with two male veterans with refractory cocaine abuse. When a CM program was initiated in which the patients could earn $25 per day to remain cocaine abstinent, cocaine use decreased significantly (Shaner et al., 1997). In another small-scale pilot study, Roll, Chermack, and Chudzynski (2004) examined the feasibility of a voucher-reinforced CM intervention for cocaine abuse in people with schizophrenia. Three male veterans with schizophrenia were enrolled in a 8-week study that used a within-subjects A B A design. In this study design, participants serve as their own control during an pretreatment baseline (no intervention) condition (A), the intervention condition (B), and a posttreatment baseline (no intervention) condition (A). The study was conducted in an outpatient day hospital program in a Veterans Administration medical center. During the two, 2-week baseline phases, participants were transported to the program daily (Monday–Friday), where they gave urine samples three times per week and were reinforced with $3 worth of VA-redeemable vouchers, regardless of immunoassay results. During the 4-week CM phase, vouchers were contingent upon a cocaine-negative urine specimen according to an escalating schedule of reinforcement. Results indicated a significant decrease in cocaine-positive samples during the intervention phase (Roll et al., 2004).

Despite the positive results in the Roll et al. (2004) study, one finding of that study was that abstinent samples were only provided during the first 2 weeks of the CM intervention. In their discussion of the findings, the investigators suggest that embedding the voucher-based reinforcement therapy (VBRT) into a more comprehensive treatment program might prolong the period of abstinence (Roll et al., 2004). Doing exactly this using a randomized controlled trial, Ries et al. (2004) demonstrated that allowing persons with SMI greater control over their own finances in a representative payee system, contingent upon drug/alcohol abstinence and treatment attendance, significantly decreased drug and alcohol use (Ries et al., 2004). In this study, the patients' clinical case managers filled out weekly logs with the patients, which included ratings of money management, treatment attendance and substance use. A logic system was attached to the log, each week providing patients with gold, silver, or red awards, each with a motivational message, but also directing the patients' study payments to be all vouchers, half voucher and half cash, or all cash (with patients receiving higher cash-voucher ratios when they accomplished treatment goals). A secondary contingent logic also directed the patients' social security disability payments to be given out in a range of frequencies (biweekly to daily) and forms (vouchers or cash) according to accumulated scores for each week, across a month of scores. Thus, drug abstinence and the accomplishment of other treatment goals were reinforced with higher degrees of freedom over one's own resources.

The advantage of the contingency reward method used in the Ries et al. (2004) study is that it includes a long-term, real-world supply of reward (i.e., the distribution of social security disability payments). Social security law mandates that patients who receive such mental disability payments and show repeated problems in managing their own assets are required to have a responsible other as payee, and Ries and Dyck (1997) found that about two-thirds of public mental health centers in Washington State did this for some of their patients. However, this system does require the mental health provider to create a banking and managing system for disability payments. In terms of substance outcomes, the results of the Ries et al. (2004) study were statistically significant but only moderate in size. It is possible that if this study had focused only on substance use in its contingency scheme, rather than also including money management and treatment attendance, a more powerful effect on drug use outcomes could have been demonstrated. This more focused type of study remains to be performed.

Another form of substance abuse that is highly prevalent among people with schizophrenia is cigarette smoking (de Leon & Diaz, 2005). A recent meta-analysis found that people with schizophrenia are three times more likely to initiate smoking and five times less likely to quit than the general population (de Leon & Diaz, 2005). Smoking leads to high rates of morbidity and mortality in these patients (Goff et al., 2005). Given CM's efficacy at promoting cigarette smoking reductions and treatment retention in nonpsychiatric smokers, a natural extension of this work was to test the efficacy of CM for smoking reductions in smokers with schizophrenia. Roll, Higgins, Steingard, and McGinley (1998) first used a within-subjects A B A design to examine the effects of contingent monetary reinforcement on abstinence. During each condition, carbon monoxide (CO) levels were measured three times per day for 5 consecutive days in subjects' homes or another agreed-on location. During the CM intervention period, CO levels < 12 parts per million (ppm) were reinforced with cash, according to an escalating schedule. Results indicated that, during the CM intervention period, the number of CO samples that met the abstinence criterion increased fourfold and average CO values decreased by more than 50%. These results were later replicated with a similar CM intervention (Tidey, O'Neill, & Higgins, 2002). In addition, results from a laboratory analogue study indicated that smokers with schizophrenia reduced their smoking by about 50% when they were given the choice between responding for monetary reinforcement and responding for cigarette puffs (Tidey, Higgins, Bickel, & Steingard, 1999). The major challenge of translating these laboratory-based or short-term CM smoking studies into viable smoking treatment programs is the high frequency of CO monitoring necessary to verify abstinence. Some researchers have switched to using urinary or salivary cotinine levels to verify abstinence. The long half-life of cotinine (16 hours or longer) reduces the frequency of monitoring to twice weekly, which makes longer interventions more feasible (e.g., Higgins et al., 2004). Although quantitative cotinine analysis presently requires expensive laboratory equipment, some laboratories have begun using inexpensive, semiquantitative dipsticks to assess cotinine level. We are presently conducting a CM smoking study in which smokers with schizophrenia are reinforced for smoking reductions that are verified with reduced urinary cotinine levels, and the preliminary results from this study are promising (Tidey, Rohsenow, Kaplan, & Swift, 2005).

Another study, which built on the promising results of CM for smoking reductions in outpatients with schizophrenia, addressed marijuana use in these patients (Sigmon, Steingard, Badger, Anthony, & Higgins, 2000). In this study, 18 outpatients who were marijuana users were enrolled into a 25-week study that included five 5-week conditions: an initial baseline condition in which participants received monetary reinforcement regardless of urinalysis results; three contingent conditions in which the amount of contingent monetary reinforcement was $25, $50, or $100 per sample; and a second noncontingent baseline condition at the end of the study. Throughout the study, participants submitted urine samples twice weekly for urinalysis. Results indicated that marijuana use responded systematically to the incentive conditions, with the $100 incentive condition producing the most abstinence. CM more than doubled the duration of continuous marijuana abstinence. However, this study had high attrition and four participants (heavier users) did not respond to the contingencies. Thus, results indicate that, in general, marijuana use in these patients responded to monetary contingencies, but heavy users may be less sensitive to these contingencies.

Finally, two studies have examined the use of CM to reduce drinking and other undesirable behaviors among veterans with schizophrenia (Peniston, 1988; Helmus, Saules, Schoener, & Roll, 2003). Using a multiple baseline design, 15 patients in an open psychiatric unit received positive reinforcement and response-cost contingency interventions to reduce verbal abuse, poor grooming, poor treatment attendance, and excessive drinking. The interventions were successful for changing most target behaviors but were less successful in the patients who had drinking behavior problems (Peniston, 1988). In a more recent study that is reviewed in the next section, Helmus et al. (2003) also investigated the effects of CM for treating alcohol abuse in patients with SMI including patients with schizophrenia and schizo-affective disorder.

Overall, the results of these studies offer consistent evidence that CM interventions reduce cigarette smoking and psychomotor stimulant use in people with schizophrenia. Few other drug disorders have been targeted in these patients. The particular challenges of using CM for these patients are stemming attrition and translating these short-term efficacy studies into sustainable treatment approaches.

Mood and Anxiety Disorders

Helmus et al. (2003) investigated the effectiveness of CM for treating alcohol abuse in patients with SMI, within a community-based dual diagnosis treatment program. Patients with MDD (35%; $n = 7$), bipolar I disorder (30%; $n = 6$), schizoaffective disorder (20%; $n = 4$) and schizophrenia (15%; $n = 3$) participated in this 20-week, A B A design study. In the first baseline phase (Weeks 1–4), patients attended twice-weekly group counseling sessions as part of the standard treatment regimen. In the CM intervention period (Weeks 5–16), patients were reinforced for on-time group attendance and alcohol-negative breathalyzer readings. This was followed by a return-to-baseline phase in Weeks 17–20. The reinforcer during the CM intervention was a $2.50 gift certificate to a local retail store. Results indicated that all breathalyzer results, regardless of phase, were negative during this study. Attendance rates significantly improved during the CM phase relative to the baseline phase, and remained elevated during the return-to-baseline phase. Average per-patient cost of the program was low: $31.50 per participant. Thus, these results indicate that a relatively low-cost and low-impact CM intervention can significantly improve treatment attendance in a community-based dual-diagnosis treatment program, and the results may extend at least 4 weeks past the incentive period.

Mental illness and SUD are associated with homelessness, which in turn can lead to less treatment for these disorders (Kushel, Hahn, Evans, Bansberg, & Moss, 2005). Milby et al. (2000) have developed for homeless, cocaine-dependent individuals, a CM intervention that includes abstinence-contingent access to rent-free housing and paid employment. In a secondary data analysis, McNamara, Schumacher, Milby, Wallace, and Usdan (2001) compared treatment outcomes in 46 (36%) participants who did not have a concurrent psychiatric diagnosis with 82 (64%) participants who had one or more psychiatric disorders (most commonly mood disorders and anxiety disorders). At baseline, the dually diagnosed participants had more severe medical, family, social, employment, and psychiatric problems and were more likely to be alcohol dependent than those with SUDs alone. However, at 6-month follow-up, both groups had made significant gains in functioning in these life areas, including significant increases in days of stable housing and days of full-time employment. Notably, the dually diagnosed patients stayed in treatment as long and did as well as the individuals who did not have an additional mental disorder.

Depression is common among people with co-occurring cocaine and opiate dependence (Rounsaville et al., 1982). Although desipramine treatment (DMI) has had mixed success in cocaine users who have comorbid depression (e.g., Ziedonis & Kosten, 1991; Kosten, Falcioni, Oliveto, & Feingold, 2004), CM procedures increased the effectiveness of desipramine in a 12-week double-blind, placebo-controlled randomized controlled trial (RCT) (Kosten et al., 2003). In that study, patients were initially stabilized with buprenorphine, and then assigned to one of four conditions: DMI (150 mg/day) + CM, DMI + yoked control (YC), placebo + CM, or placebo + YC. Clean urine samples were reinforced with vouchers of escalating value for consecutive abstinence (CM group) or were independent of voucher value (YC group). In a secondary analysis of data from the Kosten et al. (2003) study, treatment response in patients with a history of major depressive disorder (MDD; $n = 53$; 45% female) was compared to response in patients without a history of MDD (never depressed (ND); $n = 96$; 28% female; Gonzalez, Feingold, Oliveto, Gonsai, & Kosten, 2003). CM was shown to be effective for reducing drug use in both the MDD and ND patients; however, there was severe attrition in the MDD + CM group (only 31% were retained). Thus, results of this study indicate that CM may be beneficial for treating opiate and cocaine abuse in people with major depression, if these patients can be retained in treatment (Gonzalez et al., 2003).

MDD is strongly associated with higher current and lifetime rates of cigarette smoking, although not with lower quit rates (Lasser et al., 2000). We were unable to find any published reports that tested the effectiveness of CM for smoking cessation in people with a diagnosis of major depression. However, Gilbert, Crauthers, Mooney, McClernon, and Jensen (1999) examined whether trait depression affected response to monetary contingencies in a 1-month trial. Smokers ($n = 56$) who expressed a desire to quit underwent a 3-week baseline phase that involved biweekly monitoring of smoking status. The Minnesota Multiphasic Personality Inventory (MMPI; Dahlstrom, Welsh, & Dahlstrom, 1972) and the NEO-Personality Inventory (NEO-PI; Costa & McCrae, 1985) were administered during the baseline period, and scales from these measures were tested as potential moderators of outcome. Participants were then randomized to either an immediate-quit group or a delayed-quit group. In the immediate-quit group, participants were monitored biweekly and could receive $300 plus their $50 deposit only if they were abstinent (CO < 9) throughout the 31-day period. In the delayed-quit group, participants were monitored equally frequently during the 31-day period but only had to meet an abstinence contingency on days 32–33. Results indicated that 88% of the immediate-quit group and 15% of the delayed-quit group remained abstinent during the 31-day study period, indicating a strong effect of the contingency upon abstinence ($p < .001$). Abstainers in both groups relapsed equally soon after the contingency period ended. Higher scores on the NEO-PI Depression subscale significantly predicted shorter time to relapse (Gilbert et al., 1999). Thus, the effects of the CM intervention used in this study were not sustained as long in individuals with trait depression. The authors note that abstinence-provoked increases in state depressive mood may mediate the relationship between trait depression and time to relapse (Gilbert et al., 1999).

Antisocial Personality Disorder and Novelty Seeking

Antisocial personality disorder (ASPD) is strongly associated with drug and alcohol problems, and drug abusers with ASPD are more likely to engage in criminal activities, aggressive behaviors, and HIV risk behaviors than are drug abusers without ASPD (Brooner, Schmidt, Felch, & Bigelow, 1992; Compton, Cottler, Shillington, & Price, 1995). Psychosocial treatments have had little effect on SUDs in people with ASPD, leading to the recommendation of highly structured behavioral therapies, including contingent incentives, for these patients (Valliant, 1975). Accordingly, Brooner, Kidorf, King, and Stoller (1998) evaluated the effectiveness of a 28-week treatment program for 40 antisocial opioid abusers enrolled in a methadone program that included a CM intervention. During the 4-week baseline period, patients were stabilized on methadone, were assigned to a study counselor, and provided weekly, randomly scheduled urine samples that were assayed for opiates, cocaine, and other drugs. Next, patients were randomly assigned to the 6-month CM or control condition. In the CM condition, drug-negative urine specimens and counseling attendance were reinforced with methadone take-home doses, dose alterations, and more control over the frequency of counseling sessions. Patients randomized to the control arm were scheduled to attend two counseling sessions per week and had their methadone doses and schedules managed according to standard clinical practice.

Results from the first 17 weeks of this study indicated that patients in both groups had good responses to treatment during this time. These groups submitted similarly high numbers of opioid-negative and cocaine-negative urine specimens and had similarly high rates of counseling attendance during the randomized treatment period. Therefore, perhaps because of the unexpectedly good response to treatment in the control group, there was no evidence to support the greater effectiveness of the CM condition in this study, at least at the Month 3 time point (Brooner et al., 1998).

Silverman et al. (1998) compared the responses of 59 methadone-maintenance (MM) patients with ASPD (19%) and those without ASPD to VBRT with a start-up bonus, VBRT with no bonus, or control treatment. Results indicated that both of the contingent groups had higher levels of cocaine and opiate abstinence than did the control group, and that ASPD did not moderate treatment outcome. Like the Brooner et al. (1998) study, this study had a small sample size and may have been underpowered to detect differences between the ASPD and non-ASPD groups.

Low treatment retention is a significant problem in substance abuse treatment, and may be particularly challenging for treating substance abusers who are high novelty seekers (Kravitz, Fawcett, McGuire, Kravitz, & Whitney, 1999). Given that CM interventions can have a powerful effect on treatment retention, one study investigated whether VBRT could improve treatment retention in a 17-week intervention for opiate dependence that combined buprenorphine and VBRT (Helmus, Downey, Arfken, Henderson, & Schuster, 2001). Of the 68 participants enrolled, 25% met DSM criteria for ASPD and 34% met criteria for other disorders. All had a diagnosis of opiate dependence and most had other SUD diagnoses. The Tridimensional Personality Questionnaire (TPQ; Cloninger, Przybeck, & Svrakic, 1991) was administered at baseline to assess the personality dimensions of Novelty Seeking, Harm Avoidance, and Reward Dependence. During the active intervention phase, participants were randomized to one of three groups: VBRT, reduced-value VBRT, or YC. Results of this study were negative with regard to the VBRT intervention, as the overall attrition rate was high (63%) and intervention condition did not affect either retention or abstinence. ASPD diagnosis was associated with higher TPQ Novelty Seeking scale scores and high novelty seekers were more likely to drop out of treatment before 17 weeks (Helmus et al., 2001). Thus, these results suggest that when trying to improve treatment retention, substance abusers with ASPD may need a larger magnitude or frequency of reinforcement than non-ASPD substance abusers.

Finally, Messina, Farabee, and Rawson (2003) examined responses of 120 methadone-maintained, cocaine-dependent patients (44% with ASPD) to cognitive-behavioral therapy (CBT), VBRT, a combination of these therapies, or a treatment-as-usual control group (MM). The CBT intervention consisted of three group sessions per week during the 16-week intervention period. Participants in the CM group provided thrice-weekly urine samples and meet briefly with the CM technician to review the urinalysis results and receive a voucher, if earned, or an earned item. Voucher values escalated with consecutive abstinent samples and participants were given bonuses for three consecutive stimulant-negative specimens (Higgins et al., 1994). All patients received identical MM services. Results indicated no between-groups differences with regard to treatment retention or rates of missing urine samples. Surprisingly, ASPD patients had higher cocaine abstinence rates than did non-ASPD patients across all treatment conditions, with highest abstinence rates in the CM-alone and CBT + CM conditions. This pattern of response was also seen for the non-ASPD patients, but the effect of condition was not significant. At the 1-year follow-up, abstinence rates remained high for the ASPD patients throughout the follow-up period, even after the incentives were removed. In contrast, abstinence rates for the non-

ASPD patients in the CBT group had increased, but abstinence rates for patients in the other conditions had declined. These results suggest that substance abusers with ASPD may be more responsive to treatment than previously believed, particularly when that treatment includes contingent reinforcement for abstinence (Messina et al., 2003).

Overall, this review of Phase I efficacy studies indicates consistently positive outcomes for effects of CM interventions on SUD in patients with schizophrenia. Many of these studies have been of short duration and were conducted in highly controlled settings. It remains to be seen whether the positive effects of CM on smoking in these patients will be replicated by longer-term studies conducted in less intensive settings. In patients with depression, anxiety disorders, and ASPD, results of CM interventions have been more mixed. Positive effects of CM have been found on cocaine and/ or opiate abstinence (Messina et al., 2003; Silverman et al., 1998), cigarette smoking, and treatment attendance (Helmus et al., 2003), but negative effects on retention have also been reported (Gonzalez et al., 2003). Unlike the studies of CM's effects in patients with schizophrenia, the studies of CM for SUDs in mood, anxiety, and ASPD patients have been conducted in longer-term treatment programs, and this may account, at least in part, for the fact that their results have been less consistently positive. Nevertheless, results of these Phase 1 studies set the stage for conducting large-scale, Phase 2 clinical trials of CM for treating SUDs in people with SMIs. These treatment programs are subject to the same critiques as are CM treatments for SUDs in people without SMIs, such as concerns about costs and the need for specialized training. Other questions are more specific to patients with SMIs. A discussion of methods of approaching these problems follows.

FACTORS THAT MAY LIMIT THE EFFECTIVENESS OF CM FOR SUDs IN PEOPLE WITH MENTAL ILLNESS

Who Will Pay?

Interestingly enough, it is the practice of most moderate-to-large community mental health centers (CMHCs) to link with their communities and receive donations of food vouchers, clothing, household items, and even tickets to community functions such as sporting events (also see Amass & Kamien, 2004). Two CMHCs in downtown Seattle, with which we are familiar, receive over $100,000 a year in such donations. It is our experience that community businesses are much friendlier to donations if it is clear that these donations are going to patients who are actively participating in treatment. Most community businesses know that substance abuse is a serious problem for persons with SMI, because they see the evidence of this problem on their doorsteps, sidewalks, and streets. Many business donors like the idea of giving, but even more like the idea of giving when they know their gifts will result in improved health for public patients, and thus their communities. Businesses also understand the fundamental theories behind CM, as they are accustomed to rewarding employees who work harder and are more productive. However, the culture of the public mental health system has historically been more socialistic, with disability benefits going to patients for their illness, not participation in recovery; and payments to providers for service, not recovery outcomes.

Another potential source of funds, noted previously, is that many CMHCs receive a portion of their patients' social security benefit checks (Ries & Dyck, 1997). The representative payee program is part of social security law, which mandates that if a recipient with disabilities is too psychotic, confused, substance affected, or otherwise unable to make responsible use of their disability funds, then they are required to have a representative payee. Many times the payee is a family member; however, putting a family member in this role can make the family member a target for hostility and even violence. If the disability payment instead comes to the CMHC, the clinic could link the receipt of funds with participation in treatment services. CMHCs that were recently surveyed (Ries & Dyck, 1997) reported that most used some sort of contingency, such as manipulating the frequency or form of disability monies disbursement, to incentivize attendance or other target behaviors. However, they also stated that they lacked clear guidelines as how to increase the effectiveness of this system. A possible model of CM around disability monies was developed by Ries et al. (2004), and it is still functioning and self-sufficient 5 years later.

Cognitive Limitations and Complexity

One concern about using CM for treating SUDs in people with SMI is that, although the concreteness and structure of CM are advantages, the reinforcement schedules can be difficult to understand. Cognitive deficits associated with some SMI could limit patients' abilities to understand the contingencies. Certainly, reinforcement schedules that involve payment escalation and reset contingencies can be complicated to explain to both patients and staff. We have found that patients easily grasp the general essence of CM and that the more specific aspects of the reinforcement schedule become clear once the patients begin to make contact with the contingencies.

Most CMHCs see most of their patients several times per week, especially patients who are more severely ill, which often includes patients with co-occurring SUDs. Thus a potential infrastructure for a CM intervention is available. However, as noted earlier, when more complexity enters an added-on treatment, it becomes harder to incorporate. Studies will eventually need to evaluate differing degrees of complexity in the trade-off with efficacy and longevity. For example, the most simple CM paradigm we (Ries et al., 2003) have used involved donated tickets to our hospital coffee stand to reinforce thrice-weekly attendance at group treatment. The contingencies were reset each week and did not escalate due to the staff's concerns about the degree of monitoring that this would require. It is possible that a similar paradigm could be used to reinforce clean urine samples. Although CMHCs often complain that they cannot hire chemical dependency specialists, CM staff need not necessarily be certified addictions staff. What a CM interventionist does and what a chemical dependency specialist does are quite different. In fact, had we staff who were a bit more familiar with variable-magnitude schemes, our own staff could have made a slightly more complex scheme, which might have rewarded increasing levels of attendance.

High Dependence

Smokers with schizophrenia enter treatment with higher daily rates of smoking and levels of nicotine dependence than smokers without psychiatric illness (de Leon & Diaz, 2005). Given that these variables have been consistently associated with lower quit rates (e.g., Hyland et al., 2004), it is possible that patients with SMI may require longer CM intervention periods or higher reinforcer values in order to abstain from smoking. Likewise, higher reinforcer values may be necessary to retain patients with ASPD in treatment (Helmus et al., 2001). Reinforcing reductions prior to targeting abstinence is another strategy that has been promoted (McChargue, Gulliver, & Hitsman, 2002).

Limited Transportation

Some patients have difficulty accessing treatment because they do not drive, may be reluctant to take public transportation, and tend to have less social support for treatment (e.g., Alvidrez & Havassey, 2006; Magliano, Fiorillo, Malangone, De Rosa, Maj, & National Mental Health Project Working Groups, 2006). This may limit the frequency with which these patients can provide samples for the biochemical verification of abstinence. Small-scale studies have provided free taxi transportation (Tidey et al., 2005) or have traveled to the patient's homes to get the specimen (Tidey et al., 2002), but this is not feasible for longer-term treatment programs. Internet-based methods of verifying abstinence and delivering reinforcement are being developed (e.g., Dallery & Glenn, 2005) and may one day provide opportunities for reaching home-bound patients. Other options might be to provide bus tokens, to reinforce participation in phone counseling sessions, or to reinforce treatment goals that require less frequent verification (reviewed later).

OTHER TARGET BEHAVIORS

Medication Adherence

While most recent CM research has focused on rewarding drug-negative urine samples, it is clear that persons with SMI manifest other problematic behaviors which could likely benefit from treatment with CM techniques. For example, the most common reason for "revolving door" admissions to expensive psychiatric units, besides substance abuse, is medication noncompliance (Haywood et al., 1995). Nonadherence with medications in SMI ranges from 25% to 75%, is almost always underrated by clinicians, and can result in a variety of adverse outcomes (Byerly et al., 2005). Medication compliance could be monitored with pill counts and electronic MEMS (Medication Event Monitoring System) caps on pill bottles and blister packs (Haynes et al., 2005) and reinforced on a weekly basis.

Treatment Attendance

Treatment attendance is a serious problem for persons with SMI and relatively low-cost and low-impact CM interventions improve treatment attendance in people with SMI–SUDs (e.g., Helmus et al., 2003; Villano, Rosenblum, Magura, & Fong, 2002). While drug courts use negative consequences such as jailing to punish poor attendance, CM paradigms focusing on positive behavior change are more potent and more likely lead to positive longer-term behavioral change. Although the use of CM paradigms in a fee for service model might be seen as conflict of interest, many state mental health systems are not fee for service but are managed care risk contracts. Seeing patients more frequently as outpatients can potentially decrease crises for the patient, decrease costs for the payer, and increase the patient's exposure to various rehabilitative interventions.

Rehabilitation Behaviors

Mental health centers are increasingly concerned with skills training and prevocational and vocational activities. These are also goals of the 2002 President's New Freedom Commission on Mental Health (*www.mentalhealth commission.gov/reports/reports.htm*). CM techniques could be used to interest and engage patients in such activities, with actual job earnings taking over as reinforcement once employment starts. In one such model, Drebing et al. (2005) recently evaluated whether incorporating CM techniques into the VA Compensated Work Therapy (CWT) program could increase patients involvement in employment activities. The CWT program is one of the largest vocational rehabilitation programs in the United States, serving more than 13,000 veterans annually, and more than half of vocational rehabilitation participants in the VA are dually diagnosed with psychiatric disorders and/or SUDs (Drebing et al., 2002).

In an effort to improve participants' rates of competitive employment at discharge, Drebing et al. (2005) conducted a randomized controlled comparison of CWT as usual versus CWT + enhanced incentives conditions. All participants in this pilot study (*n* = 19) were dually diagnosed veterans. In the CWT-enhanced condition, participants could receive escalating payments for drug (alcohol, cocaine, opiate) abstinence based on twice-weekly variable-interval urine screens. Employment-related goals, such as creating a resume, attending a job interview, obtaining a job, and working for up to 4 consecutive weeks, were reinforced with fixed payments ranging from $20 to $70. In addition, all payments were contingent upon continued CWT enrollment, which requires on-time attendance at CWT and psychiatric appointments. The total possible payment for meeting all abstinence and job-related goals over the 16-week study period was $1,006, paid either in cash or as a voucher. Results from this study indicated that participants in the enhanced condition performed more intense job searches, earned greater wages, and had longer periods of initial abstinence (Drebing et al., 2005). Nonsignificant results from several other measures also favored the enhanced group. The study investigators note that there is a natural synergy between vocational rehabilitation (VR) programs and CM techniques: CM can improve VR attendance, particularly by reducing drug use, a frequent precipitant of VR dropout. Conversely, CWT provides naturalistic reinforcement such as social status and self-esteem. Importantly, CWT programs already contain the infrastructure and financial payments necessary to sustain CM programs (Drebing et al., 2005). Clearly, this is an arena in which incorporating CM could have a significant impact on drug use and other important behaviors in people with co-occurring disorders.

CONCLUDING COMMENTS

This review of the literature has illustrated many advantages, and no disadvantages, of including CM techniques in treatment plans for people with co-occurring SMI–SUDs. Despite this, there has been limited penetration of CM techniques into real-world treatment settings (Ries & Dyck, 1997). One way of increasing penetration is for clinics to focus on reinforcing easily verified target behaviors. Although much of recent research has focused on substance abuse, behaviors such as participation in vocational rehabilitation programs, medication adherence, and treatment engagement are equally good targets for CM techniques. Penetration can also be increased by reducing costs of CM interventions, through the use of donated reinforcers, variable-schedule ("fishbowl") reinforcement schedules (Petry, Martin,

Cooney, & Kranzler, 2000), or the representative payee strategy (Ries et al., 2004). Bringing focused CM techniques into the CMHCs might allow for these techniques to be seen as standard, to be used by any kind of clinician, rather than abstract techniques that are tested by researchers. For example, in a report on the introduction of CM interventions into the New York City Health and Hospital Addiction Treatment Service, Kellogg et al. (2005) described how the staff's initial resistance to these techniques dissipated once the staff experienced the positive effects on patient motivation, therapeutic progress, and patient and staff morale. Finally, there is a need for CM interventions to be taught as part of standard addictions counselor training, with easy-to-follow workbook schemes, documentations, and logic forms.

REFERENCES

Alvidrez, J., & Havassy, B. E. (2006, January). Clinical characteristics and service utilization patterns of clients with schizophrenia-spectrum disorders in public residential detoxification settings. *Community Mental Health Journal, 20*, 1–12.

Amass, L., & Kamien, J. (2004). A tale of two cities: Financing two voucher programs for substance abusers through community donations. *Experimental and Clinical Psychopharmacology, 12*, 147–155.

Ayllon, T., & Azrin, N. H. (1965). The measurement and reinforcement of behavior of psychotics. *Journal of the Experimental Analysis of Behavior, 8*, 357–383.

Ayllon, T., & Michael, J. (1959). The psychiatric nurse as a behavioral engineer. *Journal of the Experimental Analysis of Behavior, 2*, 323–334.

Barrowclough, C., Haddock, G., Tarrier, N., Lewis, S. W., Moring, J., O'Brien, R., et al. (2001). Randomized controlled trial of motivational interviewing, cognitive behavior therapy, and family intervention for patients with comorbid schizophrenia and substance use disorders. *American Journal of Psychiatry, 158*, 1706–1713.

Bennett, M. E., Bellack, A. S., & Gearon, J. S. (2001). Treating substance abuse in schizophrenia. An initial report. *Journal of Substance Abuse Treatment, 20*, 163–175.

Brooner, R. K., Kidorf, M., King, V. L., & Stoller, K. (1998). Preliminary evidence of good treatment response in antisocial drug abusers. *Drug and Alcohol Dependence, 49*, 249–260.

Brooner, R. K., Schmidt, C. W., Felch, L. J., & Bigelow, G. E. (1992). Antisocial behavior of intravenous drug abusers: Implications for diagnosis of antisocial personality disorder. *American Journal of Psychiatry, 149*, 482–487.

Byerly, M., Fisher, R., Whatley, K., Holland, R., Varghese, F., Carmody, T., et al. (2005). A comparison of electronic monitoring vs. clinician rating of antipsychotic adherence in outpatients with schizophrenia. *Psychiatry Research, 28*, 129–133.

Carroll, K. M. (2004). Behavioral therapies for co-occurring substance use and mood disorders. *Biological Psychiatry, 56*, 778–784.

Center for Substance Abuse Treatment. (1994). *Assessment and treatment of patients with coexisting mental illness and alcohol and other drug abuse* (Treatment Improvement Protocol [TIP] Series 9. DHHS Publication No. [SMA] 95-3061). Rockville, MD: Substance Abuse and Mental Health Services Administration.

Center for Substance Abuse Treatment. (2005). *Substance abuse treatment for persons with co-occurring disorders* (Treatment Improvement Protocol [TIP] Series 42.

DHHS Publication No. [SMA] 05-3922). Rockville, MD: Substance Abuse and Mental Health Services Administration.

Cloninger C. R., Przybeck, R. R., & Svrakic, D. M. (1991). The Tridimentional personality Questionnaire: U.S. normative data. *Psychological Reports, 69,* 1047–1057.

Compton, W. M., Cottler, L. B., Schillington, A. M., & Price, R. K. (1995). Is antisocial personality disorder associated with increased HIV risk behaviors in cocaine users? *Drug and Alcohol Dependence, 37,* 37–44.

Costa, P. T., & McCrae, R. R. (1985). *Manual of the NEO Personality Inventory.* Odessa, FL: Psychological Assessment Resources.

Dahlstrom, W. G., Welsh, G. S., & Dahlstrom, L. E. (1972). *An MMPI handbook* (rev. ed., Vol. 1). Minneapolis: University of Minnesota Press.

Dallery, J., & Glenn, I. M. (2005). Effects of an Internet-based voucher reinforcement program for smoking abstinence: A feasibility study. *Journal of Applied Behavior Analysis, 38,* 349–357.

de Leon, J., & Diaz, F. J. (2005). A meta-analysis of worldwide studies demonstrates an association between schizophrenia and tobacco smoking behaviors. *Schizophrenia Research, 76,* 135–157.

Drake, R. E., Mueser, K. T., Brunette, M. F., & McHugo, G. J. (2004). A review of treatments for people with severe mental illnesses and co-occurring substance use disorders. *Psychiatric Rehabilitation Journal, 27*(4), 360–373.

Drebing, C. E., Fleitas, R., Moore, A., Krebs, C., Van Ormer, A., Penk, W., et al. (2002). Patterns in work functioning and vocational rehabilitation associated with coexisting psychiatric and substance use disorders. *Rehabilitation Counseling Bulletin, 46,* 5–13.

Drebing, C. E., Van Ormer, E. A., Krebs, C., Rosenheck, R., Rounsaville, B., Herz, L., et al. (2005). The impact of enhanced incentives on vocational rehabilitation outcomes for dually diagnosed veterans. *Journal of Applied Behavior Analysis, 38,* 359–372.

Gilbert, D. G., Crauthers, D. M., Mooney, D. K., McClernon, F. J., & Jensen, R. A. (1999). Effects of monetary contingencies on smoking relapse: Influences of trait depression, personality, and habitual nicotine intake. *Experimental and Clinical Psychopharmacology, 7*(2), 174–181.

Goff, D. C., Sullivan, L. M., McEvoy, J. P., Meyer, J. M., Nasrallah, H. A., Daumit, G. L., et al. (2005). A comparison of ten-year cardiac risk estimates in schizophrenia patients from the CATIE study and matched controls. *Schizophrenia Research, 80,* 45–53.

Gonzalez, G., Feingold, A., Oliveto, A., Gonsai, K., & Kosten T. R. (2003). Comorbid major depressive disorder as a prognostic factor in cocaine-abusing buprenorphine-maintained patients treated with desipramine and contingency management. *American Journal of Drug and Alcohol Abuse, 29,* 497–514.

Haughton, E., & Ayllon, T. (1965). Production and elimination of symptomatic behavior. In L. P. Ullman & L. Krasner (Eds.), *Case studies in behavior modification* (pp. 94–98). New York: Holt, Rinehart & Winston.

Haynes, R., Yao, X., Degani, A., Kripalani, S., Garg, A., McDonald, H., et al. (2005, October). Interventions to enhance medication adherence. *Cochrane Database of Systematic Reviews, 19*(4), CD000011.

Haywood, T. W., Kravitz, H. M., Grossman, L. S., Cavanaugh, J. L. Jr., Davis, J. M., & Lewis, D. A. (1995). Predicting the "revolving door" phenomenon among patients with schizophrenic, schizoaffective, and affective disorders. *American Journal of Psychiatry, 152,* 856–861.

Helmus, T. C., Downey, K. K., Arfken, C. L., Henderson, M. J., & Schuster, C. R. (2001).

Novelty seeking as a predictor of treatment retention for heroin dependent cocaine users. *Drug and Alcohol Dependence, 61*, 287–295.

Helmus, T. C., Saules, K. K., Schoener, E. P., & Roll, J. M. (2003). Reinforcement of counseling attendance and alcohol abstinence in a community-based dual-diagnosis treatment program: A feasibility study. *Psychology of Addictive Behaviors, 17*, 249–251.

Higgins, S., Budney, A., Bickel, W. K., Foerg, F. E., Donham, R., & Badger, G. J. (1994). Incentives improve outcome in outpatient behavioral treatment of cocaine dependence. *Archives of General Psychiatry, 51*, 568–576.

Higgins, S. T., Heil, S. H., Solomon, L. J., Bernstein, I. M., Lussier, J. P., Abel, R. L., et al. (2004). A pilot study on voucher-based incentives to promote abstinence from cigarette smoking during pregnancy and postpartum. *Nicotine and Tobacco Research, 6*(6), 1015–1020.

Hingtgen, J. N., Sanders, B. J., & DeMeyer, M. K. (1965). Shaping cooperative responses in early childhood schizophrenics. In L. P. Ullman & L. Krasner (Eds.), *Case studies in behavior modification* (pp. 130–138). New York: Holt, Rinehart & Winston.

Hyland, A., Li, Q., Bauer, J. E., Giovino, G. A., Steger, C., & Cummings, M. (2004). Predictors of cessation in a cohort of current and former smokers followed over 13 years. *Nicotine and Tobacco Research, 6*(Suppl. 3), S363–S369.

Isaacs, W., Thomas, J., & Goldiamond, I. (1960). Application of operant conditioning to reinstate verbal behavior in psychotics. *Journal of Speech and Hearing Disorders, 25*, 8–12.

Jeffrey, D. P., Ley, A., McLaren, S., & Siegfried, N. (2000). Psychosocial treatment programmes for people with both severe mental illness and substance misuse. *Cochrane Database of Systematic Reviews, 2*, CD001088.

Kellogg, S. H., Burns, M., Coleman, P., Stitzer, M., Wale, J. B., & Kreek, M. J. (2005). Something of value: The introduction of contingency management interventions into the New York City Health and Hospital Addiction Treatment Service. *Journal of Substance Abuse Treatment, 28*, 57–65.

King, G. F., Armitage, S. G., & Tilton, J. R. (1960). A therapeutic approach to schizophrenics of extreme pathology: An operant-interpersonal method. *Journal of Abnormal and Social Psychology, 61*, 276–286.

Kosten, T., Falcioni, J., Oliveto, A., & Feingold, A. (2004). Depression predicts higher rates of heroin use on desipramine with buprenorphine than with methadone. *American Journal on Addictions, 13*, 191–201.

Kosten, T., Oliveto, A., Feingold, A., Poling, J., Sevarino, K., McCance-Katz, E., et al. (2003). Desipramine and contingency management for cocaine and opiate dependence in buprenorphine maintained patients. *Drug and Alcohol Dependence, 70*, 315–325.

Kravitz, H. M., Fawcett, J., McGuire, M., Kravitz, G. S., & Whitney, M. (1999). Treatment attrition among alcohol-dependent men: Is it related to novelty seeking personality traits? *Journal of Clinical Psychopharmacology, 19*, 51–56.

Kushel, M. B., Hahn, J. A., Evans, J. L., Bangsberg, D. R., & Moss, A. R. (2005). Revolving doors: Imprisonment among the homeless and marginally housed population. *American Journal of Public Health, 95*(10), 1747–1752.

Lasser, K., Boyd, J. W., Woolhandler, S., Himmelstein, D. U., McCormick, D., & Bor, D. H. (2000). Smoking and mental illness: A population-based prevalence study. *Journal of the American Medical Association, 284*(20), 2606–2610.

Magliano, L., Fiorillo, A., Malangone, C., De Rosa, C., Maj, M., & National Mental Health Project Working Group. (2006). Social network in long-term diseases: A comparative study in relatives of persons with schizophrenia and physical illnesses versus a sample from the general population. *Social Science and Medicine, 62*, 1392–1402.

McChargue, D. E., Gulliver, S. B., & Hitsman, B. (2002). Would smokers with schizophrenia benefit from a more flexible approach to smoking treatment? *Addiction, 97*, 785–793.

McNamara, C., Schumacher, J. E., Milby, J. B., Wallace, D., & Usdan, S. (2001). Prevalence of nonpsychotic mental disorders does not affect treatment outcome in a homeless cocaine-dependent sample. *American Journal of Drug and Alcohol Abuse, 27*(1), 91–106.

Messina, N., Farabee, D., & Rawson, R. (2003). Treatment responsivity of cocaine-dependent patients with antisocial personality disorder to cognitive-behavioral and contingency management interventions. *Journal of Consulting and Clinical Psychology, 71*(2), 320–329.

Milby, J. B., Schumacher, J. E., McNamara, C. L., Wallace, D., Usdan, S., & Michael, M. (2000). Initiating abstinence in cocaine abusing dually diagnosed homeless persons. *Journal of Drug and Alcohol Dependence, 60*, 55–67.

Peniston, E. G. (1988). Evaluation of long-term therapeutic efficacy of behavior modification program with chronic male psychiatric patients. *Journal of Behavioral Therapy and Experimental Psychiatry, 19*, 95–101.

Petry, N. M., Martin, B., Cooney, J. L., & Kranzler, H. R. (2000). Give them prizes, and they will come: Contingency management for treatment of alcohol dependence. *Journal of Consulting and Clinical Psychology, 68*, 250–257.

Regier, D. A., Farmer, M. E., Rae, D. S., Myers, J. K., Kramer, M., Robins, L. N., et al. (1990). Comorbidity of mental disorders with alcohol and other drug abuse: Results from the Epidemiologic Catchment Area (ECA) study. *Journal of the American Medical Association, 264*, 2511–2518.

Ries, R. K. (2003). *A simple contingency management paradigm to reinforce attendance at group treatment*. Unpublished raw data.

Ries, R. K., & Dyck, D. G. (1997). Representative payee practices of community mental health centers in Washington State. *Psychiatric Services, 48*, 811–814.

Ries, R. K., Dyck, D. G., Short, R., Srebnik, D., Fisher, A., & Comtois, K. A. (2004). Outcomes of managing disability benefits among patients with substance dependence and severe mental illness. *Psychiatric Services, 55*, 445–447.

Ries, R. K., Short, R. A., Dyck, D. G., & Srebnik, D. (2004). Unlinking disability income, substance use and adverse outcomes in dually diagnosed, severely mentally ill outpatients. *American Journal of Addiction, 13*, 390–397.

Roll, J. M., Chermack, S. T., & Chudzynski, J. E. (2004). Investigating the use of contingency management in the treatment of cocaine abuse among individuals with schizophrenia: A feasibility study. *Psychiatry Research, 125*, 61–64.

Roll, J. M., Higgins, S. T., Steingard, S., & McGinley, M. (1998). Use of monetary reinforcement to reduce the cigarette smoking of persons with schizophrenia: A feasibility study. *Experimental and Clinical Psychopharmacology, 6*, 157–161.

Rounsaville, B. J., Weissman, M. M., Kleber, H., & Wilber, C. (1982). Heterogeneity of psychiatric diagnosis in treated opiate addicts. *Archives of General Psychiatry, 39*, 161–166.

Shaner, A., Eckman, T. A., Roberts, L. J., Wilkins, J. N., Tucker, D. E., Tsuang, J. W., et al. (1995). Disability income, cocaine use, and repeated hospitalization among schizophrenic cocaine abusers: A government-sponsored revolving door? *New England Journal of Medicine, 333*, 777–783.

Shaner, A., Roberts, L. J., Eckman, T. A., Tucker, D. E., Tsuang, J. W., Wilkins, J. N., et al. (1997). Monetary reinforcement of abstinence from cocaine among mentally ill patients with cocaine dependence. *Psychiatric Services, 48*, 807–810.

Sigmon, S. C., Steingard, S., Badger, G. J., Anthony, S. L., & Higgins, S. T. (2000). Contingent reinforcement of marijuana abstinence among individuals with serious mental illness: A feasibility study. *Experimental and Clinical Psychopharmacology, 8*, 509–517.

Silverman, K., Wong, C., Umbricht-Schneiter, A., Montoya, I., Schuster, C., & Preston, K. (1998). Broad beneficial effects of cocaine abstinence reinforcement among methadone patients. *Journal of Consulting and Clinical Psychology, 66*, 811–824.

Swartz, M. S., Wagner, H. R., Swanson, J. W., Strouo, T. S., McEvoy, J. P., McGee, M., et al. (2006). Substance use and psychosocial functioning in schizophrenia among new enrollees in the NIMH CATIE study. *Psychiatric Services, 57*, 1110–1116.

Tidey, J. W., Higgins, S. T., Bickel, W. K., & Steingard, S. (1999). Effects of response requirement and the presence of an alternative reinforcer on cigarette smoking by schizophrenics. *Psychopharmacology, 145*, 52–60.

Tidey, J. W., O'Neill, S. C., & Higgins, S. T. (2002). Contingent monetary reinforcement of smoking reductions, with and without transdermal nicotine, in outpatients with schizophrenia. *Experimental and Clinical Psychopharmacology, 10*, 241–247.

Tidey, J., Rohsenow, D., Kaplan, G., & Swift, R. (2005, June). *Contingency management plus bupropion for smoking reductions in outpatients with schizophrenia.* Paper presented at session 24 of the annual meeting of the College on Problems of Drug Dependence, Orlando, FL.

Ullman, L. P., & Krasner, L. (1965). *Case studies in behavior modification.* New York: Holt, Rinehart & Winston.

U.S. Department of Health and Human Services. (2002). *Report to Congress on the prevention and treatment of co-occurring substance abuse and mental disorders.* Washington, DC: Author.

Valliant, G. E. (1975). Sociopathy as a human process: A viewpoint. *Archives of General Psychiatry, 42*, 1081–1086.

Villano, C. L., Rosenblum, A., Magura, S., & Fong, C. (2002). Improving treatment engagement and outcomes for cocaine-using methadone patients. *American Journal of Drug and Alcohol Abuse, 28*, 213–230.

Watkins, K. E., Burnam, A., Kung, F. Y., & Paddock, S. (2001). A national survey of care for persons with co-occurring mental and substance use disorders. *Psychiatric Services, 52*, 1062–1068.

Ziedonis, D. M., & Kosten, T. R. (1991). Pharmacotherapy improves treatment outcome in depressed cocaine addicts. *Journal of Psychoactive Drugs, 23*, 417–425.

Ziedonis, D. M., Smelson, D., Rosenthal, R. N., Batki, S. L., Green, A. I., Henry, R. J., et al. (2005. Improving the care of individuals with schizophrenia and substance use disorders: Consensus recommendations. *Journal of Psychiatric Practice, 11*(5), 315–337.

CHAPTER 12

ADOLESCENTS

Suchitra Krishnan-Sarin,
Amy M. Duhig, *and* Dana Cavallo

In his review of the current status of evidence surrounding adolescent "storm and stress," Arnett (1999) concludes that most adolescents navigate adolescence with minimal difficulties. However, for some, adolescence is a time of increased risk for a variety of issues, including, but not limited to, intensity of conflict with parents, emotional volatility, increased negative mood, increased risk-taking behavior, novelty seeking, and sensation and reward seeking (Arnett, 1999). Furthermore, many externalizing and internalizing problems, either which have not yet manifested or are evident to lesser degrees, emerge or intensify during adolescence; examples of these are eating disorders, depression, violence, and substance abuse and dependence.

Factors responsible for these changes appear to be both intrinsic and extrinsic in nature. There are intra- and interindividual changes in the biological, social, cognitive, and emotional worlds of adolescents, as well as contextual changes (i.e., time spent in school, family, and peers; Steinberg et al., 2006). Although the intricacies involved are beyond the scope of this chapter, recent research suggests that the various problems that may arise in adolescence are related to neurobehavioral changes of puberty, including changes in brain systems that regulate arousal and appetite, which then influence the intensity and duration of emotion and motivation. There are also changes associated with puberty that intensify drives relevant to reward-, novelty-, and stimulation-seeking behavior (see Steinberg et al.,

2006, for review). Other investigators have also suggested that vulnerability to high-risk behaviors such as substance use in adolescence may be mediated by an underdeveloped neural circuitry (Chambers, Taylor, & Potenza, 2003; Spear, 2000). Supporting evidence for this view comes from imaging studies which suggest that the structure of the brain in adolescence is significantly different from that in adults and that areas of the brain, such as the prefrontal cortex, that are significantly involved in mediating executive functioning and control over one's behavior are not fully developed until the early 20s (Giedd et al., 1999). The exact impact of these changes on adolescent behavior and emotional development has yet to be determined, but it has been postulated that these differences may mediate the high-risk nature of adolescence and that this may be a unique and prime period of time for prevention and intervention, particularly in the area of substance use.

OVERVIEW OF THE SUBSTANCE ABUSE PROBLEM IN ADOLESCENTS

Adolescence is a critical period when substance use begins and progresses. Early initiation of substance use is a major concern with almost one-third of teens experimenting with substances before completing the eighth grade (Johnston, O'Malley, Bachman, & Schulenberg, 2005). Some teens will experiment with nicotine and alcohol and stop, or continue to use occasionally, without significant problems. However, others will develop a pattern of regular use or a dependency, move on to use other dangerous drugs, and experience significant future health problems causing considerable harm to themselves and possibly to others.

According to a recent Youth Risk Behaviors Survey (Grunbaum et al., 2004), approximately 22% of teens reported smoking cigarettes, 45% reported drinking alcohol, and 22% have used marijuana at least once in the past month. Episodic binge drinking (5 drinks of alcohol on one drinking occasion) was reported by 28% of adolescents and marijuana use was reported by 22% of adolescents at least once in the prior 30 days. Frequent cigarette use (20–30 days in the preceding month) was reported by 10% of adolescents with 3% smoking more than 10 cigarettes per day. Furthermore, the use of other drugs is also on the rise. The 2005 Monitoring the Future survey (Johnston et al., 2005) revealed an upward trend in the use of sedatives and barbiturates among adolescents since 2001, with continued increased rates of nonmedical use of prescription medications, especially opioid painkillers.

Although rates of daily and heavy use of many of these drugs are lower than that of use by adults, adolescence is a prime period for the initiation of use of substances such as tobacco, alcohol, and marijuana. Use of these substances leads to relatively immediate adverse effects as well as continued

drug use into adulthood and associated adverse consequences and, therefore, warrants a signal for early intervention. Drug prevention programs
have long been the focus of school personnel and legal authorities, as well
as community professionals. The idea behind prevention is to intervene as
early as possible, before a significant pattern of substance abuse is established, and to discourage experimentation that may lead to progressive alcohol and drug misuse and abuse. However, the efficacy of most of the existing drug prevention programs is modest at best (Botvin, Schinke, &
Orlandi, 1989; Botvin et al., 2000; Lynam et al., 1999) and there is some
question about whether they are reaching high-risk children and adolescents.

The vast majority of treatment studies on adolescent substance abuse
have focused on psychosocial interventions, involving multiple components
derived from theories of social and learning theory and operant and classi-

Although drug prevention programs may have their place in the
schools for students as young as the third grade to thwart possible drug experimentation, a need still exists for continued intervention for the children
who have started using drugs and alcohol more regularly and are at risk for
or are currently addicted. It has been estimated that over 400,000 adolescents are in need of substance abuse treatment (Greenblatt, 2000), but only
a small number actually receive treatment, usually those with severe substance disorders, comorbid psychiatric disorders, and legal problems. Most
of the treatments currently offered to adolescents have been established by
borrowing techniques from the adult substance abuse literature, including
various behavioral therapies with and without the use of pharmacological
treatment.

Pharmacological approaches to adolescent substance abuse are not
well delineated, due to the lack of empirical data on the safety and effectiveness of these medications for youth. Preliminary evidence suggests that
antidepressants may be effective in adolescents with major depression and
alcohol use disorders (Cornelius et al., 2001). Nicotine replacement strategies have recently been used to treat adolescent smokers and although the
use of transdermal nicotine has shown some efficacy (Hurt et al., 2000;
Moolchan et al., 2005; Smith et al., 1996), end-of-treatment abstinence
rates are slightly lower than that in adult studies. In a recent clinical trial of
opioid-dependent adolescents, a multimodal approach involving an intensive behavioral therapy and vouchers to reinforce abstinence in combination with randomization to detoxification with either buprenorphine or
clonidine resulted in end of treatment abstinence rates of 64% and 32%,
respectively. Although these rates are encouraging, most clinicians are reluctant to use medications to treat substance use disorders (SUDs) in adolescents due to the lack of adequate safety/toxicity information as well as
definitive clinical treatment guidelines on the use of these medications in
this population.

The vast majority of treatment studies on adolescent substance abuse
have focused on psychosocial interventions, involving multiple components
derived from theories of social and learning theory and operant and classi-

cal conditioning, with core elements of functional analysis, coping-skills training, and relapse prevention. Some of the therapies studied include family interventions (e.g., Liddle, Rowe, Dakof, Ungaro, & Henderson, 2004; Williams & Chang, 2000), cognitive-behavioral therapy (CBT) (e.g., Curry et al., 2003; Kaminer & Burleson, 1999), and motivational enhancement therapy (MET) (e.g., Dennis et al., 2004). Family-based interventions have been shown to hold some promise for adolescents (e.g., Waldron, Slesnick, Brody, Turner, & Peterson, 2001), with significant reductions in self-reports of drug use from baseline to follow-up. Similarly, there is some evidence to suggest that motivational and other brief interventions could also be used to increase both motivation to quit and compliance with treatment in adolescents with SUDs (see Tevyaw & Monti, 2004, for review). However, most of the behavioral therapy research has been conducted with adolescents in clinical treatment facilities and a lot more work needs to be done to increase the generalizability and accessibility of these interventions to adolescents in the community.

Thus, in summary, adolescents are in need of improved treatment options with age-appropriate programs, bearing in mind the developmental issues characteristic of adolescence. Although there is a growing need for efficacious substance abuse treatment for adolescents, there is little consensus on how best to treat this population. Some of the psychosocial interventions show utility in assisting adolescents in quitting smoking or ending a drug habit. However, as discussed below, getting adolescents motivated to quit and retaining them in treatment, especially during the initial weeks of abstinence, when both the withdrawal syndrome and relapse are common, is the biggest challenge that we face in the treatment of SUDs in this high-risk population.

WHY MIGHT CONTINGENCY MANAGEMENT WORK FOR ADOLESCENT SUBSTANCE USE PROBLEMS?

One of the basic principles underlying interventions for substance users, regardless of whether they are adults or adolescents, is motivating change in behavior. Many chapters in this book cover the appropriateness and value of contingency management (CM) techniques for addressing this issue in adult substance users. In general, adult substance users who have experienced the negative consequences of their behavior are somewhat motivated to quit. However, adolescents, in general, are particularly resistant to the concept of change in behavior. Moreover, unlike adults, they typically do not find their substance use to be problematic or they may not view quitting as urgent because they have not experienced any negative consequences of their substance use due to their shorter use histories (Breda & Heflinger, 2004).

Overall, adolescents suffer from low levels of motivation to quit sub-stance-using behavior (e.g., Breda & Heflinger, 2004; Friedman, Granick, & Kreisher, 1994; Sussman et al., 1998). The few existing evaluations of motivation to change in adolescents indicate that motivation varies as a function of age, ethnicity, and legal status (Breda & Helflinger, 2004; Melnick, DeLeon, Hawke, Jainchill, & Kressel, 1997). It appears that the majority of adolescents who join treatment programs have been legally mandated to do so. In addition, if they do quit, adolescents in particular may not have a desire to remain abstinent and therefore frequently relapse (Balch et al., 2004; Dennis et al., 2000). In addition, most adolescents say that they would rather quit on their own than participate in a program (Balch et al., 2004; Leatherdale, Cameron, Brown, Jolin, & Kroeker, 2006; Leatherdale & McDonald, 2005), despite evidence suggesting that cessa-tion programs increase quit rates. Moreover, Sussman et al. (1998) also re-port that adolescent smokers have low self-efficacy of quitting. Hence, one of the basic problems facing most substance use adolescent researchers and clinicians is how to convince adolescents that they should and can quit us-ing substances.

A limited amount of research has examined cessation-related percep-tions, attitudes, beliefs, and behaviors among adolescent cigarette smokers using focus groups and other survey techniques. Most of this research has found that adolescents, although interested in quitting smoking and con-cerned about the health consequences of smoking (Balch et al., 2004; Mermelstein, 1999), did not consider their smoking behavior to be urgent enough to seek help and most of them were unaware of existing smoking-cessation programs and methods (Balch et al., 2004; Gillespie, Stanton, Lowe, & Hunter, 1995). Interestingly, adolescent smokers reported that the potential of saving money (Gillespie et al., 1995) and receiving money and small enticements or incentives (Balch, 1998) were features that would draw them to a cessation program. The concept of using rewards or incen-tives to increase motivation in adolescents is certainly not a novel one and a large body of school-based literature suggests that incentives/rewards can be used to motivate change in a number of behaviors in children. While there is an ongoing debate about the influence of different kinds of rewards on perceived self-determination and competence over a particular behavior (e.g., Deci, Koestner, & Ryan, 1999; Eisenberger, Pierce, & Cameron, 1999) it appears that performance-contingent rewards are particularly ef-fective at increasing both intrinsic motivation and perceived autonomy over behavior change (Eisenberger et al., 1999; Eisenberger & Rhoades, 2001).

Interestingly, as discussed in other chapters, CM interventions, which are based on the principle of providing tangible reinforcers contingent upon achieving certain performance or target behaviors such as drug abstinence or clinic attendance, are remarkably effective at motivating and maintaining abstinence and increasing retention in programs targeting substance use. Therefore, CM interventions, and the behavioral economic theory on which they are based, may be particularly suitable for adolescents, given their focus on the use of rewards to increase engagement in particular behaviors. For instance, when examining the progression of smoking behavior in high school-age adolescents, recent evidence indicates that the availability of alternative reinforcers, such as school-related activities and perceived academic performance, decreased the odds of progression of smoking behavior (Audrain-McGovern et al., 2004). Although these naturally occurring sources of reinforcement are somewhat distinct from the reinforcement of abstinence using vouchers or money, they provide evidence that adolescents are amenable to reinforcers other than the effects of a substance. CM interventions may also help with treatment retention, which is particularly important given that a recent review suggests that with an increasing number of sessions attended, there is a greater likelihood of smoking cessation in adolescents (Sussman, 2002).

Finally, a significant advantage of CM procedures that reinforce abstinence is that CM not only strives for achieving total and immediate abstinence but can do so more reliably than other treatments, which may significantly enhance the chances of long-term abstinence. For example, the AHCPR Clinical Practice Guidelines for smoking cessation (Fiore et al., 2000) emphasize that for a quit attempt to be successful, total abstinence (i.e.,"Not even a puff after the quit date") is essential. Rates of relapse to smoking during the first few days of a quit attempt are very high and it has been suggested that smoking on the first day of a quit attempt may predict failure to maintain abstinence (Westman, Behm, Simel, & Rose, 1997). Eighty percent of relapses occur during the first 1–2 weeks of a quit attempt (Kenford et al., 1994). Therefore, achieving immediate abstinence using CM techniques significantly enhances the possibility of sustained abstinence in adolescent smokers.

CM FOR SUBSTANCE USE IN ADOLESCENTS

While evaluations of the use of CM for adolescent substance use have been limited, the existing studies vary widely in methodological issues, including different treatment targets ranging from reinforcement of attendance, drug abstinence, or non-drug-related activities, as well as different types of adult involvement and settings, including parents, clinicians, researchers, substance use clinics, private homes, and schools (e.g., Azrin, Donohue, Besalel, Kogan, & Acierno, 1994; Corby, Roll, Ledgerwood, & Schuster, 2000; Hanson, Allen, Jensen, & Hatsukami, 2003; Kamon, Budney, & Stanger, 2005; Krishnan-Sarin et al., 2006; Marsch et al., 2005; Roll, Chudzynski, & Richardson, 2005; Weissman, Glasgow, Biglan, & Lichtenstein, 1987). In all these programs, CM procedures are used in combination with other behavioral or pharmacological therapies.

Azrin, Donohue, et al. (1994) studied 26 adolescents who had used illegal drugs (other than alcohol). They were referred to treatment by an agency, school, or family and then randomized to receive either a general supportive therapy or an enhanced treatment consisting of individualized plans addressing stimulus and urge control and contracting with parents to achieve social control. Drug-incompatible behaviors were reinforced by parents with increased allowance, special gifts of clothing/recreational items, increased transportation by parents or use of a family car, later curfew, or telephone/stereo/television privileges. Significant reductions in targeted drug use, confirmed by urine-toxicology levels, were observed in the last month of the 6-month treatment period in the enhanced treatment group (73%) compared with the control group (9%). The enhanced treatment also resulted in improved school/work attendance, youth–parent relationships, and conduct ratings, as well as decreased depression. Number of months used and mean number of days used continued to be significantly lower in the enhanced treatment condition compared to those treated with supportive therapy during the follow-up period.

Marsch et al. (2005) used procedures similar to those used in the enhanced intervention provided by Azrin, Donohue, et al. (1994) in a 28-day, outpatient, parallel-group randomized trial of buprenorphine or clonidine-assisted withdrawal in 36 adolescents who were opiate dependent. Although the study was not designed to isolate the efficacy of the CM intervention, the results suggest that combining buprenorphine with CM was more efficacious than CM combined with clonidine. The contribution of CM to outcomes using this combined buprenorphine + CM treatment will have to be determined in future studies.

Kamon et al. (2005) also conducted a study involving abstinence-contingent vouchers but with a research design that did not permit their effect to be isolated from that of other components of a multielement treatment intervention. It was a pilot study with 19 adolescent marijuana users all of whom received an individualized 14-week intervention with MET and CBT components in combination with a clinician-administered abstinence-based voucher program, a family management parent-training curriculum, and a parent reward component for motivating parental participation. The adolescents could earn up to $590 in vouchers over the treatment period for biochemical evidence of abstinence from marijuana at twice-weekly urine testings. The program was found to be feasible and acceptable to participants and parents and abstinence rates were enhanced from 34% at intake to 74% at the end of treatment. An ongoing randomized clinical trial is further examining the efficacy of this intervention.

The use of CM techniques has also been evaluated in the area of adolescent tobacco cessation. Weissman et al. (1987) reported on an uncontrolled smoking-cessation study conducted with 11 adolescents smoking 8–35 cigarettes per day. This program had five phases: baseline (normal smoking), gradual reduction (33% reduction in carbon monoxide levels in first week and additional 25% reduction in second week), cessation (preset quit date), maintenance and follow-up (5 months). Results indicated that of the six male subjects, five quit smoking and four maintained abstinence at the follow-up appointment, while all five female subjects dropped out of the program. Corby et al. (2000) conducted a within-subjects feasibility study examining the use of progressive contingent reinforcement procedures to motivate abstinence in non-treatment-seeking adolescent tobacco users; results indicated that when adolescents were reinforced for not smoking, there was an increase in the total number of abstinences (breath carbon monoxide [CO] < 8 ppm) and number of consecutive abstinences compared to baseline conditions, where payments were delivered independent of smoking status.

More recent evidence from Roll (2005) and our group suggests that CM procedures can be used successfully to initiate and maintain a period of abstinence in treatment-seeking adolescent smokers. In Roll's study, 22 adolescent smokers were randomly assigned to receive either CM for abstinence (determined by daily breath CO levels) or CM for attendance (based on daily attendance) on an escalating magnitude schedule of reinforcement. Participants received a total of $230 in vouchers in either condition. The results indicated that while CM reinforcement for abstinence and CM reinforcement for attendance were equally effective at retaining participants in treatment, the former was more effective at enhancing biochemically-verified end-of-treatment abstinence rates (50% in abstinence condition versus 10% in attendance condition).

Our group (Krishnan-Sarin et al., 2006) also studied the use of an escalating magnitude schedule of reinforcement with adolescent smokers as part of a formal smoking-cessation program conducted in a school setting. We randomized 28 adolescent smokers to receive weekly CBT sessions with either CM for abstinence or attendance. Abstinence was determined using breath CO and urine cotinine levels and participants could receive approximately $300 for staying abstinent. Figure 12.1 indicates that 53% of adolescent smokers in the CM-for-abstinence condition were abstinent at the end of the 1-month intervention period compared to 0% in the control condition.

Taken together, these preliminary studies suggest that CM techniques show promise for use with adolescent cigarette smokers. However, continued work is needed in this area to evaluate the long-term effectiveness of CM-based interventions in randomized clinical trials with larger samples and longer follow-up periods.

In summary, a limited literature provides an initial signal that CM-based interventions may increase retention in treatment and abstinence

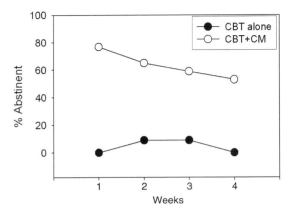

FIGURE 12.1. Point prevalence abstinence rates in adolescent smokers participating in a 1-month smoking-cessation program and receiving either CM + CBT ($n = 17$) or CBT alone ($n = 11$). From Krishnan-Sarin et al. (2006). Copyright 2006 by the American Psychological Association. Reprinted by permission.

rates in adolescent SUDs. However, more research needs to be done to evaluate the efficacy of these interventions in the short and long term and also evaluate methods to maintain abstinence upon removal of the contingencies. Moreover, as with any intervention, it is also very important to increase generalizability and feasibility of these interventions and for this we need to develop a better understanding of the barriers related to the use of these interventions in adolescent populations.

BARRIERS/ISSUES RELATED TO USING CM IN THIS POPULATION

As suggested in the earlier section, CM interventions have significant potential for the treatment of SUDs; however, it is important to keep in mind certain barriers that might arise when using these intensive interventions for adolescent smokers. Some of these barriers are more general, such as parental consent, confidentiality, and increasing access and are applicable to any substance use interventions. Others are more specific to CM approaches, such as variable smoking patterns and the use of biochemical indicators of smoking status, as well as potential problems using money as a reinforcer with this population. These issues are discussed in more detail below.

General Issues

One of the most important considerations about the use of CM or any formal intervention with adolescent smokers is how to ensure accessibility of the intervention to a large number of adolescents. One effective way to increase accessibility is by conducting the intervention in a setting in which many adolescents are present (e.g., local health clinics or schools). A review by Sussman (2002) of 66 adolescent and young-adult smoking-cessation studies, conducted over the last decade, noted that programs delivered in school-based clinical and medical/recovery clinical settings achieved the highest percentage reductions. However, the development of a school-based intervention is fraught with many challenging, but not insurmountable, problems including the recruitment of school participation. In most instances, involvement is contingent upon a mutual decision made by the school principals and local school superintendents who have to keep the school's, students' and parents' interests in mind in making such decisions. Similarly, the development of an intervention in a medical clinic involves a significant amount of upfront work on establishing relationships with clinic personnel and ensuring appropriate training/education to make sure that the study boundaries/parameters are maintained and that the research is being conducted within the guidelines of the clinic/school.

Specific attention needs to be given to issues of confidentiality and coercion. All schools have strict rules and punitive consequences for the use of substances on school premises and, therefore, researchers have to make sure that these consequences do not extend to CM interventions that involve biochemical testing. Researchers and treatment providers need to exercise caution to ensure that adolescents are not being coerced into participating by school personnel or parents and need to put procedures into place to maintain the privacy of the participant. Moreover, if the adolescent is participating in an intervention study in the school, there is always the possibility of loss of confidentiality because teachers, students, and other school personnel could become aware of their involvement and subsequently of their drug use status.

Another issue that often arises with the use of any intervention with adolescents is that of transportation. Unlike adults, most adolescents have to depend on others for transportation unless they live in an urban area with access to buses, trains, or other forms of mass transit. This is a very important consideration for substance use CM interventions, many of which involve frequent appointments for the purpose of biochemical testing. Transportation can be somewhat less of an issue when parents/guardians are involved because they can provide needed transportation. Establishing the intervention in a school-based setting (e.g., Krishnan-Sarin et al., 2006) where all appointments and counseling sessions can be conducted in the school surmounts at least some of these logistical challenges.

Another significant barrier to adolescent substance use interventions, including those involving CM, is the requirement of parental permission. While existing studies have demonstrated how CM-based programs could use parents as gatekeepers for the provision of rewards and suggest that interventions that involve parents have better outcome rates, one needs to cautiously weigh the risks and benefits of parental involvement. In our experience with CM in the school setting, a number of adolescents either indicate that their parents do not know about their substance use and/or do not want their parents involved in the treatment process. Similarly, Balch (1998) found that adolescent smokers seeking cessation services reported that keeping their smoking confidential would be extremely important. Parental involvement could also lead to adolescent misrepresentation of substance use status as well as quantity/frequency of use (e.g., Frissell et al., 2004). Thus, the involvement of parents in these kinds of programs could increase rates of refusal or the validity of self-reports obtained from adolescents as well as decrease rates of participation. To increase the generalizability of an intervention, it would be desirable to obtain waiver of parental permission provided the research or clinical intervention being provided has minimal risk (see Tillett, 2004, for review). However, CM-based interventions, even if they represent minimal risk of physical or psychological harm, could raise significant concerns because of the provision of monetary and other material reinforcement. One way to avoid these concerns would be to focus on other kinds of reinforcers instead of monetary-based rewards, such as enhanced school or clinic privileges, but these would need to be developed under careful consideration and collaboration with school and clinic authorities. Conversely, parental involvement may not be a significant issue with adolescents who are mandated to treatment or referred by agencies or family members. A parent-based intervention may be more appropriate in situations in which the parents are already aware of the adolescent's substance use problem and are also involved in treatment. However, it may not be appropriate to require parental permission in situations in which adolescents express hesitation about parental involvement. Thus, the pros and cons should be weighed in choosing one kind of intervention versus another. It is important to keep in mind that decisions about the use of parental permission should be made after consultations with local institutional review boards as well as school boards.

Barriers Related to Use of CM Techniques

One of the problems with CM interventions focusing on achieving and maintaining abstinence from drug use stems from the inherent requirement of obtaining objective evidence of abstinence. Objective evidence of abstinence is best obtained using biochemical methods (e.g., urine-toxicology testing). Adolescent self-reports of substance use can be unreliable, especially when potential rewards are dependent on the outcome of these reports. However, the use of biochemical measures raises the question of how to quantify and establish baseline levels of use in this population, as most adolescent substance users have less regular and less intensive use patterns compared with adults. This is somewhat less of a problem for substances such as marijuana where use can be detected easily in urine samples for a prolonged period of time. However, biochemical verification is more difficult when the indicator has a relatively short half-life, like for tobacco or alcohol use. For example, tobacco use is often quantified using a breath CO level, which has a very short half-life of approximately 2 hours. Because many adolescent smokers have irregular use patterns, it is hard to establish use by means of these indicators. The use of indicators with short half-lives also requires that abstinence be determined multiple times per day, which also decreases the feasibility of this intervention.

An alternative is to use biochemical indicators that have longer half-lives and that can be easily detected in urine or saliva samples. For example, for use in CM-based program, our group has developed the use of cotinine assessments. Cotinine, a by-product of nicotine, has a longer half-life (of approximately 20 hours) as well as superior sensitivity and specificity in measuring tobacco use when compared with CO levels (Gariti, Alterman, Ehrman, Mulvaney, & O'Brien, 2002). Until recently, cotinine levels were measured using laboratory-based gas-chromotographic quantitative techniques which were expensive, required special equipment, and decreased the feasibility of using cotinine as a marker for immediate reinforcement of abstinence as required by CM principles. However, the recent availability of semiquantitative urine cotinine immunoassay test strips has provided the CM field with an alternative method of verifying abstinence. The semiquantitative test strips are easy to implement, do not require special equipment, and, most important for use with CM procedures, provide the immediate verification of abstinence within a 10–20-minute incubation period. Our findings suggest that the immunoassay test strips were moderately sensitive and highly specific at detecting abstinence; however, sensitivity was low during the first few days of a quit attempt and improved over time, suggesting that during the first few days of a quit attempt, it would be advisable to continue to use daily multiple CO measurements to verify abstinence. However, as soon as abstinence is achieved, once-daily urine cotinine tests (determined using immunoassay test strips levels) could be used for continued monitoring. The use of cotinine as an abstinence indicator could also significantly enhance the feasibility and utility of CM-based interventions for smoking cessation by reducing the number of appointments required per day to verify abstinence.

However, the use of cotinine to determine adolescent tobacco use is not without problems. First, the immunoassay test strips are expensive (approximately $10 each) and can significantly add to the cost of the program. Second, although most adult smokers experience steady increases in cotinine levels throughout the day which corresponds to their continuous smoking pattern, it is not uncommon to find very low levels of these substances in an adolescent smoker who has spent the entire day in a nonsmoking environment (i.e., school) and tends to smoke later in the evening. Therefore, unlike the adult smoker, an adolescent smoker may not experience continual increases in cotinine and it may be necessary to obtain cotinine levels at the most common smoking times of the day, such as late evening or early morning, in order to obtain levels that reflect actual use patterns.

While most of our work has focused on tobacco use, similar work to determine optimal abstinence indicators needs to be conducted in the area of alcohol use. Because a majority of adolescents report binge drinking on weekends with little if any use of alcohol during weekdays, breath alcohol levels, which also have a relatively short half-life, may not be the optimal method of determining use or abstinence status. Therefore, the use of alternative markers of alcohol use such as fatty acid ethyl esters, ethyl glucuronide (Borucki et al., 2005), or the electronic transdermal alcohol sensor (Swift, Martin, Swette, LaConti, & Kackley, 1992) needs to be evaluated in adolescent drinkers. Alternatively, an abstinence-based CM program for adolescent drinkers may wish to consider targeting reinforcements to fit the adolescent's alcohol use profile (e.g., weekends for alcohol use) or an increase in non-alcohol-related behaviors.

Finally, one has to consider the ethical issues of providing monetary and other rewards to adolescents and ask the question, "How much is too much?" While the literature in this area would suggest that developmentally it is appropriate for children this age to have access to small amounts of cash, one needs to ensure that compensation levels are not overly coercive. For example, compensation levels could be developed to be equivalent to an income an adolescent could typically earn for working at a part-time job. Interestingly, research by Furnham (1999) indicates that most parents believe that it is important for children this age to have access to small amounts of money so that they begin to learn money-management skills. Moreover, ethicists such as Hoagwood, Jensen, and Fischer (1996) generally agree that children and adolescents should be fairly compensated for time spent on research activities. Researchers and clinicians who use CM could consider the inclusion of educational information for teens about money management and maybe even a brief intervention to help adolescents come up with a list of prosocial activities to achieve with the money they earn.

CONCLUDING COMMENTS

Although there has been progress toward the advancement of CM-based interventions for adolescent substance use, a significant amount of work still needs to be conducted in this area. To date, CM interventions for adolescents have focused on providing tangible reinforcers for abstinence, attendance, or engagement in behaviors incompatible with drug use. A majority of these studies, including our own, have focused on methods to reduce tobacco and marijuana use and future research needs to focus on other substances that are used by adolescents, including alcohol. Moreover, although the existing literature suggests that CM-based interventions significantly increase retention in treatment and abstinence rates for adolescent smokers, larger efficacy/effectiveness studies are needed to confirm these findings. Research also needs to be conducted to optimize both the duration of treatment and schedule of reinforcement that should be used with this population. Furthermore, we also need to conduct policy-related research to determine where the money to be used in CM-based programs is going to come from; that is, who is going to pay for such treatments in adolescents. And, finally, we also need to find ways to overcome some of the logistical, technical, and other barriers to the use of CM interventions with adolescents as discussed earlier. Thus, we have only just begun this exciting journey into developing efficacious CM interventions for adolescent SUDs with an overall goal of assisting more adolescents in navigating successfully through these challenging years.

REFERENCES

Arnett, J. J. (1999). Adolescent storm and stress, reconsidered. *American Psychologist, 54*(5), 317–326.

Audrain-McGovern, J., Rodriguez, D., Tercyak, K. P., Epstein, L. H., Goldman, P., & Wileyto, E. P. (2004). Applying a behavioral economic framework to understanding adolescent smoking. *Psychology of Addictive Behaviors, 18*(1), 64–73.

Azrin, N. H., Donohue, B., Besalel, V. A., Kogan, E. S., & Acierno, R. (1994). Youth drug abuse treatment: A controlled outcome study. *Journal of Child and Adolescent Substance Abuse, 3*(3), 1–16.

Balch, G. I. (1998). Exploring perceptions of smoking cessation among high school smokers: Input and feedback from focus groups. *Preventive Medicine, 27*(5), A55–A63.

Balch, G. I., Tworek, C., Barker, D. C., Sasso, B., Mermelstein, R., & Giovino, G. A. (2004). Opportunities for youth smoking cessation: Findings from a national focus group study. *Nicotine and Tobacco Research, 6*(1), 9–17.

Borucki, K., Schreiner, R., Dierkes, J., Jachau, K., Krause, D., Westphal, S., et al. (2005). Detection of recent ethanol intake with new markers: Comparison of fatty acid ethyl esters in serum and of ethyl glucuronide and the ratio of 5–hydroxytryptophol to 5-hydroxyindole acetic acid in urine. *Alcoholism: Clinical and Experimental Research, 29*, 781–787.

Botvin, G. J., Griffin, K. W., Diaz, T., Scheier, L. M., Williams, C., & Epstein, J. A. (2000). Preventing illicit drug use in adolescents: Long-term follow-up data from a randomized control trial of a school population. *Addictive Behaviors, 25*(5), 769–774.

Botvin, G. J., Schinke, S. P., & Orlandi, M. A. (1989). Psychosocial approaches to substance abuse prevention: Theoretical foundations and empirical findings. *Crisis, 10*(1), 62–77.

Breda, C., & Heflinger, C. A. (2004). Predicting incentives to change among adolescents with substance abuse disorder. *American Journal of Drug and Alcohol Abuse, 30*(2), 251–267.

Chambers, R. A., Taylor, J. R., & Potenza, M. N. (2003). Development neurocircuitry of motivation in adolescence: A critical period of addition vulnerability. *American Journal of Psychiatry, 160*(6), 1041–1052.

Corby, E. A., Roll, L. M., Ledgerwood, D. M., & Schuster, C. R. (2000). Contingency management interventions for treating the substance abuse of adolescents. *Experimental and Clinical Psychopharmacology, 8*(3), 371–376.

Cornelius, J. R., Bukstein, O. G., Lynch, K., Birmaher, B., Gershon, S., & Clark, D. B. (2001). Fluoxetine in adolescents with major depression and an adolescent alcohol use disorder: An open label trial. *Addictive Behaviors, 26,* 735–739.

Curry, S. J., Hollis, J., Bush, T., Polen, M., Ludman, E. J., Grothaus, L., et al. (2003). A randomized trial of a family-based smoking prevention intervention in managed care. *Preventive Medicine, 37*(6), 617–626.

Deci, E. L., Koestner, R., & Ryan, R. M. (1999). A meta-analytic review of experiments examining the effects of extrinsic rewards on intrinsic motivation. *Psychological Bulletin, 125*(6), 627–668.

Dennis, M., Godley, S. M., Diamond, G., Tims, F. M., Babor, T., Donaldson, J., et al. (2004). The cannabis youth treatment study: Main findings from two randomized trials. *Journal of Substance Abuse Treatment, 27*(3), 197–213.

Eisenberger, R., Pierce, W. D., & Cameron, J. (1999). Effects of reward on intrinsic motivation—negative, neutral and positive: Comment on Deci, Koestner, and Ryan (1999). *Psychological Bulletin, 125*(6), 677–691.

Eisenberger, R., & Rhoades, L. (2001). Incremental effects of reward on creativity. *Journal of Personality and Social Psychology, 81*(4), 728–741.

Fiore, M. C., Bailey, W. C., Cohen, S. J., Dorfman, S. F., Goldstein, M. G., Gritz, E. F., et al. (2000). *Treating tobacco use and dependence: Clinical practice guideline.* Rockville, MD: U.S. Department of Health and Human Services, Public Health Service.

Friedman, A., Granick, S., & Kreisher, C. (1994). Motivation of adolescent drug abusers for help and treatment. *Journal of Child and Adolescent Substance Abuse, 3*(1), 69–88.

Frissell, K. C., McCarthy, D. M., D' Amico, E. J., Metrik, J., Ellingstad, T. P., & Brown, S. A. (2004). Impact of consent procedures on reported levels of adolescent alcohol use. *Psychology of Addictive Behaviors, 18*(4), 307–315.

Furnham, A. (1999). Economic socialization: A study of adults' perceptions and uses of allowances (pocket money) to educate children. *British Journal of Developmental Psychology, 17,* 585–604.

Gariti, P., Alterman, A. I., Ehrman, R., Mulvaney, F. D., & O'Brien, C. P. (2002). Detecting smoking following smoking cessation treatment. *Drug and Alcohol Dependence, 65*(2), 191–196.

Giedd, J. N., Blumenthal, J., Jeffires, N. O., Castellanos, F. X., Liu, H., Zijdenbos, A., et al. (1999). Brain development during childhood and adolescence: A longitudinal MRI study. *Nature Neuroscience, 2*(10), 861–863.

Gillespie, A., Stanton, W., Lowe, J. B., & Hunter, B. (1995). Feasibility of school-based smoking cessation programs. *Journal of School Health, 65*(10), 432–437.

Greenblatt, J. C. (2000). *Patterns of alcohol use among adolescents and associations with emotional and behavioral problems* (Office of Applied Studies Substance Abuse and Mental Health Services Administration, Rockville, MD).

Grunbaum, J. A., Kann, L., Kinchen, S., Ross, J., Hawkins, J., Lowry, R., et al. (2004, May 21). Youth risk behavior surveillance—United States, 2003. *Morbidity and Mortality Weekly Report. Surveillance Summaries/DC, 53*(2), 1–96.

Hanson, K., Allen, S., Jensen, S., & Hatsukami, D. (2003). Treatment of adolescent smokers with the nicotine patch. *Nicotine and Tobacco Research, 5*(4), 515–526.

Hoagwood, K., Jensen, P. S., & Fischer, C. B. (Eds.). (1996). *Ethical issues in mental health research with children and adolescents.* Mahway, NJ: Erlbaum.

Hurt, R. D., Croghan, G. A., Beede, S. D., Wolter, T. D., Croghan, I. T., & Patten, C. A. (2000). Nicotine patch therapy in 101 adolescent smokers. *Archives of Pediatric and Adolescent Medicine, 154*(1), 31–37.

Johnston, L., O'Malley, P., Bachman, J., & Schulenberg, J. (2005). *Monitoring the future national results on adolescent drug abuse: Overview of key findings* (NIH Publication No. 05-5726). Bethesda, MD: National Institute on Drug Abuse.

Kaminer, Y., & Burleson, J. (1999). Psychotherapies for adolescent substance abusers. *American Journal of Addictions, 8*(2), 114–119.

Kamon, J., Budney, A., & Stanger, C. (2005). A contingency management intervention for adolescent marijuana abuse and conduct problems. *Journal of the American Academy of Child and Adolescent Psychiatry, 44*(6), 513–521.

Kenford S. L., Fiore, M. C., Jorenby, D. E., Smith, S. S., Wetter, D., & Baker, T. B. (1994) Predicting smoking cessation. Who will quit with and without the nicotine patch. *Journal of the American Medical Association, 271,* 589–594.

Krishnan-Sarin, S., Duhig, A., McKee, S., McMahon, T. J., Liss, T., McFetridge, A., et al. (2006). Contingency management for smoking cessation in adolescent smokers. *Experimental and Clinical Psychopharmacology, 14*(1), 306–310.

Leatherdale, S. T., Cameron, R., Brown, K. S., Jolin, M. A., & Kroeker, C. (2006). The influence of friends, family, and older peers on smoking among elementary school students: Low-risk students in high-risk schools. *Preventive Medicine, 6,* 218–222.

Leatherdale, S. T., & McDonald, P. W. (2005). What smoking cessation approaches will young smokers use? *Addictive Behaviors, 30*(8), 1614–1618.

Liddle, H., Rowe, C., Dakof, G., Ungaro, R., & Henderson, C. (2004). Early intervention of adolescent substance abuse: Pretreatment to post-treatment outcomes of a randomized, clinical trial comparing multidimensional family therapy and peer group treatment. *Journal of Psychoactive Drugs, 36*(1), 49–63.

Lynam, D. R., Milich, R., Zimmerman, R., Novak, S. P., Logan, T. K., Martin, C., et al. (1999). Project DARE: No effects at 10-year follow-up. *Journal of Consulting and Clinical Psychology, 67*(4), 590–593.

Marsch, L. A., Bickel, W. K., Badger, G. J., Stothart, M. A., Quesnel, K. J., Stanger, C., et al. (2005). Comparison of pharmacological treatments for opioid-dependent adolescents. *Archives of General Psychiatry, 62*(10), 1157–1164.

Melnick, G., De Leon, G., Hawke, J., Jainchill, N., & Kressel, D. (1997). Motivation and readiness for therapeutic community treatment among adolescents and adult substance abusers. *American Journal of Drug and Alcohol Abuse, 23*(4), 485–506.

Mermelstein, R. (1999). Ethnicity, gender, and risk factors for smoking initiation: An overview. *Nicotine and Tobacco Research, 1*(2), 539–543.

Moolchan, E. T., Robinson, M. L., Ernst, M., Cadet, J. L., Pickworth, W. B., Heishman, J., et. al. (2005). Safety and Efficacy of the nicotine patch and gum for the treatment of adolescent tobacco addiction. *Pediatrics, 115*(4), e407–e414.

Roll, J. M. (2005). Assessing the feasibility of using contingency management to modify cigarette smoking by adolescents. *Journal of Applied Behavior Analysis, 38*(4), 463–467.

Smith, T. A., House, R. F., Croghan, I. T., Gauvin, T. R., Colligan, R. C., Offord, K. P., et al. (1996). Nicotine patch therapy in adolescent smokers. *Pediatrics, 98*(4), 659–667.

Spear, L. P. (2000). The adolescent brain and age-related behavioral manifestations. *Neuroscience and Biobehavioral Reviews, 24*(4), 417–463.

Steinberg, L., Dahl, R. E., Keating, D., Kupfer, D. J., Masten, A. S., & Pine, D. (2006). The study of developmental psychopathology in adolescence: Integrating affective neuroscience with the study of context. In D. Cicciretti (Ed.), *Handbook of developmental psychopathology* (pp. 1–96). New York: Wiley.

Sussman, S. (2002). Effects of sixty six adolescent tobacco use cessation trials and seventeen prospective studies of self initiated quitting. *Tobacco Induced Diseases, 1*(1), 35–81.

Sussman, S., Dent, C. W., Nezami, E., Stacy, A. W., Burton, D., & Flay, B. R. (1998). Reasons for quitting and smoking temptation among adolescent smokers: Gender differences. *Substance Use and Misuse, 33*(14), 2703–2720.

Swift, R. M., Martin, C. S., Swette, L., LaConti, A., & Kackley, N. (1992). Studies on a wearable, electronic, transdermal alcohol sensor. *Alcoholism: Clinical and Experimental Research, 16*, 721–725.

Tevyaw, T. O., & Monti, P. M. (2004). Motivational enhancement and other brief interventions for adolescent substance abuse: Foundations, applications, and evaluations. *Addiction, 99*(Suppl. 2), 63–75.

Tillett, J. (2004). Adolescents and informed consent. *Journal of Perinatal and Neonatal Nursing, 19*(2), 112–121.

Waldron, H. B., Slesnick, N., Brody, J. L., Turner, C. W., & Peterson, T. R. (2001). Treatment outcomes for adolescent substance abuse at 4- and 7-month follow-up assessments. *Journal of Consulting and Clinical Psychology, 69*(5), 802–813.

Weissman, W., Glasgow, R., Biglan, A., & Lichtenstein, E. (1987). Developmental and preliminary evaluation of a cessation program for adolescent smokers. *Psychology of Addictive Behaviors, 1*, 84–91.

Westman, E. C., Behm, F. M., Simel, D. L., & Rose, J. E. (1997). Smoking behavior on the first day of a quit attempt predicts long-term abstinence. *Archives of Internal Medicine, 157*, 335–340.

Williams, R. J., & Chang, S. Y. (2000). A comprehensive review of adolescent substance abuse treatment outcome. *Clinical Psychology, 7*, 138–166.

PART III

DISSEMINATION

CHAPTER 13

LARGE-SCALE DISSEMINATION EFFORTS IN DRUG ABUSE TREATMENT CLINICS

Maxine L. Stitzer *and* Scott Kellogg

Contingency management (CM) interventions have demonstrated efficacy in the treatment of drug abuse, as amply documented in this volume and elsewhere. However, these interventions have not as yet become part of mainstream substance abuse treatment delivered in this country. This chapter reviews the progress to date in dissemination and the adoption of CM within the larger drug abuse treatment community.

As a precursor to dissemination and adoption, it is important to ascertain the effectiveness of CM interventions when implemented at real-world community treatment programs. Such research was recently undertaken within the National Institute on Drug Abuse's Clinical Trials Network (CTN), where the largest study undertaken to date designed to test the effectiveness of a CM intervention in a drug-abusing population was completed. This chapter describes the protocol development process and study outcomes for the multisite CTN trial. In addition to documenting the effectiveness of a particular abstinence incentive protocol, the CTN study development process highlighted some of the barriers that need to be overcome as well as the decisions that clinicians face in designing and implementing a CM program. Further, the CTN protocol development process illustrates how the issues can be resolved by striking a balance between clinical

acceptability/feasibility considerations and fidelity to research-based methods previously shown to be efficacious.

The demonstration of effectiveness in a large-scale community-based
study paves the way for more widespread dissemination and adoption of
these techniques in clinical practice. In a second section of the chapter, we
describe selected dissemination and adoption initiatives that have been undertaken following the CTN clinical trial. These descriptions provide an example of how CM interventions will most likely be adopted by clinicians
who devise their own unique programs rather than copying any particular
protocol that has been developed and tested in controlled research. Thus,
the purpose of the chapter is to summarize recent support for effectiveness,
to highlight some of the complex decisions that need to be made prior to
adoption, and to illustrate several possible pathways to more widespread
adoption of CM interventions by community treatment providers.

MOTIVATIONAL INCENTIVES FOR ENHANCED DRUG ABUSE RECOVERY: THE CTN CM STUDY

The opportunity to implement a large-sample multisite effectiveness study
of CM was afforded when the CTN was established in 1999. A sobering
study had been published by the Institute of Medicine (IOM; Lamb,
Greenlick, & McCarty, 1998), which pointed out the chasm that existed
between new treatments developed and tested for efficacy by researchers
working at academic centers and the real-world practices ongoing at drug
abuse treatment programs operating in the community. Based on recommendations from the IOM study, a CTN was established that would help
to foster the adoption of evidence-based practices in community treatment
programs while verifying the effectiveness of the new practices when implemented in those treatment programs.

The CTN is comprised of several regionally diverse centers where experienced treatment researchers working at some of the leading academic
institutions in this country have formed a coalition with local community
treatment providers. Communication and collaboration between researchers and treatment providers is fostered within the CTN through a unique
governance structure in which academic researchers and community program directors are equally represented and equally involved in the decision-
making processes of the network, including selection and design of research
projects.

The first job of the newly formed CTN governance structure was to
choose and develop the initial research studies that would be conducted.
Based in part on the very strong evidence base that had accumulated from
efficacy research with CM, a decision was made to develop a CM protocol
as one of the first-wave studies, with all details to be worked out as a col-

laborative effort between the designated lead investigator (Stitzer) and her support team. The protocol was given a name, Motivational Incentives for Enhanced Drug Abuse Recovery (MIEDAR), that would serve to emphasize the clinical intent and utility of the intervention.

Research–Practice Considerations in Design of the MIEDAR Study

Development of the MIEDAR protocol took place through a process that involved input from both researchers and clinicians. It was recognized from the start that the protocol needed to make sense from a clinical perspective, to be feasible to implement in community programs, and to be potentially sustainable in these programs. As a result, protocol development was an instructive exercise that brought into focus the diverse perspective of researchers and clinicians and the need for adjustment and compromise on the part of both parties in the research-to-practice translation. Further, to establish the broadest possible generality of CM effects, it was decided early on that two types of outpatient clinics would participate—those that delivered methadone maintenance for opioid dependence and those that delivered only psychosocial counseling support for patients abusing a variety of drugs. Thus, in designing the protocol, tailoring was also needed to accommodate differences in characteristics of the patients treated and/or in clinical operation of these two treatment modalities.

Modality tailoring considerations were most clearly apparent in selection of study inclusion and exclusion criteria. In methadone clinics, where patients may remain in treatment for long periods of time but exhibit ongoing patterns of therapeutically undesirable behaviors, patients were invited for study participation after they had become medically stabilized and based on documented evidence of the target behavior (stimulant drug use). In contrast, because of the known problem with treatment dropout in the psychosocial counseling modality, it was important to enroll patients into the CTN study as soon as possible after clinical intake, thus exposing the maximum number of new treatment patients to the intervention. Further, in this modality, there was more reliance on self-report of recent drug use in qualifying patients for study participation.

Clinical versus Research Considerations in Choice of a Behavioral Target

A decision was made early on in protocol development that the target of the intervention should be abstinence from drugs rather than some other behavioral target such as attendance at therapy sessions or accomplishment of treatment plan goals. While some of the latter behaviors may be easier to target, it was deemed important to emphasize and reinforce drug abstinence as the primary outcome of interest in drug abuse treatment. It was then necessary to decide which drug or drugs to incorporate in the contingency. Much of the previous research documenting efficacy for CM interventions had been conducted using single drug targets, particularly cocaine. Some of this research had demonstrated that there were secondary gains in the reduction of nontargeted drug use when the intervention focused only on one drug. For example, reductions in opiates had been consistently demonstrated when CM interventions targeted cocaine use (Silverman et al., 1996; Silverman, Robles, Mudric, Bigelow, & Stitzer, 2004). Similarly, reductions in cocaine use have been apparent when opiates were the target of intervention (Robles, Stitzer, Strain, Bigelow, & Silverman, 2002). However, other research has suggested that efficacy of a CM intervention is reduced when multidrug targets are employed (see Lussier, Heil, Mongeon, Badger, & Higgins, 2006).

The scientific data and their implications were in conflict with the practices and goals of the community treatment programs. On the one hand, it was desirable to maintain close adherence to methods used in efficacy research, which suggested that a single drug target should be employed. On the other hand, a focus on abstinence from all drugs of abuse as well as alcohol was the most common usual-care practice in community treatment programs. A balanced compromise was reached on this point. Stimulants would be the primary target drug of the intervention, acknowledging that stimulants are the most prevalent drug of abuse (after alcohol) among individuals entering drug abuse treatment programs (Community Epidemiology Work Group [CEWG], 2006). Further, behavioral interventions are especially needed to address the use of these drugs for which no pharmacotherapy has yet been identified. Importantly, both cocaine and methamphetamine would be incorporated into the drug target in order to account for regional diversity in the specific type of stimulants abused.

Consideration was also given, however, to the clinically important goal of stopping all types of drug use. Given the association between stimulant and alcohol use (Brady, Sonne, Randall, Adinoff, & Malcolm, 1995; Heil, Badger, & Higgins, 2001), it was deemed clinically important to prevent any patient who came to the clinic intoxicated on alcohol from receiving a reinforcer. Thus, alcohol use to intoxication was included as part of the primary drug target such that delivery of a reinforcer would require both a stimulant negative urine and a negative alcohol breathalyzer. Interestingly, the subsequent data showed that alcohol intoxication at the clinic was a rare event in our study population, with alcohol being detected in 0.5% of all samples tested in psychosocial counseling patients (Petry, Peirce, et al., 2005) and in 1% of samples tested among methadone-maintenance patients enrolled in the study (Peirce et al., 2006).

Two additional drug classes, opiates and cannabinoinds (marijuana), were also incorporated into the protocol as secondary targets for which stimulant-abstinent participants could earn extra reinforcement. This was a place where tailoring was needed to accommodate the clinical perspective of the two treatment modalities. In psychosocial counseling programs, where total abstinence was typically a strong emphasis of treatment, both drugs were included as secondary targets. However, in methadone-maintenance programs, clinicians felt that marijuana should not be included as a target drug as clinical attention to this substance was inconsistent, with some methadone programs not routinely testing for this substance or incorporating abstinence from marijuana in the treatment plan.

Thus, selection of drug target(s) was an area in which clinical-research compromise was needed, as well as tailoring to meet the needs of different treatment modalities. While designed to acknowledge the importance of stopping the use of drugs from multiple classes, the protocol was structured in such a way that use versus abstinence from the secondary drugs did not have an impact on the participants' ability to earn reinforcers for primary target drug abstinence (negative stimulants and alcohol). This is important because if all drugs are included in the primary target, the ability of a given patient to earn incentives may depend on the number of drugs he or she is using, with the likelihood of having any positive impact on behavior being reduced for patients who are using more than one drug, where the task of stopping use is presumably more difficult.

Cost Considerations and Solutions

A serious concern of clinicians about the sustainability of contingent incentive procedures is related to their cost. The strongest evidence for efficacy of these interventions resided in voucher incentive studies where patients were offered up to $1,000 over a 3-month intervention for submitting continuously cocaine-negative urine specimens (e.g., Higgins et al., 1994; Silverman et al., 1996). Despite evidence that the extent of behavior change obtained with CM procedures is positively related to the magnitude of reinforcement provided (see Lussier et al., 2006), this level of incentive payment was deemed by CTN clinicians to be patently unsustainable and not worth investigating if part of the goal was to develop protocols that could potentially be adopted by community programs.

One innovation that could be brought into play to address the cost concern was a recently developed "fishbowl" method (Petry & Martin, 2002; Petry, Martin, & Simcic, 2005; Petry, Martin, Cooney, & Kranzler, 2000; Petry et al., 2004) that utilizes principles of intermittent reinforcement to reduce cost of CM interventions (see Petry & Alessi, Chapter 14, this volume, for full description of research using the "fishbowl" technology). In the fishbowl method, submission of a drug-free urine sample results in the opportunity to draw tokens from a bowl, on which prize winnings are designated. Intermittent reinforcement is accomplished by having only half the tokens in the bowl result in prizes. Cost is further reduced by including prizes of varying value and by adjusting the number of tokens in the bowl such that the probability of winning is inversely related to the value of the prize. The CTN study utilized the fishbowl technology, with 50% of chips resulting in a "good job!" (no prize) message, 42% of chips resulting in a prize worth about $1 (e.g., sodas, candy bars, and toiletries), 8% of chips resulting in a "large" prize worth about $20 (e.g., cordless phones, CDs, pots, and pans), and a single chip indicating that a "jumbo" prize worth about $100 (e.g., TV and VCR) had been won. To increase their saliency, prizes were kept onsite in a lockable cabinet so that participants could view their potential earnings and ask for prizes they wanted to be stocked.

Because previous research had indicated the importance of escalating schedules for promoting sustained periods of abstinence (Roll, Higgins, & Badger, 1996), an escalation feature was built into the prize draw (fishbowl) intervention by increasing the number of draws that could be taken from the bowl with each consecutive week in which stimulant- and alcohol-negative samples had been submitted, and resetting the number of draws to the original low value (one draw) in the event that a positive urine was submitted or an entire week passed with no sample submitted. Two bonus draws could also be taken following the submission of stimulant- and alcohol-negative samples provided that the participant's urine sample also tested negative for marijuana and/or opiates.

With study visits scheduled twice weekly, total possible value of the prizes that could be won over 12 weeks was $400 on average. While this total earning value is less than half the total earnings possible in previous voucher incentive programs, it is consistent with values used in several small-scale studies previously published by Petry and colleagues that demonstrated the efficacy of the prize draw (fishbowl) procedure (Petry & Martin, 2002; Petry et al., 2000, 2004; Petry, Martin, & Simsic, 2005). Notably, positive findings from the CTN study would provide important support for lower-cost methods that represent a breakthrough in the feasibility and sustainability of abstinence incentive programs overall.

The staffing of a urinalysis-based incentive intervention is a related concern and potential feasibility barrier for dissemination because the collection and the testing of urine samples is labor intensive and costly. A twice-weekly urine collection schedule was adopted in the MIEDAR study to accommodate the short-acting drugs targeted for intervention, recognizing that this was a greater frequency of urine testing than could probably be sustained in community treatment programs due to cost. While sustainability of the intervention would most likely have been enhanced if counselors were taught how to implement the contingency program, the protocol development team elected to use research staff to collect and test urines. This strategy was expected to enhance fidelity with the research protocol.

More importantly, the use of research staff would free counselors to focus on other important aspects of their job.

Clinical Concerns about Adverse Effects

Another feasibility concern raised during development of the CTN protocol was related to the possibility that participation in a protocol that involved chances of winning or not winning prizes would have an adverse impact on (i.e., stimulate) gambling behavior among participants. This concern was addressed in several ways. First, any study applicant who admitted to being in recovery from a gambling problem was excluded (although no such participants were actually found). Second, increased gambling was defined as a study-related adverse event and tracked throughout the protocol (however, no study-related incidences were ever identified). Finally, data about gambling were collected from all participants at baseline, 1, 3, and 6 months. Analysis of these data has revealed that at any given time point, about 15% of psychosocial counseling patients and 20–25% of methadone patients reported any gambling. However, amounts spent were quite modest ($10–$20 per month on average) and there were no differences either during or after treatment between participants exposed to incentive and control conditions (Petry et al., 2006). Thus, the study was able to collect evidence indicating that exposure to a prize draw incentive procedure had no adverse effects on gambling behavior among stimulant abusers.

Overall, CTN clinicians raised a variety of concerns about incentive interventions during the protocol development phase of the project, and they raised issues that will need to be faced by any program looking to adopt these methods. All the concerns were addressed by reasonable compromise in a manner that remained sensitive to both research integrity and clinical feasibility considerations. Table 13.1 summarizes the resulting protocol methods.

Sample Characteristics

Development of the MIEDAR protocol took about 1 year, and the study was launched in the spring of 2001. Study participants were recruited from six methadone-maintenance and eight psychosocial counseling programs in regionally diverse areas. The sample sizes accrued into this study were substantial, with 388 stimulant abusers enrolled in methadone-maintenance and 415 enrolled in psychosocial counseling programs, making this the largest evaluation of contingent incentive interventions ever undertaken. Table 13.2 shows demographic and drug use characteristics for the stimulant abuser study samples drawn from the two types of treatment programs. Participant characteristics were quite similar across the two modalities ex-

TABLE 13.1. MIEDAR Methods

Study design	Randomized 2-group: usual care with and without incentives
Participants	Stimulant abusers (cocaine or methamphetamine)
Inclusion criteria	Methadone: stimulant-positive urine submitted within 2 weeks of study start; in treatment 1–36 mos Counseling: stimulant use reported within 2 weeks of treatment entry; in treatment < 1 month
Exclusion criteria	Provides no recent evidence of stimulant use In recovery from a gambling problem
Intervention duration	12 weeks
Expected study visits	24 (twice weekly)
Primary drug targets	Stimulant-negative urine test Negative breath alcohol test
Secondary drug target(s)	Opiates (methadone and psychosocial counseling) Marijuana (psychosocial counseling only)
Reinforcement method	Drawing for prizes
Drawing schedule	Draws escalate once per week for consecutive stimulant- (and alcohol-) negative samples 2 bonus draws if also negative for secondary drug(s)
Total possible draws	205
Average max prize value	$400

cept that psychosocial counseling patients were younger than methadone patients and more likely to be referred from the criminal justice system. However, ongoing drug use at the start of the study was markedly different for the two samples, with methadone patients submitting 75% stimulant-positive samples at their first study visit compared to 25% stimulant-positive samples submitted by the psychosocial counseling patients. This is consistent with study entry criteria and reflects large behavioral differences in ongoing drug use among these samples that were apparent both at the time of study entry and during treatment.

Main Study Outcomes

Outcomes from the MIEDAR studies have been published in a prominent psychiatry journal, with results published separately for the parallel studies conducted in psychosocial counseling (Petry, Peirce, et al., 2005) and methadone-maintenance (Peirce et al., 2006) programs. Both studies showed significant positive benefits for the abstinence incentive program, although outcomes patterns differed across the two modalities.

TABLE 13.2. MIEDAR Participant Demographics

	Methadone maintenance ($n = 388$)	Psychosocial counseling ($n = 415$)
Female (%)	45	55
Minority (%)	49	58
Age (mean years)	42	36
Education (mean years)	12	12
Employed at study start (%)	32	35
Criminal-justice-involved (%)	16	36
Methadone dose (mean mg)	86	—
Months in treatment at study start	9	1
First study urine (% stimulant positive)	75	25

Psychosocial Counseling Study

As shown in Figure 13.1, the ability to earn incentives for drug abstinence resulted in a significant improvement in retention for patients in psychosocial counseling programs. Overall, 50% of those exposed to usual care + incentives were retained for 12 weeks compared with 35% of those in usual care without incentives (hazard ratio = 1.60; confidence interval [CI] = 1.23–2.07). Interestingly, there was little evidence of during-treatment drug use for psychosocial counseling patients, with approximately 90% of all samples delivered testing negative for stimulants and alcohol. In part because of this low overall rate of during-treatment drug use, incentives were

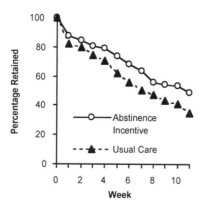

FIGURE 13.1. Percent of participants retained over a 12-week incentive intervention. Data are shown for two groups of stimulant abusers enrolled in psychosocial counseling treatment randomly assigned to receive usual care treatment with ($n = 209$) or without ($n = 206$) a prize-based abstinence-incentive intervention. Adapted from Petry, Peirce, et al. (2005). Copyright 2005 by the American Medical Association. Adapted by permission.

not demonstrated to have a direct impact on the rates of stimulant-positive versus -negative samples delivered during treatment. Nevertheless, the longest duration of documented abstinence (LDA) was significantly greater for incentive than for control participants (4.4 vs 2.6 week, respectively; $p <$ .001), suggesting that abstinence was prolonged via increased duration of treatment retention (and assuming that treatment dropout is associated at least in some cases with relapse to drug use). A nearly fourfold increase was observed in the percentage of participants who achieved 12 weeks of sustained abstinent treatment participation (18.7% of incentive vs. 4.9% of control participants; odds ratio = 4.48; CI = 2.17–9.23).

For dissemination purposes, it is instructive to examine the impact of incentive interventions at individual clinics, even though the study was not powered to test effects at the individual clinic level. In five of eight programs, retention increased by at least 1 week (mean increase = 2.1 weeks) in patients exposed to incentive compared with control interventions. Clinics that showed improved retention were those that had relatively poorer mean baseline retention durations ranging from 3.6 to 6.8 weeks (mean = 5.5 weeks). In contrast, those clinics that failed to show a benefit from incentives were already keeping patients in treatment for 8 weeks on average. These observations suggest that abstinence incentives may be most effectively employed to boost retention duration in clinics in which retention has historically been relatively low. However, in deciding when and where to implement incentive programs, additional research would be helpful. Given the low rates of during-treatment drug use observed, it would be useful to determine whether similar results on retention could be obtained in psychosocial counseling programs by targeting treatment attendance rather than abstinence, because incentives targeted on attendance could potentially be less costly and labor-intensive to implement. Also, it will be important to establish the conditions under which improved retention in community programs achieved through use of incentive procedures translates into better long-term outcomes on other measures of drug use and psychosocial adjustment.

Methadone-Maintenance Study

Contrasting results were obtained in the methadone-maintenance sample. In this modality, abstinence incentives had no impact on retention, a result that is expected because retention is quite good in usual care methadone treatment. Overall, about 70% of participants were retained in the study for the full 12 weeks. (Note that methadone patients may have dropped out of the study while still remaining in usual care treatment at their clinic.) However, as shown in Figure 13.2, incentives produced a significant reduction in rates of ongoing stimulant use during treatment, doubling the odds that a stimulant- and alcohol-negative urine would be

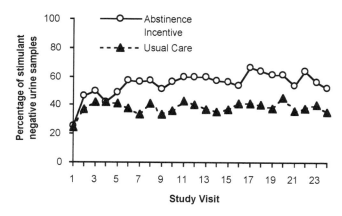

FIGURE 13.2. Percent of submitted samples testing negative for stimulants and alcohol. Data are shown for two groups of stimulant abusers enrolled in methadone-maintenance treatment and randomly assigned to receive usual care with (*n* = 198) or without (*n* = 190) a prize draw abstinence-incentive intervention. The intervention was implemented over a 12-week period with two study visits scheduled per week. From Peirce et al. (2006). Copyright 2006 by the American Medical Association. Reprinted by permission.

delivered at any given urine collection time point (OR = 1.98; CI = 1.42–2.77).

Longest duration of abstinence (LDA) was also significantly increased for incentive versus control participants in the methadone study (3 weeks vs. 1 week, respectively; $p < .001$). In this case, the effect on LDA appeared to reflect a direct impact on drug use rather than an indirect effect mediated through improved retention. A 2.5-fold increase was observed in the percentage of participants who achieved 10 or more weeks of sustained abstinence (21% of incentive vs. 8% of control participants; $p < .001$). Higher rates of stimulant- and alcohol-negative urines were seen for incentive compared to control patients in all clinics, and these improvements were substantial (greater than 10 percentage points) in four of six clinics.

DISSEMINATION AND ADOPTION

The CTN MIEDAR study resulted in convincing evidence for the effectiveness of abstinence-contingent incentives when delivered in community treatment programs. This new evidence provides an important springboard for further dissemination and adoption of incentive-based interventions by community treatment providers. Nevertheless, uncertainties remain about exactly what should be adopted as well as practical considerations about the barriers that need to be overcome in order to promote adoption. In this section, we provide two examples of how those barriers have been over-come in order to implement incentive procedures at community treatment programs.

Dissemination in the Mid-Atlantic Node

The CTN infrastructure provides the opportunity to begin exploring adoption methods and models that may help introduce incentive procedures more widely in community-based treatment programs. Six community treatment programs affiliated with the Mid-Atlantic node of the CTN, two of which participated in the MIEDAR study, have initiated an incentive adoption project using no-cost or low-cost prizes. With the help of a node dissemination coordinator, these programs are developing their own incentive procedures tailored to the unique clinical priorities of their program and the specific needs of their own patient populations.

Interestingly, each clinic was able to arrive quickly at a clear consensus on the behavioral target. One methadone-maintenance clinic chose fee payments that resulted in a zero balance as their behavioral target and called the program "Pay to Play." The remaining programs chose therapy group attendance as their target—a behavior considered especially important for early engagement and retention—in most cases, electing to provide incentives to new patients for attendance at their first 4–8 sessions. Clinicians became actively involved in designing the details of these programs including exactly what the incentives would be, what rules for earning prizes made most sense for their situation, and where incentives would be obtained, stored, displayed and distributed. Clinicians recognized the benefits of a raffle-type system in order to control costs, while building in motivation for sustained behavior change. In a raffle system, the more times the patient performs the behavior (attend group, pay fees), the more tickets he or she would get in the bowl, with increased chance to win a prize. The dissemination coordinator brought examples of no-cost prizes (laminated cards with the serenity prayer; achievement certificates), provided information about low-cost prizes that can be purchased online, and displayed low-cost prizes from dollar stores and drugstores. Clinical staff came up with creative ideas about where to obtain moderate-cost prizes in the community and, in some cases, volunteered to donate prizes themselves.

Importantly, the model of dissemination being used is experiential rather than didactic, with the dissemination coordinator providing onsite monitoring and feedback to clinicians. This process should result in a rich array of insights about what works and what interferes with effective adoption of incentives at each site. Ideally, clinical data will be collected on the target behavior selected before and during the intervention to provide feedback that can be used as the basis for determining whether the intervention worked at the site. After an initial 3-month experience, the staff and program director can look at the data, then make a joint decision about whether to continue, what changes to make, if any, and where the funding would come from for continuing with incentives.

The Mid-Atlantic dissemination initiative grew out of experience with incentive procedures derived originally from participation in CTN effectiveness research. Other models are also available for the introduction of CM or incentive procedures into clinical practice. One of the most remarkably effective examples to date is described in the section that follows.

Dissemination: Experience from the New York City Health and Hospitals Corporation

The largest and most exciting dissemination project to date is that launched by the New York City Health and Hospitals Corporation (HHC; Kellogg et al., 2005). HHC is a large municipal health care system providing care to substance abusers in over 40 different treatment settings in New York City. In the years 1998–2000, HHC received funding from the city as well as the New York State Office of Substance Abuse Services to enhance the vocational rehabilitation counseling component in five of its methadone clinics. This infusion of funding sparked a broadly based change process that included systems reorganization at the clinics and adoption of a new philosophy that embraced rehabilitation, recovery, and self-sufficiency as primary treatment goals for the patients.

As part of this change initiative, HHC developed and launched in 2001 a "Patient Recognition and Motivation Initiative" based on research that supported the utility of contingent incentives to encourage and motivate patients to attain treatment goals. Although the initiative was devised and promoted from the top by the HHC organization leaders, clinics that wished to participate were asked to develop and submit their own individualized implementation plans. Start-up of the initiative was facilitated when HHC leadership met and formed a collaboration with faculty members from the CTN. The collaboration resulted in a series of onsite consultation meetings between CTN faculty (Kellogg) and participating clinics in order to help the clinics develop their incentive implementation plans.

The specific incentive procedures developed and implemented at the five clinics that initially participated in the project are described in more detail by Kellogg et al. (2005). Consistent with the Mid-Atlantic node project discussed earlier, most of the programs focused initially on group therapy attendance as the primary intervention target and used a variety of token reward systems to reinforce this behavior. Several of the programs subsequently expanded the focus of their incentive plan to incorporate the delivery of reinforcers when patients attained various objective treatment plan goals. The types of reinforcers offered included transportation vouchers ("metro cards"), movie passes, and gift certificates to department stores, music stores, and fast-food restaurants. Tangible prizes were also used in-cluding clothing items, date books, water bottles, sunglasses, toiletries, food, and candy. In addition, many programs expanded on their awards ceremonies, at which patients exhibiting behavior change were honored with the presentation of certificates.

Lessons Learned from the HHC Experience

REWARD VERSUS REINFORCEMENT

The opportunity to engage in training with front-line clinicians provided in-valuable insights into the issues that need to be addressed in adoption of in-centive programs by community treatment providers. One critical issue that emerged early in the process was the importance of making a distinction for the clinicians between reward and reinforcement. The natural inclination of line staff was to invoke a doctrine of "fairness" and to set up a program that offered incentives to every patient. In fact, this approach is less than ideal for inculcating behavior change, because clinic resources end up being used to reward patients who are already doing well rather than to reinforce behavior change in those who are not doing particularly well. Further, the inclusion of patients who are already doing well tends to focus attention on long-term achievements (e.g., finishing a vocational training program and keeping a job for 30, 60, or 90 days) rather than focusing on the smaller incremental steps of behavior change that may lead to the larger more sus-tained changes. Thus, it was important to teach clinicians the value of set-ting up contingencies that reinforced smaller behavior changes so that more troubled and/or more severely addicted patients would have the opportu-nity to benefit.

The focus on rewarding short-term gains is one that can change the en-tire outlook of clinical staff. Thus, this approach encourages staff members to focus on the good things that patients did, not on their failings. The ap-proach trains clinicians to understand that any steps in the right direction are a cause for celebration and that in the face of setbacks, patients should be encouraged to try harder, not criticized. In keeping with the importance of an enthusiastic and celebratory staff attitude, any staff members who were not enthusiastic about or were opposed to the intervention were in-vited to exclude themselves from the distribution of reinforcers to patients.

CLIENT AND STAFF REACTIONS

Typically, counseling staff was resistant to the new intervention at first. Consistent and supportive local clinic leadership was an important factor that helped to combat this tendency, and providing opportunities to staff to air their concerns seemed to help. However, the most salient factor in changing staff attitudes was observing the beneficial effects of the intervention and the reaction of patients to it. Patients, many of whom came from profoundly deprived backgrounds where they had never been recognized for anything positive, were more than enthusiastic about the incentive program; they could hardly believe that they were being singled out to receive prizes and rewards. Patients who received incentives appeared to improve in self-esteem, to become more socially integrated and participatory at the clinic, and to begin talking about longer-term goals. These general impressions, as well as examples of individual patients who turned around their behavior abruptly in a more positive direction, had a strong impact on counselors. In addition, some patients began to express gratitude to counselors for their help. Thus, counselors' positive attitudes were shaped when they began to feel that they were more effective at their job, and when they began to receive direct reinforcement through patient statements of gratitude.

CLINIC CULTURE CHANGE

The description provided here of the HHC initiative suggests that there was a fairly profound change in the operation and culture of the clinics as a result of participating in the incentives program, and this was indeed the case. Instead of viewing the intervention as an add-on to usual care, some of the clinics began to see incentives as the centerpiece of the psychosocial counseling part of their treatment. The shift from punitive to a celebratory attitude toward clients was a beneficial change that raised staff morale and reduced conflict at the clinic sites. The fact that counselors designed and operated their own incentive programs and directly experienced the benefits of those programs was no doubt important in their enthusiastic adoption. Overall, although objective evidence of effectiveness was not a central focus, the HHC project can be seen as an enormous success from a process perspective, and one that can serve as a model for future dissemination efforts.

OVERCOMING ADOPTION BARRIERS

Both the CTN and HHC projects highlight important barriers to adoption and how experience with CM interventions can help overcome these barriers. This section reviews two of the most salient barriers: negative attitudes and cost, with some additional speculations on how these barriers may be overcome in the future.

Negative Attitudes

Clinician attitudes continue to be a barrier to more widespread adoption of CM techniques. McGovern, Fox, Xie, and Drake (2004) surveyed clinicians in 24 New Hampshire treatment programs about their attitudes toward several evidence-based treatment approaches. The survey revealed that CM was infrequently used and rated as less likely to be adopted than other therapies such as motivational interviewing, cognitive-behavioral therapy, and 12-Step facilitation. Nearly half the clinicians (48%) said they were unfamiliar with CM, suggesting yet another barrier to adoption. Another recent study conducted at the clinical programs affiliated with CTN (D. McCarty et al., 2007) suggested that there is little support among staff at community programs for paying patients to attend sessions or provide drug-free urines. This skepticism about the clinical value of incentive procedures appears to be widespread, and was even reflected during the initial phases of study planning within the CTN.

Both the CTN and HHC experiences testify to the fact that attitudes of clinicians can change. This change, as with any attitudinal change, occurred gradually and required multiple sources of input. Within the CTN, it appeared important for clinicians to gain an appreciation of the clinical flexibility of CM interventions and, in particular, to understand that they are best used as an add-on to usual care. Thus, incentive interventions did not pose a threat to the basic operation of the clinic or require a major change in existing practices. On the contrary, CM interventions that "jump-start" the abstinence process could be viewed as helpful to counselors in doing their most important job of promoting and teaching lifestyle change for long-term stability and abstinence. Further, clinicians could appreciate the role of CM in fostering a more positive clinic culture that focuses on rewarding and celebrating success—"catching people being good" rather than taking success for granted and focusing clinical attention primarily on crises and failures.

Underlying the clinician reluctance to support incentives is the concern that the provision of "artificial" external reinforcers might have a negative impact on the development of internal motivation to abstain from drugs. The evidence in this point that swayed opinions within the CTN was delivered at a meeting held early on in the protocol development process. Here, testimonials from a panel of clinicians and patients who had previously participated in Dr. Petry's incentive-based interventions at community clinics were presented. The patients interviewed said that it made them feel proud to be able to stay off drugs. Further, although they might have been working for the prizes at first, at some point they began appreciating the benefits of abstinence and wanted to continue maintaining abstinence for their own personal welfare and that of their families. The fact that these patients could articulate experiencing a switch from external to internal motivation offered powerful and impressive evidence that the receipt of incentives is not necessarily a deterrent to internal motivation and in fact may facilitate its development.

As attitudes change, there may be increasing demand for training in the principles and techniques of CM, which in turn could help to spur adoption. Fortunately, there are many continuing education opportunities for counselors, sponsored by a variety of local, state, and national organizations and agencies, with web-based training becoming increasingly popular and available on a variety of topics (see, e.g., *www.nattc.org*). Thus, an infrastructure exists to provide needed training in new evidence-based treatments, and the availability of explicit training in reinforcement-based interventions is likely to increase as interest and demand from the field rises.

Incremental Cost

The costs associated with the implementation of contingent incentive interventions continue to be perceived as a barrier. In calculating the costs of incentive interventions, it should be noted that actual costs of prizes or vouchers earned by participants are typically about 50% or less of the total possible earnings, depending on the number of patients who are able to earn incentives under whatever specific program is offered. Thus, in the CTN MIEDAR study, actual average incentive earnings were about 50% of possible earning in the psychosocial counseling study ($198 per patient enrolled) and only about one-quarter of possible earnings ($119 per patient enrolled) in the methadone-maintenance study, where fewer participants were abstinent for prolonged periods of time and fewer prizes were earned overall.

While the costs of prize draws may be less than anticipated, other costs of operating the program must be added onto the basic cost of prizes. This includes staff time to purchase and inventory prizes and to implement the intervention at the clinic. In the case of abstinence-based incentive programs, there is also a substantial time and materials cost involved in the frequent urinalysis collection and testing needed to operate the contingency intervention. The cost of urinalysis testing poses a more significant barrier to abstinence-based incentives than is the case for incentives targeting other behaviors, and this may account in part for the choice of group attendance and other nonabstinence targets by community programs that have adopted these interventions so far. Cost-benefit and/or cost-effectiveness analyses of a variety of CM interventions will provide an important perspective for informing the future course of adoption, including the most cost-effective behaviors to target.

Ultimately, the costs of contingent incentive interventions will most likely be covered in a variety of ways at individual treatment programs. For example, private programs that operate on patient fees may increase charges to cover incentive costs or provide fee payment rebates to patients as an incentive for meeting intervention targets (see Amass & Kamien, Chapter 15, this volume). Public programs that operate with block grant funds may begin including incentive costs as a line item in their budget, justified by the desire of state and local oversight agencies to incorporate more evidence-based treatments into usual-care practice. Finally, programs that operate on fee-for-service reimbursement from insurance providers may be able to increase their income sufficiently to cover or exceed costs of incentives if the incentives effectively increase patient attendance rates and retention. Other strategies to fund incentive programs may include grants from local philanthropic agencies and donations solicited from businesses or individuals in the community (Amass & Kamien, 2004; see Amass & Kamien, Chapter 15, this volume). Overall, although cost has been perceived as a barrier, it is likely that this barrier will be overcome by a variety of creative funding strategies once there is either a grass-roots desire or mandate from above for programs to initiate incentive interventions.

CONCLUDING COMMENTS

This chapter has reviewed protocol development and outcomes for MIEDAR, the largest study of CM conducted to date, which was made possible through the National Drug Abuse Treatment CTN. The study, which enrolled approximately 800 stimulant abusers in a regionally diverse set of community treatment programs, provided convincing evidence for the effectiveness of a contingent incentive intervention targeted on stimulant and alcohol abstinence when delivered in community treatment programs. This data, in conjunction with findings from a host of smaller-scale efficacy studies conducted over the years, clearly supports more widespread adoption of CM interventions in community programs. However, barriers to adoption remain that include negative staff attitudes, lack of training, and cost.

The chapter also documents important recent advances in the dissemination and adoption of CM interventions that are proceeding both within and outside the CTN. Development of the CTN protocol was instructive in pointing out several areas in which compromise may be needed between research fidelity and clinical acceptability/feasibility. However, the protocol development process also illustrates that adequate and sensible compromise can be reached that resulted in an effective intervention. Subsequent initiatives at community programs in Baltimore and New York are heartening in that they demonstrate clinical enthusiasm for the adoption of these novel and well-supported interventions, and in the case of the HHC project, a gratifying positive response on the part of both patients and clinical staff. As evidenced by the CTN and HHC dissemination examples, clinician attitudes are likely to become more positive through training, through the experience of others who have adopted the new interventions, and, most important, through their own direct experience with the interventions.

Because the drug abuse treatment field is just on the verge of more widespread adoption of CM interventions, there is much need and substantial opportunity to conduct important research that will guide and support future dissemination efforts. For example, most research studies have examined relatively short-term intervention with incentive procedures. Dissemination studies would be welcome that examine intervention fidelity, intervention effectiveness, and staff attitudes about the use of incentive interventions when these are implemented over lengthy periods of time as part of usual-care clinical practice. Research on different methods of staff training and different methods of funding incentive interventions would be valuable. Also important would be research on the cost-effectiveness of incentive programs when they use different levels of incentive payout and when they focus on different behavioral outcome targets such as clinic attendance versus drug abstinence.

While future dissemination efforts will be aided through additional research, the success of the CTN effectiveness study as well as subsequent adoption initiatives described here provides a strong and promising foundation for further adoption of these novel and effective interventions into community treatment practice.

REFERENCES

Amass, L., & Kamien, J. (2004). A tale of two cities: Financing two voucher programs for substance abusers through community donations. *Experimental and Clinical Psychopharmacology, 12,* 147–155.

Brady, K. T., Sonne, E., Randall, C. L., Adinoff, B., & Malcolm, R. (1995). Features of cocaine dependence with concurrent alcohol use. *Drug and Alcohol Dependence, 39,* 69–71.

Community Epidemiology Work Group. (2006). Epidemiologic trends in drug abuse. *Proceedings of the CEWG, June, 2005* (NIH Publication No. 06-5281).

Heil, S. H., Badger, G. J., & Higgins, S. T. (2001). Alcohol dependence among cocaine-dependent outpatients: Demographics, drug use, treatment outcome and other characteristics. *Journal of Studies on Alcohol, 62,* 14–22.

Higgins S. T., Budney A. J., Bickel, W. K., Foerg, F. E., Donham, R., & Badger, G. J. (1994). Incentives improve outcome in outpatient behavioral treatment of cocaine dependence. *Archives of General Psychiatry, 51,* 568–576.

Kellogg, S. H., Burns, M., Coleman, P., Stitzer, M., Wale, J. B., & Kreek, M. J. (2005). Something of value: The introduction of contingency management interventions into the New York City Health and Hospitals Addiction Treatment Service. *Journal of Substance Abuse Treatment, 28,* 57–65.

Lamb, S., Greenlick, M. R., & McCarty, D. (Eds.). (1998). *Bridging the gap between practice and research.* Washington, DC: National Academy Press.

Lussier, J. P., Heil, S. H., Mongeon, J. A., Badger, G. J., & Higgins, S. T. (2006). A meta-analysis of voucher-based reinforcement therapy for substance use disorders. *Addiction, 101,* 192–203.

McCarty, D., Fuller, B. E., Arkken, C., Miller, M., Nunes, E. V., Edmundson, E., et al.

(2007). Direct care workers in the national drug abuse treatment Clinical Trials Network: Characteristics, opinions, and beliefs. *Psychiatric Services, 58*(2), 181–190.

McGovern, M. P., Fox, T. S., Xie, H., & Drake, R. E. (2004). A survey of clinical practices and readiness to adopt evidence-based practices: Dissemination research in an addiction treatment system. *Journal of Substance Abuse Treatment, 26,* 305–312.

Peirce, J. M., Petry, N. M., Stitzer, M. L., Blaine, J., Kellogg, S., Satterfield, F., et al. (2006). Lower-cost incentives increase stimulant abstinence in methadone maintenance community treatment: Results of the national drug abuse treatment Clinical Trials Network multi-site study. *Archives of General Psychiatry, 63,* 201–208.

Petry, N. M., Kolodner, K. B., Li, R., Peirce, J. M., Roll, J. M., Stitzer, M. L., et al. (2006). Prize-based contingency management does not increase gambling. *Drug and Alcohol Dependence, 83,* 269–273.

Petry, N. M., & Martin, B. (2002). Low-cost contingency management for treating cocaine- and opioid-abusing methadone patients. *Journal of Consulting and Clinical Psychology, 70,* 398–405.

Petry, N. M., Martin, B., Cooney, J. L., & Kranzler, H. R. (2000). Give them prizes and they will come: Variable-ratio contingency management for treatment of alcohol dependence. *Journal of Consulting and Clinical Psychology, 68,* 250–257.

Petry, N. M., Martin, B., & Simcic, F. (2005). Prize reinforcement contingency management for cocaine dependence: Integration with group therapy in a methadone clinic. *Journal of Consulting and Clinical Psychology, 73,* 354–359.

Petry, N. M., Peirce, J. M., Stitzer, M. L., Blaine, J., Roll, J. M., Cohen, A., et al. (2005). Prize-based incentives improve outcomes of stimulant abusers in outpatient psychosocial treatment programs: A national drug abuse treatment Clinical Trials Network study. *Archives of General Psychiatry, 62,* 1148–1156.

Petry, N. M., Tedford, J., Austin, M., Nich, C., Carroll, K. M., & Rounsaville, B. J. (2004). Prize reinforcement contingency management for treating cocaine users: How low can we go, and with whom? *Addiction, 99,* 349–360.

Robles, E., Stitzer, M. L., Strain, E. C., Bigelow, G. E., & Silverman, K. (2002). Voucher-based reinforcement of opioid abstinence during methadone detoxification. *Drug and Alcohol Dependence, 65,* 179–189.

Roll, J., Higgins, S. T., & Badger, G. J. (1996). An experimental comparison of three different schedules of reinforcement of drug abstinence using cigarette smoking as an exemplar. *Journal of Applied Behavior Analysis, 29,* 495–505

Silverman, K., Higgins, S. T., Brooner, R. K., Montoya, I. D., Cone, E. J., Schuster, C. R., et al. (1996). Sustained cocaine abstinence in methadone maintenance patients through voucher-based reinforcement therapy. *Archives of General Psychiatry, 53,* 409–415.

Silverman, K., Robles, E., Mudric, T., Bigelow, G. E., & Stitzer, M. L. (2004). A randomized trial of long-term reinforcement of cocaine abstinence in methadone-maintained patients who inject drugs. *Journal of Consulting and Clinical Psychology, 72,* 839–854.

CHAPTER 14

LOWERING COSTS IN DRUG ABUSE TREATMENT CLINICS

Nancy M. Petry *and* Sheila M. Alessi

OVERVIEW OF RATIONALE FOR LOWERING COSTS OF CONTINGENCY MANAGEMENT

An extensive body of literature demonstrates the efficacy of contingency management (CM) for improving outcomes in substance abuse treatment patients. The most widely studied CM procedure uses vouchers as the reinforcers, which are provided to patients whenever they demonstrate objective evidence of a target behavior, such as abstinence or treatment attendance. Vouchers have a monetary value and can be exchanged for retail items or services.

As noted throughout this book, voucher CM has demonstrated efficacy for improving outcomes in many treatment populations and settings (see also Higgins & Silverman, 1999; Higgins, Alessi, & Dantona, 2002, for reviews). A primary advantage of voucher CM is that it can complement essentially any treatment program and structure. That is, voucher CM can be integrated into methadone treatment programs, drug-free treatment settings that do not use maintenance medications, dual-diagnosis programs, and even specialty clinics, as described by Drebing, Rounsaville, and Rosenheck (Chapter 16, this volume) and Donlin, Knealing, and Silverman (Chapter 7, this volume). Vouchers are widely effective in part because they can accommodate personal preferences, and patients may request that their vouchers be used for such items as clothing, hobby equipment, or restaurant gift certificates. Vouchers, in essence, are like money, but money is not directly handed to patients such that voucher items may be less readily exchanged for drugs or other items inconsistent with treatment goals, like weapons or cigarettes.

Typically, voucher CM programs contain several key elements. Amounts of vouchers escalate for consecutive occurrences of the behavior, bonus vouchers may be available for sets of behavior (e.g., three negative toxicology screens in a row), and values reset to an initially low value whenever the target behavior does not occur (Higgins et al., 1991). For example, patients may receive a $2.50 voucher for the first negative urine-toxicology test, $3 for the second negative test, and $3.50 for the third negative test plus a $10 voucher bonus for three negative tests in a row. If the fourth test is positive, the voucher amount would reset to $2.50 for the next negative test provided.

Despite the demonstrated efficacy of voucher-based CM, a disadvantage of voucher CM programs from the perspective of sustainability in community-based treatment settings is the costs associated with administration and management. About $1,200 in vouchers is typically available during a 12-week treatment period, with average earnings of about $600 (Bickel, Amass, Higgins, Badger, & Esch, 1997; Higgins et al., 1993, 1994; Higgins, Wong, Badger, Ogden, & Dantona, 2000; Silverman et al., 1996). Not only must the costs of the vouchers be considered but so must the staff time to track earnings and purchase and dispense items. These costs may be prohibitive in already financially strapped treatment settings. Most publicly supported substance abuse treatment programs, and even private and for-profit programs, do not have financial or staff resources available to implement voucher-based CM programs as described and tested in research settings. Adaptations or novel applications of these procedures to make them self-sustaining are necessary as this empirically based intervention is brought to the context of community-based settings.

CM INTERVENTIONS THAT HAVE ADDRESSED LOWERING COSTS

Several methods have been used to address the issue of costs associated with CM procedures. Some options are reviewed briefly herein, with an emphasis on the prize CM system.

Clinic Privileges

Treatment programs incur relatively few costs when clinic privileges, rather than vouchers, are used to reinforce target behaviors. These procedures are most often utilized in methadone or other maintenance medication settings, because these drugs have reinforcing properties of their own that can be garnered to alter patient behavior. Some privileges that have been utilized to reinforce abstinence are changes in methadone dose (Calsyn & Saxon, 1987; Preston, Umbricht, & Epstein, 2000; Stitzer, Bickel, Bigelow, & Liebson, 1986), take-home dosing privileges (e.g., Stitzer, Iguchi, & Felch, 1992), alternate-day dosing options with buprenorphine (Bickel et al., 1997), and continued treatment as opposed to discharge from treatment (Dolan, Black, Penk, Robinowitz, & DeFord, 1985; McCarthy & Borders, 1985). Epstein and Preston (Chapter 3, this volume) further describe some of these procedures and studies.

While privileges can be efficacious in altering behavior, some issues limit their widespread applicability. First, federal laws regulating methadone administration mandate that patients need to be in treatment for at least 3 months before they are eligible for take-home doses. Hence, behavioral principles for minimizing delay between the behavior (e.g., drug abstinence) and reinforcer (e.g., take-home dose) cannot be invoked early in the treatment process. Second, the efficacy of CM also relies on frequent monitoring of the target behavior so that opportunities to detect the behavior and reinforce it are maximized. Unfortunately, state and federal regulations require (and some may only reimburse for) infrequent testing. Practices that are currently in place (e.g., monitoring urine samples only monthly and providing take-home doses once 3 months of testing fails to uncover drug use) go against many of the principles of behavioral modification. Inconsistent monitoring and reinforcing procedures can decrease the efficacy of CM (Griffith, Rowan-Szal, Roark, & Simpson, 2000). Finally, most of these types of privileges are only applicable in methadone or other maintenance medication settings.

Stars Exchangeable for Retail Goods and Services and Point Systems

Rowan-Szal, Joe, Chatham, and Simpson (1994) provided methadone patients with stars for attending counseling sessions and submitting cocaine-negative urine specimens; stars could be exchanged for retail items at a clinic store. Similar CM interventions have been described in non-methadone settings, in which for example, pregnant women can earn and exchange stars or points for baby items and clothing kept at an onsite store sustained by community donations (see Amass & Kamien, Chapter 15, this volume). These systems are similar to token economies, and they have the advantage of being applicable in a variety of clinical settings. However, while the use of onsite stores may reduce some costs associated with individualized purchases, solicitations for donations may also involve substantial staff time and effort. Further, if the magnitudes of items associated with the star or point system are too low, these systems may not be sufficient to alter behavior.

Fishbowl/Prize Incentives

About 8 years ago, we first developed an alternative to the voucher system that awards chances to win prizes, rather than guaranteed vouchers, as the reinforcers for each occurrence of a target behavior (e.g., negative urine-toxicology test) (Petry, Martin, Cooney, & Kranzler, 2000). Instead of earning a voucher worth a set monetary amount, patients earn the opportunity to draw from a fishbowl, and each draw is associated with the possibility of winning prizes of varying magnitudes. There are typically 500 slips of paper in the bowl, and about half of them are associated with a prize. The other half say "good job!" but do not result in a tangible reward. Among the winning slips, most of them (e.g., 219 of the 500 slips, or 45%) state "small" prize, a relatively small proportion state "large," and one is a "jumbo" prize. Small prizes are things such as bus tokens, $1 gift certificates to fast-food restaurants, toiletries, and so on; typically, they cost about $1. Large items are things such as sweatshirts, hand-held CD players, watches, and gift certificates to stores or restaurants, and they usually cost about $20. The jumbo prize is worth up to $100, and popular jumbos are televisions, DVD players, or PlayStations. Chances of winning prizes are inversely related to the prizes' magnitudes.

The prize system may be considered a type of variable-ratio reinforcement schedule because not every occurrence of a target behavior (e.g., submitting a negative sample) is followed by tangible reinforcement (i.e., a prize). Rather, whether the behavior is followed by receipt of a prize varies from event to event as a function of some draws being associated with an affirmative statement only and not a prize. By comparison, the voucher system may be described as a fixed-ratio reinforcement schedule because every occurrence of a target behavior is followed by receipt of a voucher (i.e., whether a voucher is received following a target behavior is fixed or certain). All other things being equal, variable-ratio schedules generate high rates of sustained behavior relative to fixed-ratio schedules. By capitalizing on this characteristic of variable-ratio schedules, the prize system may sustain high rates of behavior at reduced costs.

DESIGNING A PRIZE CM SYSTEM

Selecting a Behavior

In designing a prize CM system, some important behavioral principles should be kept in mind, and these are reviewed more thoroughly by Petry (2000). First, one needs to select a behavior to reinforce that can be objectively verified. Good examples of objectively verifiable behaviors are abstinence from a particular drug (which can be determined by urine-toxicology screens) or attendance at group or individual therapy sessions (which can be verified by therapists or group leaders). Other behaviors of substance abusers can also be problematic but are probably not well suited for a CM procedure because of difficulties in obtaining objective verification of their presence or absence. For example, "good attitude in group sessions" may be a goal that therapists try to achieve, but a good attitude is not a yes–no phenomenon, and any individual patient may demonstrate attitudes and verbal behaviors ranging from excellent to very poor within the same 1-hour session. Different therapists and even different group participants may disagree on their overall ratings of any individual patient's attitude in the group. Therefore, the behavior targeted by a CM intervention should be selected carefully.

The behavior should also be one that occurs relatively frequently. If a patient only uses cocaine once or twice a year, there would be little point in reinforcing him for cocaine abstinence. Similarly, if patients are in aftercare phases of treatment and only attend monthly, such a patient population may not be best suited for CM procedures. At the other extreme, attempting to reinforce behaviors that occur all the time or that are not within the patients' own ability to change is also inappropriate. Thus, a methadone patient who is positive 100% of the time for cocaine and 40% of the time for opioids may best be served by a CM intervention that targets opioid use alone initially. Opioid use may be easier to change than cocaine use, as it is not occurring daily. Requiring this patient to achieve abstinence from both opioids and cocaine simultaneously to earn reinforcement would be particularly challenging and may result in the patient not earning any reinforcement (Griffith et al., 2000).

Developing a Monitoring and Reinforcement Schedule

Once a behavior is selected for reinforcement, the monitoring and reinforcement schedule should be designed. The monitoring schedule needs to be fairly frequent (at least twice a week is recommended, with three times weekly preferred). It should also follow as closely as possible potential occurrences of the behavior. Because most urine-toxicology screens can assess any use versus abstinence over 48–72 hours, most CM procedures collect specimens two to three times per week. The reinforcement needs to come as soon as possible after the target behavior occurs. So, urine-toxicology testing needs to be done onsite, with results relayed to patients more or less immediately (5 minutes after sample submission). If reinforcing attendance at group sessions, the reinforcement should be provided in the group session itself, not delayed until the patient has attended groups for a month in a row, for example.

While frequent monitoring and closely thereafter reinforcing patients is ideal from a behavioral modification perspective, including escalating reinforcers or bonuses may further improve the efficacy of the CM intervention (Roll & Higgins, 2000; Roll, Higgins, & Badger, 1996). In most prize CM studies, increasing draws from the fishbowl are provided for sustained behavior. For example, if providing a negative urine-toxicology screen is the target behavior, the patient gets one draw for the first negative sample submitted, two draws if two samples in a row are negative, three draws for three negative samples in a row, and so on. Increasing reinforcers or bonuses is important because if the patient relapses (provides a positive sample or fails to provide a sample at all), not only does he or she not earn any draws that day, but the number of draws earned resets back to the initially low level of one draw once the appropriate behavior again occurs, thus discouraging relapse. Using an escalating-reinforcement schedule or bonuses, however, also increases costs. We have often capped the number of draws per target behavior to 10 draws maximum to provide a balance between the benefits of increasing reinforcement and offsetting costs.

Duration of Intervention

The duration of the intervention also needs to be decided. Usually, one wants to implement a CM procedure for a long enough time period to engender sustained behavioral change, with a minimum of 8 to 12 weeks of reinforcement for abstinence recommended. The general consensus in the field is that if the intervention is much shorter, patients may not grasp the procedures or may have only started to succeed when the intervention is discontinued. On the other hand, indefinite exposure is probably not necessary and would become very costly. In designing CM systems, one should be conscious of costs and consider the expected earnings for a patient who has perfect performance over the duration of the planned intervention.

Calculating Costs

A number of parameters will affect costs. Figure 14.1 shows an example allowing for imputation of various parameters. One can see how alteration of any of the parameters noted at the top (duration, frequency of monitoring, start and cap on the number of draws, and manner in which draws escalate) would influence the total number of draws possible.

Once an initial decision is made on these variables, one should calculate costs of the prize bowl to ascertain if it is within the allotted budget. Again, an algorithm with the total number of slips; number of small, large, and jumbo slips; total draws; and dollar value of smalls, larges, and jumbos calculates average prize costs. Cost per draw is a little under $2 for the typical fishbowl described earlier: 250 no wins, 219 ($1) smalls, 30 ($20) lar-

Duration of intervention:	12 weeks
Times monitored/week:	2
Draws start at:	1 draw
Draws escalate by:	1 draw
Draws cap at (if applicable):	10 draws

Week	Consecutive times behavior is monitored	Draws for each behavior
1	1	1
	2	2
2	3	3
	4	4
3	5	5
	6	6
4	7	7
	8	8
5	9	9
	10	10
6	11	10
	12	10
7	13	10
	14	10
8	15	10
	16	10
9	17	10
	18	10
10	19	10
	20	10
11	21	10
	22	10
12	23	10
	24	10
Total draws possible		195

FIGURE 14.1. Example of monitoring and reinforcement schedule for perfect performance.

ges, and 1 ($100) jumbo. Thus, with a total 195 draws in the example in Figure 14.1, expected maximal earnings per patient would be a little under $400. Most patients do not have perfect performance, and typically earnings are about one-half the arranged maximums (Higgins et al., 1994; Petry et al., 2000, 2004).

If the amount of reinforcement is too high from a practical standpoint, one could reduce any one or more of the parameters discussed previously, but there are always trade-offs to consider. If duration of the intervention is reduced, patients may not have the opportunity to achieve enough sustained behavior to generate long-term behavior change. If the cap on maximum draws is decreased to 5, the total number of draws possible would be 110, effectively almost reducing costs in half. However, a reset to 1 draw from 5 draws may not have as salient an influence on behavior as a reset to 1 draw from 10 draws. Also in this scenario, one would achieve the maximum draws at only 3 weeks into the program, and 3 weeks of escalating incentives may have a less pronounced effect on behavior than 5 weeks of escalating incentives.

It is tempting to alter the magnitude or probabilities of slips in the bowl to reduce the costs of prize rewards. Eliminating or reducing the value of the jumbo prize is a common reaction to calls to decrease costs. However, the availability of a $100 jumbo prize adds only $0.20 to each draw at a 1/500 probability. Reducing the magnitude of the jumbo to a $50 item would only save $0.10/draw, and may have a very negative impact on salience, as the presence of a $100 jumbo prize appears to drive a lot of patient behavior. The $20 large prizes, in contrast, contribute $1.20 to the costs of each draw at a probability of 30/500. Reducing the number of large slips in the bowls decreases costs but also the frequency of obtaining valuable prizes during treatment. At a 30/500 proportion of large slips, patients, on average, earn a large prize by about Week 3 in treatment, and every other week once they are earning the maximal number of draws. The consequences of parameter changes such as those described earlier require further investigation in clinical trials. In designing a prize CM system for use in clinical practice, prize costs and the potential consequences of reducing costs need to be carefully considered as they are likely to impact effectiveness.

Ethical Issues

There are also some ethical issues that should be thought through in developing and implementing prize CM. First, the prize system has an element of chance associated with it, and a related concern is that exposure to the procedure may increase gambling in some individuals. Comorbid pathological gambling and substance use disorders is prevalent (Shaffer, Hall, & Vanderbilt, 1999; Petry, Stinson, & Grant, 2005). Most prize CM studies have excluded patients who endorse being in recovery for gambling problems from participating in these interventions, but less than 1% of patients have been excluded for this reason. In addition, gambling behavior has been closely monitored in patients who do participate in prize CM. There is no evidence of an increase in gambling participation or problems among substance abusers assigned to prize CM conditions (Petry, Alessi, Marx, Austin, & Tardif, 2005; Petry et al., 2004, 2006; Petry & Martin, 2002; Petry, Martin, & Simcic, 2005).

Another consideration is the possibility that prizes will be sold for other goods or drugs. This issue is no different from that associated with voucher purchases, except that prize CM has the possibility, albeit low, of awarding a high-magnitude reward to a patient in the early stages of treatment, whereas in voucher CM patients must sustain long periods of abstinence prior to earning large voucher amounts. While this is a consideration, the escalating nature of the reinforcement system, in both prize and voucher CM, wards against exchanging items earned for drugs. If the patient sold items and used drugs, he or she would present positive at the next testing session and experience a reset in the voucher or draws available.

Although the concern that nonmonetary rewards may be used to purchase drugs is somewhat tempered when reinforcers are made contingent upon abstinence, these issues may emerge if reinforcement is used simply to reinforce attendance. That is, if a patient earns all the reinforcement for attendance, the exchange of prize or voucher items would not invoke reset contingencies if the patient continued attending treatment while using drugs. Such a situation could be handled clinically, or by increasing the frequency of urine sample testing and invoking natural contingencies for repeated positive samples, such as a step up to a higher level of care.

SCIENTIFIC EVIDENCE OF EFFICACY OF PRIZE CM

Nonmethadone (Drug-Free) Clinics

The first prize-based CM study (Petry et al., 2000) was conducted with alcohol-dependent patients beginning intensive outpatient treatment at a veteran's administration hospital. Forty-two patients, most of whom had other drug use disorders as well as alcohol dependence, were randomly assigned to standard care or standard care plus chances to win prizes for submitting breath samples that tested negative for alcohol and for completing goal-related activities (e.g., attending Alcoholics Anonymous and going to a job interview [see section "Compliance with Goal-Related Activities"]). Retention was almost fourfold higher in the CM condition, with 84% of CM patients remaining in treatment for 8 weeks versus 22% in standard care. By the end of treatment, 61% of those in standard care self-reported alcohol use or had provided a positive breath sample, compared with only 31% in the CM condition. Rates of illicit drug use were also suppressed in CM patients, even though alcohol was the only substance upon which draws were contingent.

While this study had very good effects on both retention and substance use outcomes, breath alcohol testing is not a very sensitive or specific measure for assessing alcohol use. Thus, we sought to evaluate the efficacy of prize CM in decreasing use of a drug for which better monitoring systems are available. Petry et al. (2004) randomly assigned 120 cocaine-abusing patients into a standard care condition, the same standard care plus our usual prize-based CM with a maximum of about $240 in prizes for urine samples that tested negative for cocaine and opioids, or the same standard care + prize-based CM with a maximum of about $80 in prizes for negative samples. CM patients were also required to provide a breath sample each time urine samples were submitted, and the breath sample had to read alcohol negative to receive any reinforcement. In that study, as in the original study with alcohol-dependent patients, the $240 CM procedure was successful in decreasing drug use overall, as well as enhancing durations of abstinence achieved. For example, the longest duration of abstinence achieved by patients in standard care was only 2.5 ± 2.6 weeks; patients in the $240 prize CM condition achieved abstinence for almost twice as long, 4.9 ± 4.4 weeks. Patients in the $80 CM condition had intermediary durations of abstinence, 3.7 ± 4.2 weeks. Thus, the prize CM procedure impacted cocaine use, similarly to alcohol, but costs are also important with prize CM.

These results were replicated in an even larger, multicenter study that was part of the National Institute on Drug Abuse's Clinical Trials Network (CTN). Petry, Peirce, et al. (2005) randomly assigned 415 stimulants abusers to standard care or standard care + prize CM for 12 weeks. Patients needed to test negative for alcohol as well as stimulants (amphetamine, cocaine, methamphetamine) to earn reinforcement. Draws increased by one for each consecutive week in which all samples tested negative for alcohol and stimulants. Additional draws (two per negative sample) were arranged for patients who also tested negative for opioids and marijuana. This study engendered similar results to earlier ones, with retention and longest durations of abstinence significantly enhanced in the prize CM condition.

Nevertheless, few individuals in these outpatient clinics submitted positive samples while engaged in treatment. The beneficial effects of CM on drug use outcomes related to durations of abstinence achieved and total number of negative samples submitted. These outcomes are affected by retention, as samples are considered missing and break the string of abstinence once patients withdraw from treatment. Benefits of CM on proportions of negative samples are not as persistently reported in drug-free treatment programs, in part because of a ceiling level of proportions of negative samples in some drug-free treatment settings. That is, the proportion of negative samples submitted during treatment was about 88% even in the standard care condition in the CTN study (Petry, Peirce, et al., 2005). Hence, there was little room for improvement in terms of percent negative samples with CM. This is not the case in studies in methadone clinics, which tend to retain patients in treatment equally well in CM and non-CM conditions. In these settings, CM is highly efficacious not only in engendering longer durations of abstinence but also in increasing the proportions of negative samples submitted, as detailed below.

Methadone Clinics

Drug use in patients attending methadone clinics is common, and three studies have now demonstrated that prize CM is efficacious in methadone patients. In the first of these studies, Petry and Martin (2002) provided the chance to win prizes contingent upon abstinence from either cocaine or opioids, with bonus draws contingent upon abstinence from both substances concurrently. The system was implemented with cocaine-abusing methadone patients who had significant continued use of opioids while maintained on stable methadone doses. The prize CM system not only significantly enhanced durations of cocaine/opioid abstinence but also significantly decreased proportions of samples submitted that were positive for cocaine and opioids. The effects were not confounded by retention or sample submission rates, as over 85% of patients in both conditions remained in treatment and the study for the 12-week trial.

A second study in a methadone clinic was recently published in which both cocaine abstinence and attendance at group therapy sessions were independently reinforced (Petry, Martin, & Simcic, 2005). That is, patients received draws from the fishbowl both for attending weekly groups and for submitting twice-weekly cocaine-negative samples. While retention in methadone treatment and the study was high in both conditions, attendance at group therapy sessions increased from a mean of 3.0 sessions in the standard condition to 6.6 sessions in the CM condition. The proportion of samples negative for cocaine was 16.8% in the standard condition and 34.6% in the CM condition, and these effects also differed significantly between conditions.

Finally, the CTN study also evaluated the efficacy of prize CM in six methadone clinics, from which 388 stimulant abusers were recruited and randomly assigned to treatment as usual or treatment as usual plus prize CM (Peirce et al., 2006). In the prize CM condition, prize draws were contingent upon submission of urine and breath samples negative for cocaine, amphetamine, methamphetamine, and alcohol, with bonus draws for opioid-negative samples. CM patients were twice as likely as usual-care patients to submit negative samples, and they also achieved longer durations of sustained abstinence than did patients in the usual-care condition. Treatment and study participation did not significantly differ between groups.

Which Behaviors Are Best to Reinforce?

Attendance

Treatment retention is a long-standing problem in community-based drug-free treatment programs (Harris, 1998; Hubbard et al., 1989; Simpson, Joe, & Brown, 1997; Simpson & Sells, 1982). Attendance rates at therapy sessions are also low in methadone clinics. CM can be used to target attendance at individual and group therapy (e.g., Stitzer et al., 1977; Carey & Carey, 1990; Helmus, Saules, Schoener, & Roll, 2003; Rhodes et al., 2003; Petry, Martin, & Finocche, 2001; Petry, Martin, & Simcic, 2005; Alessi, Hanson, Wieners, & Petry, in press).

We conducted a demonstration project among substance abusers at an HIV drop-in center (Petry, Martin, & Finocche, 2001), and this study included an even lower-cost alternative to our usual draws from the fishbowl procedure. Initially, we simply monitored attendance at groups, and fewer than two patients attended group per week on average. Once we implemented prize CM with increasing draws for successive attendance, an average of 12 patients attended group per week. However, the drawing procedure (sometimes > 10 draws/patient with over 20 patients in groups) was taking the bulk of group session time. We subsequently developed a system in which patients' names went into a hat, and the number of times one's name was placed in the hat was based on consecutive attendance. Then, just five names were drawn from the hat each group session, with those five individuals getting to draw from the fishbowl for prizes. This modification not only reduced the time of the intervention but also the costs as only five draws occurred daily. Still, this system was effective in enhancing attendance in that project (Petry et al., in press) as well as in another larger, multisite study (Alessi et al., in press).

Compliance with Goal-Related Activities

Substance abuse patients typically present to treatment with problems in a variety of life domains such as family relationships, employment, and medical issues. A comprehensive treatment plan involves not only establishing and maintaining abstinence but also developing long-term goals in the other domains. CM can be used to target activities that are steps toward treatment goals (Petry, 2000; Petry, Martin, & Finocche, 2001; Petry, Tedford, & Martin, 2001). When prize CM is used to reinforce completion of activities related to treatment goals, patients typically select three activities each week such as going to the movies with a son or daughter, preparing a resume, or scheduling a doctor's appointment. A receipt verifying completion of each activity is required, and patients earn a draw for each activity accomplished, with escalating draws for successful completion of all activities each week. In one study, prize CM for goal-related activities doubled compliance rates (Petry, Martin, & Finocche, 2001).

We recently completed a study in which 131 patients beginning intensive outpatient substance abuse treatment were randomly assigned to receive standard outpatient treatment alone, standard treatment plus prize CM for completing activities related to treatment goals, or standard treatment plus prize CM for abstinence (Petry et al., 2006). Samples were collected regularly from all patients throughout the 12-week trial, and overall amount of reinforcement available for activities and abstinence was equated across the two CM conditions. Patients in standard, CM activity, and CM abstinence conditions completed medians of 4.0, 6.0, and 10.5 weeks in treatment, respectively. While CM as a whole significantly improved retention relative to standard care, patients in the CM abstinence condition were retained significantly longer than patients in the CM activities condition. In terms of drug use outcomes, patients receiving CM for activities also performed intermediary between standard treatment and CM for abstinence. Thus, results from this study suggest that arranging some reinforcement contingent upon abstinence should be considered, even when other behaviors are targeted.

Abstinence (Single and Multiple Target Drugs)

The majority of substance abuse treatment patients are polydrug abusers (Substance Abuse and Mental Health Services Administration, 2003). Problems related to a primary drug are not addressed in isolation of difficulties related to other drug use, but the efficacy of CM for abstinence has been demonstrated primarily in studies that made reinforcement contingent upon abstinence from a single drug (e.g., Higgins et al., 1994). There are circumstances in which targeting a single drug may be appropriate. The most obvious is the case of the individual with a history of using only one drug. There may also be situations that warrant targeting a single drug in a polydrug abuser; this approach is often taken with methadone patients. If poly-drug-using patients are required to work too hard to earn a reinforcer (e.g., abstinence from multiple types of drugs), amounts of reinforcement need to be increased or the success of the program is likely to be diminished. Hence, in methadone settings in particular, we recommend targeting only a single drug at a time.

Although no known CM study targeting a single drug has shown increases in other drug use, providers often express concern about CM systems that reinforce abstinence from only one drug. While it may appear reasonable on the surface to mandate abstinence from all substances, one serious concern about this procedure when using CM is that some patients may never earn any reinforcement if total abstinence is required. In fact, among methadone patients for whom drug use is regular and quite high, many patients fail to earn a reinforcer when only *one* drug is targeted (Silverman et al., 1996; Stitzer, Iguchi, & Felch, 1992). Clearly, reinforcement rates will be even lower if complete abstinence is mandated (e.g., Downey, Helmus, & Schuster, 2000).

There are several adaptations to standard CM procedures that can be made to address concerns associated with targeting one drug at a time, while retaining essential behavior modification procedures. One approach is to make access to an initial reinforcer contingent upon abstinence from a single substance, and access to bonus escalating reinforcers contingent upon abstinence from at least one other drug. This was the approach taken by Petry and Martin (2002), when poly-drug-using cocaine-dependent methadone patients were evaluated. Another possibility is to provide an escalating rate of reinforcement for consecutive tests that indicate abstinence from a primary target drug, and additional draws at a fixed and low rate (e.g., two per negative test) for abstinence from all supplementary drugs. This approach was utilized in the CTN studies (Petry, Peirce, et al., 2005; Peirce et al., 2006) and may be well suited for methadone clinics in which polydrug use is common. In treatment programs in which positive samples are rarely submitted (e.g., some drug-free treatment programs), it may be appropriate to require abstinence from all substances for access to any prize reinforcement, as most patients in these settings are able to earn reinforcers and benefit from CM systems (Petry, Alessi, et al., 2005; Petry, Peirce, et al., 2005; Petry et al., 2004).

Importance of Magnitude of Reinforcement Even with Prizes

Although prize CM was developed to address cost issues, magnitude of reinforcement is still directly related to efficacy with the prize procedure. In the Petry et al. (2004) study, patients who were assigned to a CM procedure that provided an average maximum of $80 in prizes had worse abstinence outcomes (i.e., percent negative samples and durations of sustained abstinence) than those in the usual $240 prize CM condition. Thus, we advise against developing a prize CM system that awards prizes of less than $240/patient if abstinence is being reinforced. However, as noted by Petry, Martin, and Finocche (2001) and Alessi et al. (2007), reinforcing attendance may be possible at lower costs than reinforcing abstinence.

We recently completed a study comparing voucher and prize CM directly (Petry, Alessi, et al., 2005). Outpatients ($n = 142$) in non-methadone settings were randomly assigned to 12 weeks of usual care, usual care + voucher CM with a maximum of $882 in vouchers, or usual care + prize CM with expected earnings of on average $240 per patient. Patients in the prize and voucher CM conditions achieved longer durations of abstinence than did those in the usual-care condition (7.8 ± 4.2 weeks, 7.0 ± 4.2 weeks, and 4.6 ± 3.4 weeks, respectively). Longest duration of abstinence predicted objectively confirmed abstinence at 6-month and 9-month follow-up evaluations. Maximum incentives in the voucher condition were arranged to be higher than expected earnings in the prize condition, but the actual amount of actual reinforcement earned did not differ between conditions, in part because of trends toward improved outcomes in the prize CM condition. Therefore, more research on parameters of prize and voucher reinforcement is needed, but results across these studies consistently point toward an association between magnitudes of reinforcement and beneficial outcomes. Although it is not surprising that higher costs can exact more behavioral change, Stitzer and Kellogg (Chapter 13, this volume), Drebing, Rounsaville, and Rosenheck (Chapter 16, this volume), and Donlin, Knealing, and Silverman (Chapter 17, this volume) also speak to how some of the costs of prize or voucher CM may be sustained by existing treatment and employment systems.

CONCLUDING COMMENTS

The efficacy of CM for treatment of substance use disorders has been steadily gaining support by researchers, but adoption of these procedures by the treatment community has been slow. Cost is often cited as an obstacle, and the prize CM system was designed to address this barrier. In a series of systematic studies, prize CM has improved retention and increased abstinence from single and multiple substances in samples that represent those predominating in substance abuse treatment programs. These effects have been accomplished at relatively lower costs than those typically provided in voucher CM studies. The cost savings result from the use of a variable-reinforcement schedule that also includes escalating incentives, resets, and access to large-magnitude incentives, elements known to be important to the efficacy of voucher CM.

Beyond cost benefits, another advantage of prize CM is that prizes are kept onsite, although this characteristic need not be unique to prize CM (see Amass & Kamien, Chapter 15, this volume). The delay between completion of a target behavior and delivery of reinforcement is minimized with prize CM compared to systems that entail purchasing items after a behavior occurs. Prize CM can also be administered in either individual or group format (Alessi et al., 2007; Petry, Martin, & Finocche, 2001), perhaps facilitating its adoption, as group therapy predominates in practice.

There are also some disadvantages of prize CM. As with other CM interventions, design and implementation of an effective prize CM system depend on familiarity with and proficiency in certain techniques and principles of behavior modification. These include behavioral contracting, consistently applying contingencies, frequently monitoring and reinforcing behaviors, integrating escalating or bonus reinforcers, and providing adequate reinforcement magnitude (Petry, 2000). Developing comprehensive training procedures for community-based treatment staff is no doubt a large undertaking, but efforts toward dissemination are under way.

Another disadvantage of prize CM are the costs, albeit lower than with some other CM procedures. The ability of a treatment system that is under tight fiscal restraints to absorb additional costs is understandably met with skepticism. Reducing reinforcement magnitudes to under $240 for prize CM may compromise efficacy, but it may be possible to offset costs in part or full via fund-raising or other strategies including clinic privileges (see Stitzer & Kellogg, Chapter 13, and Amass & Kamien, Chapter 15, this volume). Furthermore, immediate costs of CM may pale in comparison to societal and individual costs of continued drug abuse. A comprehensive cost-effectiveness analysis is needed to accurately evaluate the position of this intervention relative to other modalities for treating substance abuse.

Thus, many factors contribute to the sustainability of a treatment innovation, including the soundness of forged research–treatment partnerships and the readiness of communities to accept an innovation. The financial resources needed to sustain an innovative intervention are another consideration. Prize-based CM was designed to be a relatively low-cost CM system. More research is required to fully evaluate this system, but research to date supports the efficacy of prize CM for improving retention and abstinence compared to usual care in substance abuse community-based treatment programs.

REFERENCES

Alessi, S. M., Hanson, T., Tardif, M., & Petry, N. M. (2007). Low-cost contingency management in community substance abuse treatment settings: A transition to delivering incentives for attendance in group therapy. *Experimental and Clinical Psychopharmacology, 15*, 293–300.

Bickel, W. K., Amass, L., Higgins, S. T., Badger, G. J., & Esch, R. (1997). Behavioral treatment improves outcomes during opioid detoxification with buprenorphine. *Journal of Consulting and Clinical Psychology, 65*, 803–810.

Calsyn, D. A., & Saxon, A. J. (1987). A system for uniform application of contingencies for illicit drug use. *Journal of Substance Abuse Treatment, 4*, 41–47.

Carey, K. B., & Carey, M. P. (1990). Enhancing treatment attendance of mentally ill chemical abusers. *Journal of Behavior Therapy and Experimental Psychiatry, 21*, 205–209.

Dolan, M. P., Black, J. L., Penk, W. E., Robinowitz, R., & DeFord, H. A. (1985). Contracting for treatment termination to reduce illicit drug use among methadone maintenance failures. *Journal of Consulting and Clinical Psychology, 53*, 549–551.

Downey, K. K., Helmus, T. C., & Schuster, C. R. (2000). Treatment of heroin-dependent poly-drug abusers with contingency management and buprenorphine maintenance. *Experimental and Clinical Psychopharmacology, 8*(2), 176–184.

Griffith, J. D., Rowan-Szal, G. A., Roark, R. R., & Simpson, D. D. (2000). Contingency management in outpatient methadone treatment: A meta-analysis. *Drug and Alcohol Dependence, 58*, 55–56.

Harris, P. M. (1998). Attrition revisited. *American Journal of Evaluation, 19*, 293–305.

Helmus, T. C., Saules, K. K., Schoener, E. P., & Roll, J. M. (2003). Reinforcement of counseling attendance and alcohol abstinence in a community-based dual-diagnosis treatment program: A feasibility study. *Psychology of Addictive Behaviors*, *17*, 249–251.

Higgins, S. T., Alessi, S. M., & Dantona, R. L. (2002). Voucher-based incentives: A substance abuse treatment innovation. *Addictive Behaviors*, *27*(6), 887–910.

Higgins, S. T., Budney, A. J., Bickel, W. K., Foerg, F. E., Donham, R., & Badger, G. J. (1994). Incentives improve outcome in outpatient behavioral treatment of cocaine dependence. *Archives of General Psychiatry*, *51*(7), 568–576.

Higgins, S. T., Budney, A. J., Bickel, W. K., Hughes, J. R., Foerg, F., & Badger, G. (1993). Achieving cocaine abstinence with a behavioral approach. *American Journal of Psychiatry*, *150*, 763–769.

Higgins, S. T., Delaney, D., Budney, A. J., Bickel, W. K., Hughes, J. R., Foerg, F., et al. (1991). A behavioral approach to achieving initial cocaine abstinence. *American Journal of Psychiatry*, *148*, 1218–1224.

Higgins, S. T., & Silverman, K. (1999). *Motivating behavior change among illicit-drug abusers: Research on contingency management interventions*. Washington, DC: American Psychology Association.

Higgins, S. T., Wong, C. J., Badger, G. J., Ogden, D. E., & Dantona, R. A. (2000). Contingent reinforcement increases cocaine abstinence during outpatient treatment and 1 year of follow-up. *Journal of Consulting and Clinical Psychology*, *68*, 64–72.

Hubbard, R. L., Marsden, M. E., Rachal, J. V., Harwood, H. J., Cavanaugh, E. R., & Ginzburg, H. M. (1989). *Drug abuse treatment: A national study of effectiveness*. Chapel Hill: University of North Carolina Press.

McCarthy, J. J., & Borders, O. T. (1985). Limit setting on drug abuse in methadone maintenance patients. *American Journal of Psychiatry*, *142*, 1419–1423.

Peirce, J. M., Petry, N. M., Stitzer, M. L., Blaine, J., Kellogg, S., Satterfield, F., et al. (2006). Lower-cost incentives increase stimulant abstinence in methadone maintenance treatment: A national drug abuse treatment Clinical Trials Network study. *Archives of General Psychiatry*, *63*, 201–208.

Petry, N. M. (2000). A comprehensive guide to the application of contingent management procedures in general clinic settings. *Drug and Alcohol Dependence*, *58*, 9–25.

Petry, N. M., Alessi, S. M., Carroll, K. M., Hanson, T., MacKinnon, S., Rounsaville, B., et al. (2006). Contingency management treatments: Reinforcing abstinence versus adherence with goal-related activities. *Journal of Consulting and Clinical Psychology*, *74*, 592–601.

Petry, N. M., Alessi, S. M., Marx, J., Austin, M., & Tardif, M. (2005). Vouchers versus prizes: Contingency management treatment of substance abusers in community settings. *Journal of Consulting and Clinical Psychology*, *73*(6), 1005–1014.

Petry, N. M., Kolodner, K. B., Li, R., Peirce, J. M., Roll, J. M., Stitzer, M. L, & Hamilton, J. A. (2006). Prize-based contingency management does not increase gambling: Results of the National Drug Abuse Treatment Clinical Trials Network multisite study. *Drug and Alcohol Dependence*, *83*, 269–273.

Petry, N. M., & Martin, B. (2002). Low-cost contingency management for treating cocaine- and opioid-abusing methadone patients. *Journal of Consulting and Clinical Psychology*, *70*(2), 398–405.

Petry, N. M., Martin, B., Cooney, J. L., & Kranzler, H. R. (2000). Give them prizes, and they will come: Contingency management for treatment of alcohol dependence. *Journal of Consulting and Clinical Psychology*, *68*(2), 250–257.

Petry, N. M., Martin, B., & Finocche, C. (2001). Contingency management in group treatment: A demonstration project in an HIV drop-in center. *Journal of Substance Abuse Treatment, 21*(2), 89–96.

Petry, N. M., Martin, B., & Simcic, F., Jr. (2005). Prize reinforcement contingency management for cocaine dependence: Integration with group therapy in a methadone clinic. *Journal of Consulting and Clinical Psychology, 73*(2), 354–359.

Petry, N. M., Peirce, J. M., Stitzer, M. L., Blaine, J., Roll, J. M., Cohen, A., et al. (2005). Prize-based incentives improve outcomes of stimulant abusers in outpatient psychosocial programs: A national drug abuse treatment Clinical Trials Network study. *Archives of General Psychiatry, 62*(10), 1148–1156.

Petry, N. M., Stinson, F. S., & Grant, B. F. (2005). Comorbidity of DSM-IV pathological gambling and other psychiatric disorders: Results from the National Epidemiologic Survey on Alcohol and Related Conditions. *Journal of Clinical Psychiatry, 66,* 564–574.

Petry, N. M., Tedford, J., Austin, M., Nich, C., Carrol, K. M., & Rounsaville, B. J. (2004). Prize reinforcement contingency management for treatment of cocaine abusers: How low can we go, and with whom? *Addiction, 99*(3), 349–360.

Petry, N. M., Tedford, J., & Martin, B. (2001). Reinforcing compliance with non-drug related activities. *Journal of Substance Abuse Treatment, 20,* 33–44.

Preston, K. L., Umbricht, A., & Epstein, D. H. (2000). Methadone dose increase and abstinence reinforcement for treatment of continued heroin use during methadone maintenance. *Archives of General Psychiatry, 57*(4), 395–404.

Rhodes, G. L., Saules, K. K., Helmus, R. C., Roll, J., Beshears, R. S., Ledgerwood, D. M., et al. (2003). Improving on-time counseling attendance in a methadone treatment program: A contingency management approach. *American Journal of Drug and Alcohol Abuse, 29*(4), 759–773.

Roll, J. M., & Higgins, S. T. (2000). A within-subject comparison of three different schedules of reinforcement of drug abstinence using cigarette smoking as an exemplar. *Drug and Alcohol Dependence, 58,* 4103–4109.

Roll, J. M., Higgins, S. T., & Badger, G. J. (1996). An experimental comparison of three different schedules of reinforcement of drug abstinence using cigarette smoking as an exemplar. *Journal of Applied Behavior Analysis, 29,* 495–505.

Rowan-Szal, G., Joe, G. W., Chatham, L. R., & Simpson, D. D. (1994). A simple reinforcement system for methadone clients in a community-based treatment program. *Journal of Substance Abuse Treatment, 11,* 217–223.

Shaffer, H. J., Hall, M. N., & Vanderbilt, J. (1999). Estimating the prevalence of disordered gambling behavior in the United States and Canada: A research synthesis. *American Journal of Public Health, 89,* 1369–1376.

Silverman, K., Higgins, S. T., Brooner, R. K., Montoya, I. D., Cone, E. J., Schuster, C. R., et al. (1996). Sustained cocaine abstinence in methadone maintenance patients through voucher-based reinforcement therapy. *Archives of General Psychiatry, 53,* 409–415.

Simpson, D. D., Joe, G. W., & Brown, B. S. (1997). Treatment retention and follow-up outcomes in the Drug Abuse Treatment Outcome Study (DATOS). *Psychology of Addictive Behaviors, 11,* 294–307.

Simpson, D. D., & Sells, S. B. (1982). Effectiveness of treatment for drug abuse: An overview of the DARP research program. *Advances in Alcohol and Substance Abuse, 2,* 7–29.

Stitzer, M. L., Bickel, W. K., Bigelow, G. E., & Liebson, I. A. (1986). Effects of methadone dose contingencies on urinalysis test results of polydrug-abusing methadone-maintenance patients. *Drug and Alcohol Dependence, 18,* 341–348.

Stitzer, M. L., Bigelow, G., Lawrence, C., Cohen, J., D'Lugoff, B., & Hawthorne, J. (1977). Medication take-home as a reinforcer in a methadone maintenance program. *Addictive Behaviors, 2,* 9–14.

Stitzer, M. L., Iguchi, M. Y., & Felch, L. J. (1992). Contingent take-home incentive: Effects on drug use of methadone maintenance patients. *Journal of Consulting and Clinical Psychology, 60,* 927–934.

Substance Abuse and Mental Health Services Administration. (2003). *Treatment Episode Data Set (TEDS): 1992–2001. National Admissions to Substance Abuse Treatment Services* (DASI Series: S-20, DHHS Publication No. [SMA] 03-3778). Rockville, MD: Office of Applied Studies.

CHAPTER 15

FUNDING CONTINGENCY MANAGEMENT IN COMMUNITY TREATMENT CLINICS

Use of Community Donations and Clinic Rebates

Leslie Amass *and* Jonathan B. Kamien

ISSUES FOR TRANSPORTING CONTINGENCY MANAGEMENT INTO COMMUNITY CLINICS

The adoption of contingency management (CM) by community treatment programs has been limited by factors such as lack of clinicians' training in CM, philosophical and/or political barriers, and the cost of implementing CM programs (see Kirby, Amass, & McLellan, 1999, for a review). Lack of adequate clinician training can lead to misapplication of aspects of CM, such as poor choice of reinforcers and/or target behaviors or inconsistent application of contingencies. Development and distribution of training manuals and guidelines for clinicians on the use of CM procedures should help in this regard (e.g., Petry, 2000), as well as involving community treatment providers in ongoing research efforts such as the National Institute on Drug Abuse's Clinical Trials Network (Hanson, Leshner, & Tai, 2002; Kellogg et al., 2005; Peirce et al., 2006; Petry et al., 2005; Roll et al.,

2006). Philosophical and political barriers often arise from the idea that is inappropriate to offer drug users additional incentives for abstinence when not using drugs is something they should be doing anyway. Perhaps placing contingencies on reinforcers that are already present in patients' lives, rather than providing novel incentives such as cash and goods, may be viewed as more acceptable. Efforts in special populations to reward clients' behavior change with reinforcers previously provided noncontingently, such as housing (see Milby & Schumacher, Chapter 9, this volume) or access to a workplace (see Donlin, Knealing, & Silverman, Chapter 17, this volume) or other entitlements such as disability benefits (see Tidey & Ries, Chapter 11, this volume) might reduce philosophical and political objections. Another strategy for dissipating philosophical and political barriers may be to apply CM procedures programs outside traditional drug treatment clinics, such as hospitals (see Drebing, Rounsaville, & Rosenheck, Chapter 16, this volume), workplaces (see Donlin et al., Chapter 17, this volume) and the criminal justice system (see Marlowe & Wong, Chapter 18, this volume). However, the cost of CM programs is most widely considered the biggest barrier to its adoption by community treatment programs.

REDUCING THE COST OF CM

Naturally Occurring Incentives

One strategy for reducing CM program cost is to use naturally occurring incentives rather than vouchers for hard goods or money. Using naturally occurring incentives is limited only by clinicians' creativity in recognizing what might serve as an effective incentive and their ability to control delivery of the incentives to patients. For example, making access to clinic privileges such as methadone take-home doses contingent upon counseling attendance (Stitzer et al., 1977) or methadone dose adjustments contingent upon drug abstinence (Stitzer, Bickel, Bigelow, & Liebson, 1986) have successfully modified these target behaviors. Surveys of patients and staff have suggested that items such as public recognition of achieving treatment goals and providing greater control over medication dosing might also be effective incentives (Amass, Bickel, Crean, Higgins, & Badger, 1996; Roll, Chudzynski, & Richardson, 2005; Stitzer & Bigelow, 1978). Although using naturally occurring, nonmonetary incentives can be effective, the surveys agree that cash rewards and vouchers exchangeable for goods and services are the incentives that are among the most highly valued and are those that are likely to be among the most effective (Amass et al., 1996; Roll et al., 2005; Stitzer & Bigelow, 1978). Although one concern with using cash incentives is that giving cash to drug users will precipitate drug use, controlled research suggests that is not necessarily so (Festinger et al., 2005).

Less Costly Incentives

Another strategy for reducing CM program cost focuses on reducing incentive values and/or changing the schedule of reinforcement so that incentives are delivered intermittently rather than every time a behavior occurs (see Petry & Alessi, Chapter 14, this volume). These techniques have great promise for decreasing the cost of providing CM incentives without compromising their efficacy, although there is probably a lower limit below which incentives become ineffective (Jones, Haug, Stitzer, & Svikis, 2000; Petry et al., 2004; Silverman, Chutaupe, Bigelow, & Stitzer, 1999; Stitzer & Bigelow, 1983, 1984). However, even when the cost of the incentives is reduced, finding the funds to pay for incentives within the tight budgets of community treatment providers may be very difficult. To date, almost all research investigating CM for treating substance use disorders has relied on governmental research grants to supply the funds for purchasing or providing incentives. Another approach would move beyond just reducing the cost of incentives and actually use community- or patient-provided resources to finance the incentives.

SUPPORTING CM THROUGH DONATIONS

Acquiring Donated Incentives

Soliciting the community for donations to use as incentives in CM programs is feasible and can accumulate sufficient resources to initiate and sustain CM programs, as demonstrated in studies targeting smoking cessation (Amass & Kamien, 2004; Donatelle, Prows, Champeau, & Hudson, 2000; Elder, Campbell, Mielchen, Hovell, & Litrownik, 1991; Lando, Pirie, Dusich, Elsen, & Bernards, 1995). For example, two donation solicitation campaigns were conducted to acquire incentives for a randomized controlled trial of CM to help pregnant, postpartum, and parenting women to reduce or quit smoking (Amass & Kamien, 2004; Amass, Kamien, & Samiy, 2003). The campaigns used targeted direct mailings to solicit a wide variety of donations from a variety of potential donors. Overall, the campaigns required about 2 days per week of one staff person's time. These campaigns, in Toronto, Canada, and Los Angeles, California, were able to acquire an average of over $4,000 per month in donated goods and services while solicitation was ongoing. The donors ranged from large, national corporations to local individuals, charitable groups, and retailers. Donated items were diverse and ranged from gift certificates to local grocery stores, fast-food restaurants, and movie theatres to clothing, toys, diapers, baby wipes, and myriad other items. Surprisingly, the positive response rates of 19% in Toronto and 25% in Los Angeles exceeded the 10%–15% usually expected for direct-mail fund-raising campaigns (Henderson, 1984). Other donated incentives used in smoking-cessation studies have been similarly diverse and have included cash (Donatelle et al., 2000)—$3,000 worth of prizes including a trip to Hawaii, athletic equipment, free dental services, and baseball game tickets (Elder et al., 1991) and a trip to Las Vegas, bicycles and in-line skates (Lando et al., 1995). These successful experiences suggest that acquiring donations to serve as incentives may be a way community-based organizations can afford to implement CM programs for substance abuse treatment.

CM Studies Using Donated Incentives

Results from studies that used donated goods and services to reinforce behavior change are promising. The donations acquired in the aforementioned Los Angeles solicitation campaign were used as incentives in a randomized controlled clinical trial for pregnant and postpartum smokers (Amass, Kamien, & Samiy, 2003). Women smokers who were pregnant or had a child living with them and provided a breath sample containing at least 8 parts per million (ppm) carbon monoxide (CO) at baseline were eligible to participate while being treated in one of two community substance abuse treatment clinics. During the 30-week intervention period, participants met with a research assistant during three data visits per week to provide breath samples analyzed for CO and complete research questionnaires. Participants also provided a urine sample on one randomly chosen day per week that was analyzed for the presence of illicit drugs or their metabolites (urinalysis [UA]; propoxyphene, codeine, methadone, morphine, alcohol, cocaine, amphetamine, methamphetamine, phenobarbital, pentobarbital, secobarbital, benzodiazepines, and THC). Ninety participants were randomly assigned to one of three groups (CO only, CO + UA, and control). The CO only and CO + UA groups received 10 voucher points for each breath sample that measured less than 8 ppm CO. The CO + UA group received an additional 10 voucher points for each weekly urine sample that tested negative for all illicit drugs. The control group did not receive voucher points contingent upon breath CO or urinalysis results. All participants received 3 voucher points for each completed data visit. The maximum number of voucher points available during the study was 1,170 points for the CO only group, 1,470 points for the CO + UA group, and 270 points for the control group. Voucher points could be spent in onsite stores stocked with the donated items discussed earlier and each point could purchase about $2 of donated goods or services. Figure 15.1 shows the average percent decrease from baseline in CO level during the 30-week intervention. The two groups receiving vouchers contingent upon CO levels decreased their CO levels more than 35% relative to baseline while the control group reduced their CO level by only about 12%. This approximately threefold greater smoking reduction by the CM groups was statistically sig-

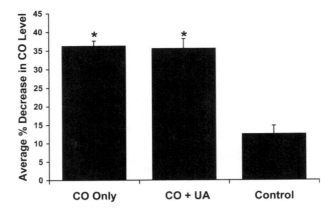

FIGURE 15.1. Average percent decreases in CO levels during a CM intervention using donated incentives. Vertical lines show the standard error of the mean. Asterisks denote significant difference from control group.

nificant ($p < 0.0001$). Illicit drug use during the study was very infrequent and did not differ among the groups. Voucher points awarded to the CO only and CO + UA groups averaged 243 ± 43 and 420 ± 48 voucher points, while the control group received an average of 83 ± 16 voucher points. Because each point was worth about $2, a total value of about $500–$800 worth of donated goods was awarded per patient in the groups receiving CM. The donations accumulated during the 27-month fund-raising campaign were more than sufficient to sustain this voucher reinforcement program and significantly reduce smoking in these pregnant, postpartum, and parenting women.

Another report that used donated cash incentives describes a randomized controlled trial of 220 pregnant smokers (Donatelle et al., 2000). In this study, businesses, foundations, and health care organizations donated the incentives, which were provided as vouchers redeemable at local stores. Smoking status was assessed monthly during pregnancy and 2 months postpartum for all participants through self-report; reports of quitting were verified through salivary thiocyanate analysis. One group was randomly assigned to receive a smoking cessation information kit designed for pregnant women. The other group was randomly assigned to receive this kit and vouchers contingent upon smoking abstinence. The group receiving vouchers also identified a significant other to serve as a social supporter who also received vouchers when the pregnant women did not smoke. Vouchers were awarded monthly throughout pregnancy (an average of 6 months) and for the first 2 months postpartum for tests that biochemically verified smoking abstinence (saliva thiocyanate < 100 ng/ml). The pregnant women received $50 vouchers for each test and their significant others received a

$50 voucher for the first and last tests and $25 vouchers for each intervening test. At the end of pregnancy, 32% of the group receiving vouchers was abstinent compared to only 9% of the group without vouchers. At 2 months postpartum, 21% of the voucher group remained abstinent compared to 6% of the nonvoucher group. The dollar amount of the donated incentives actually paid to participants was not provided in this report. The results provide additional support for the viability and effectiveness of using donated incentives in CM programs.

Finally, donated incentives, as well as donated recruiting announcements in local print and broadcast media, were used in two "Quit and Win" smoking-cessation contests (Elder et al., 1991; Lando et al., 1995). Briefly, Quit and Win contests recruit broadly from the community for individuals who may be interested in quitting smoking. Participants return registration cards that indicate that they are current smokers, intend to quit smoking on a specified quit date, and intend to remain abstinent for 1 month. Registered participants receive smoking-cessation literature and tips to help them quit. A lottery is then held to award the donated prizes to participants who report smoking abstinence at 1 month. Typically, smoking abstinence is verified biochemically before awarding prizes. One study that used donated incentives reported 46% self-reported abstinence at 1 year after the contest ended (Lando et al., 1995). The other study reported 35% self-reported abstinence 2 months after the contest ended (Elder et al., 1991). Although these were uncontrolled studies and abstinence after the contest ended was not confirmed biochemically, the donated incentives seemed to be effective for decreasing smoking. Overall, research to date has shown that local communities and organizations are willing to donate a range of commodities, including cash, for use in CM programs targeting smoking cessation and these donated incentives were effective reinforcers.

Advantages of Donated Incentives

Conducting CM programs using donated incentives may have several advantages beyond simple cost reductions compared to CM programs that use governmental grants or other outside funding sources to acquire incentives. First, relapse to drug use once a CM program ends and incentives are no longer awarded is most common, suggesting that CM interventions might be best used as long-term maintenance treatments (Crowley, 1999; e.g., Silverman et al., 2002). Using donated incentives accumulated on an ongoing basis through inexpensive donation-solicitation campaigns may provide a means for providing a CM intervention over longer periods than those that rely on outside funding to provide incentives. Second, soliciting donations involves a community in supporting addiction treatment and emphasizes the community's involvement in and support for clients' substance abuse treatment, perhaps contributing to making the clients feel less marginalized. This may yield benefits when patients frequent the stores and venues that donated the incentives, knowing that those entities supported their efforts to reduce substance use.

Limitations of Donated Incentives

Although the results from CM programs using donated incentives are promising, this approach has some limitations. First, CM programs using donated incentives have been reported only for the behavior of smoking cessation (Elder et al., 1991; Lando et al., 1995) and the only controlled trials involved pregnant women (Amass, Kamien, & Samiy, 2003; Donatelle et al., 2000). Whether similar success could be achieved in soliciting donations for other substance abuse problems and for other substance-using populations is unknown. Second, higher incentive values yield better results in CM programs (Lussier, Heil, Mongeon, Badger, & Higgins, 2006). When using donated incentives, both their magnitude and nature are limited by who the donors were and what products were donated. Finally, soliciting donations from the community requires personnel and resources such as stationery and postage that community programs may not be able to spare. Thus, cost-effectiveness analyses are needed to evaluate whether acquiring incentives through donations actually costs less than buying incentives outright.

SUPPORTING CM THROUGH PATIENT RESOURCES

Alternative sources of incentives for CM may come from the clients themselves. Using client resources for incentives precludes the need for external funds or extra clinic resources and has the potential to provide incentives in the long term. These incentives may come from contracts that specify punishments to be delivered in the case of drug use, deposits that clients provide at the outset of the intervention, or rebates of portions of fee payments in fee-for-service treatment programs.

Punishment Contracting

Crowley (1999) describes several cases in which drug users contract with a therapist to give up something of significant value in their life as a consequence of drug use. As examples, a cocaine user agreed to forfeit his house if he tested positive for cocaine, and health care professionals agreed to surrender their licenses if they tested positive for drugs. Although the studies were uncontrolled, results were promising, with large percentages of clients remaining abstinent while the contingency contracts were in effect. Although published reports of the efficacy of these types of arrangements are rare, many states have programs in which doctors and other health care workers with substance abuse problems can be mandated to treatment. Failure to comply and cease drug use leads to loss of licenses and/or employment. While these types of contracts can no doubt be effective, their use would be limited to clients with something of value to lose, and to those who could be convinced to enter into such contracts.

Deposit Contracting

An older literature describes CM procedures using "deposit contracting," which involves clients posting a deposit that serves as an incentive during the treatment. For example, patients deposited money with the clinic that could be earned back on meeting previously specified therapeutic goals, such as reliably taking disulfiram for the treatment of alcoholism (Bigelow, Strickler, Liebsen, & Griffiths, 1976) or reducing smoking (Tighe & Elliot, 1968). If the goals are not met, the deposited money is forfeited, typically to a charity of the client's choice.

In the report describing contingency contracting for disulfiram treatment, clients deposited a negotiated amount averaging $71 and forfeited from $5–$10 each time they failed to attend the clinic to receive a scheduled disulfiram dose during a 3-month period (Bigelow et al., 1976). During this procedure, 95% of patients were validated as being alcohol abstinent for the first 2 months of treatment enrollment and 80% of the participants exceeded the greatest amount of continuous abstinence they had achieved during the 3 years preceding treatment. These abstinence rates greatly exceeded those reported in other disulfiram treatment programs at that time.

Several studies have demonstrated that deposit contracting procedures are effective for short-term (e.g., 2 months) smoking reduction with self-reported abstinence rates ranging from 50 to 84% (Elliott & Tighe, 1968; Paxton, 1980, 1981, 1983; Spring, Sipich, Trimble, & Goeckner, 1978; Winett, 1973; Lando, 1977). In studies that compared groups with deposit contracts to those without, rates of smoking abstinence were significantly higher in subjects with deposit contracts (Spring et al., 1978; Paxton, 1980; Winett, 1973). Given the encouraging efficacy of deposit contract programs in smoking reduction, the dearth of CM research using this source of incentives to address substance abuse problems is surprising. Perhaps this is at least partially due to the inherent limitation of deposit contracting programs to those patients willing and able to provide enough of a deposit to serve as a meaningful incentive. Regardless, deposit contracting deserves more attention as a possible source of incentives in CM programs for substance abuse.

Fee Rebates

Because the majority of outpatient community substance abuse treatment organizations require clients to remit fees for services, using client fees as a source of incentives may be a viable, practical, and easily adopted way to finance CM procedures in drug abuse treatment. As an example, methadone-maintenance treatment (MMT) financing across the United States suggests the viability of patient fees as a source for incentives. Over 30% of MMT clients are expected to pay for at least a portion of MMT costs. This figure increases dramatically in private, for-profit facilities, with over three-quarters of patients funding their own treatment (Rettig & Yarmolinsky, 1995). Although regional variability exists, in many states, MMT patients pay for a substantial amount of their treatment and a portion of the fees they pay can be used as a source of incentives for a CM program as discussed further later. Under this system, part of a patient's fees is returned to the patient in the form of a cash rebate when specified behavioral requirements are met. Although fee rebates have only recently been applied to substance abuse treatment, at least one report exists of using this technique successfully outside the substance abuse arena, to improve dental hygiene (Iwata & Becksfort, 1981).

Two randomized controlled trials have investigated contingent fee rebates for reducing drug use in MMT patients (Amass, Kamien, Samiy, Reiber, Noe, et al., 2005). Participants were fee-paying patients receiving MMT at two private, for-profit clinics in Southern California who had submitted at least one opioid-positive urine sample within the 90 days before enrollment. Procedures common to both studies were as follows. Every participant met with a research assistant to answer questions and submit a urine sample for drug urinalysis on one randomly chosen day per week during these 12-week studies. All participants received similar written feedback regarding urinalysis results and a $2 fast-food gift certificate for completing each data visit. In both studies, rebates were only awarded to participants who were up to date on their fee payments as of Friday of each week.

In Study 1, 48 participants were randomized to one of three groups. One group (continuous reinforcement, or FR1; $n = 16$) received 15% of their weekly fee as a cash rebate each week that their urine sample tested negative for all illicit drugs or their metabolites (cocaine, amphetamine, methamphetamine, THC, methadone, opiates, PCP, barbiturates, and benzodiazepines). Weekly rebates averaged $8.70. In addition, a bonus rebate of 40% of their weekly fee was awarded whenever four consecutive urine samples tested negative for all illicit drugs (bonus rebates averaged $23.22). A second group (variable ratio 3, or VR3; $n = 16$) received 15% of their weekly fee as a cash rebate during each of the first 2 weeks if their samples tested negative for all illicit drugs. During the subsequent 10 weeks, participants in the VR3 group received weekly rebates of 67% of their weekly fee for negative urine samples according to a VR3 schedule (weekly rebates averaged $40.20). This schedule awarded rebates after an average of three negative samples was submitted. That is, rebates were delivered sometimes after only one negative sample, sometimes after two or three negative samples, and at other times only after four negative samples. Although the amount of each rebate was much greater than under the FR1 schedule, only four rebates could be earned during the 12 weeks. A variable-reinforcement schedule was studied because variable schedules generate higher rates of behavior than do fixed schedules and should sustain unreinforced behavior much longer (Ferster & Skinner, 1957). Under this arrangement, the total value of rebates available to the FR1 and VR3 groups were equal and the maximum value of rebates available to either group was 25% of the fees paid during the study. A third group (control; $n = 16$) did not receive fee rebates.

In Study 2, 60 participants were randomized to three groups. One group (continuous reinforcement, or FR1; $n = 21$) had the same schedule of contingent fee rebates as described above for Study 1's FR1 group (weekly rebates averaged $8.70; bonus rebates averaged $23.50). Another group (Gradual; $n = 20$) received rebates contingent upon urinalysis requirements that gradually became more stringent as the study progressed (weekly rebates averaged $8.59). During Weeks 1–3, participants received 15% of their weekly fee as a cash rebate if their urine sample tested negative for opiates. During Weeks 4–6, participants received 15% rebates if their urine tested negative for opiates and stimulants. During the remainder of the trial (Weeks 7–12), rebates were awarded for each weekly urine sample that tested negative for all illicit drugs or their metabolites (cocaine, amphetamine, methamphetamine, THC, methadone, opiates, PCP, barbiturates, and benzodiazepines). In addition, bonus rebates of 40% of their weekly fee were awarded any time four consecutive samples tested negative for the targeted drugs (bonus rebates averaged $22.75). The maximum value of rebates available to either group was again 25% of the fees paid during the study. A third group (control; $n = 19$) did not receive fee rebates.

Results were similar in the two studies and suggest that the fee rebates used were effective incentives for behavior change. Figure 15.2 shows the percentage of urine samples that were negative for all illicit drugs during baseline (Week 0) and each of the 12 weeks during which rebates were available. Overall, groups receiving fee rebates submitted a higher percentage of drug-free urine samples. This conservative analysis assumes that any sample not submitted would have tested positive for illicit drugs and may confound abstinence with attendance. However, simply counting the number of negative samples submitted during the study revealed that the rebate

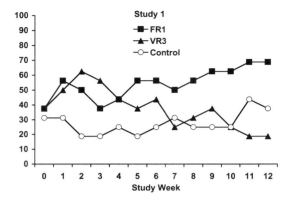

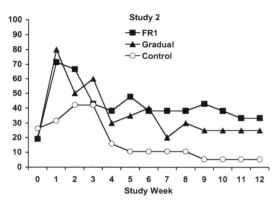

FIGURE 15.2. Percentage of urine samples that tested negative for all illicit drugs at baseline (Week 0) and the 12 weeks during which rebates were available. Filled symbols represent the groups receiving contingent fee rebates; open circles represent the control groups.

groups submitted an average of 72 (VR3), 89 (gradual), and 109 (FR1) negative samples, almost twice the number of negative samples submitted during the study compared to the control groups (44). Moreover, the fee-rebate groups also had significantly longer periods of continuous opioid abstinence than did the control groups ($p < .05$; data not shown). Simple continuous-reinforcement schedules produced slightly more drug abstinence compared to the more complicated VR3 and gradual schedules. Participants receiving contingent fee rebates attended from 35% to 68% more data visits than did controls, retention increased by 37% to 72%, and significantly more clients receiving fee rebates completed the study. Taken together, these results suggest that the fee rebate incentives used in this study

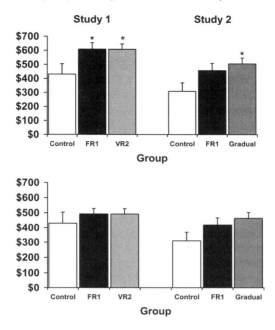

FIGURE 15.3. Top panel: Average total fees received during the 12-week intervention. Vertical lines represent standard errors of the mean. Asterisks (*) designate significant differences from control groups. Bottom panel: Average net income during the 12-week intervention (rebates paid subtracted from fees received). Vertical lines represent standard errors of the mean.

effectively reduced drug use and increased retention in these MMT patients.

A critical issue in using fee rebates for CM incentives is whether a program would lose income by providing them. In the studies described earlier, the value of the rebates actually delivered per participant across groups was rather low, averaging $9.72/week in Study 1 and $3.25/week in Study 2. Figure 15.3 shows the amount of fees collected and the net clinic revenue after the rebates were paid for each group. The clinics collected from 41% to 63% more fees from the groups receiving rebates than from the control groups. This increased compliance with fee payments is not surprising, given the added contingency that patients had to be up to date on their fee payments in order to receive any rebates. Once the rebates paid were subtracted from the fees collected, the clinics' net income was still 14–50% higher from the groups receiving rebates than from the control groups. This finding replicated a similar increase in program income reported in an earlier pilot study in Denver, Colorado (Amass, Ennis, Mikulich, & Kamien,

1998). These results strongly suggest that contingent fee rebates will not result in decreased clinic income and are a practical source for incentives for CM interventions in community-based substance abuse treatment programs.

Strengths of Fee Rebates

Fee rebates seem to offer several advantages as a source for CM incentives. First, fee rebates tap into an existing revenue stream that exists within most community-based substance abuse treatment organizations, eliminating the need for an external source for incentives. Second, cash is a preferred and flexible reinforcer. Cash leads directly to a range of possible alternative reinforcers and may therefore be a more attractive incentive for behavior change than vouchers exchangeable for goods and services. Importantly, cash also represents a nondrug reinforcer readily available within all communities that will continue to be available once treatment is completed. Thus, using cash to reinforce behavior change in CM programs represents a highly generalizable CM dissemination strategy. Third, this approach is attractive from a staffing perspective. Health care personnel in substance abuse treatment are already accustomed to handling and tracking patient fee payments. Cash is easier for staff to manage than vouchers and requires less program overhead because money does not need to be exchanged by staff for goods or services, nor does staff have to spend time storing or managing goods, prizes, or donations. Importantly, the increased fee-payment compliance that resulted from this procedure will also be attractive from a staffing perspective. In fee-for-service clinics, a lot of effort goes into making sure clients pay their fees and staff have to spend time imposing sanctions when clients fall behind in payments, including procedures for withdrawing treatment and withholding or reducing medication when pharmacotherapy is involved. Obviously, reducing staff effort around fee collections would give them more time to focus on treating patients. Finally, fee rebates as a source for incentives offers a win–win approach for both providers and patients. During the fee-rebate programs, providers collected more fees and the net clinic revenue increased. Moreover, retention also increased, giving providers more time to treat the patients. Patients also benefited from the procedure, because it decreased their drug use and they stayed in treatment longer.

Limitations of Fee Rebates

Several variables may limit using fee rebates as a source for incentives in CM programs. First, fee-rebate incentives do not seem feasible for patients who pay little or no fees—for example, in areas in which substance abuse treatment is heavily funded by third-party sources or is subsidized by state benefits. Second, supplying cash incentives may also raise an ethical concern because providing cash to drug-dependent individuals may risk precipitating new drug use. Whether this concern is reasonable, however, when the cash incentive is actually money returned to the clients from their own fees, and when no cash is given if fees have not been paid first, is debatable. Further, when incentives are made contingent upon drug abstinence, using the cash for drug use is self-limiting because new or continued drug use will prevent additional cash from being delivered. However, the concern remains if contingencies are applied to other behaviors such as counseling attendance. A recent trial directly examined whether providing larger cash incentives for completing follow-up visits precipitated more drug use than smaller incentives (Festinger et al., 2005). No evidence was found that up to $70 payments precipitated new drug use, an amount that far exceeds the typical fee rebates clients received in the two studies described earlier. Nonetheless, future studies should specifically demonstrate that providing cash rebates does not precipitate drug use or increase adverse events. Third, the fee-rebate approach has only been tested in patients receiving MMT in opioid treatment programs. Further research should test fee-rebate incentives in drug-free treatment settings and by placing contingencies on behaviors other than drug abstinence, such as counseling attendance. Finally, an ethical issue related to fee rebates is whether they would constitute "fee forgiveness," a prohibited practice of collecting fees only from the insurance company but not from the client. To avoid this issue, rebates should amount to only a relatively small percentage of clients' payments. A client's payments may or may not represent the total cost of treatment (e.g., the client's payment may be a copayment that supplements fees paid by a third party). Therefore, in no case should a rebate exceed or match a client's payments or copayments, no fees collected from third parties should be given to clients, and in no case should client's fees ever be under- or overreported to third-party payers. Moreover, to ensure that the incentives are always coming from the patient's own fee payments, rebates should only be awarded if the patient is up to date with his or her fee payments. In prior research (Amass et al., 1998), discussions with major third-party payors revealed that they viewed patient copayments as belonging to the clinics, supported using fee rebates for substance abuse treatment, and did not foresee any ethical or legal issues arising from using fee rebates to reinforce drug abstinence.

CONCLUDING COMMENTS

Barriers to the dissemination of CM techniques into community-based substance abuse treatment organizations include a lack of clinician training, philosophical barriers, and cost issues. Ideally, this volume will help provide important background to help clinicians implement CM programs and provide evidence and suggestions to help break down philosophical barriers. The current chapter, along with Chapter 14 (Petry & Alessi, this volume), addressed the cost of incentives, one of the most significant barriers to the dissemination of CM to community-based organizations.

This chapter focused on moving beyond just reducing the cost of incentives and examined the use of community- or patient-provided resources to finance the incentives used in CM. Examples were reviewed in which donations of cash, goods, and services were solicited from the community in sufficient amounts and for long enough to initiate and sustain CM programs for smoking cessation. Using donated incentives may offer advantages for the longevity of the program and involving the community in substance abuse treatment. However, the success of securing donations for these CM programs may very well have been related to the fact that two of these programs were for pregnant or postpartum women. After all, the health of pregnant mothers and unborn babies can provide compelling reasons to donate. Whether communities will donate to CM programs targeting other substance abuse problems is an empirical question. Moreover, all the examples of the efficacy of donated incentives were for reducing smoking. Whether donated incentives will be effective for reducing other drug use similarly awaits further research. Finally, the cost of conducting a donations-solicitation campaign must be recognized. Although Amass and Kamien (2004) reported that such a campaign does not need to be very costly or require a lot of time, the cost and staff effort were not zero and may be beyond what is available in many community-based organizations.

Using patient resources to provide incentives is promising. Punishment and deposit contracts where patients agree to give up something significant if drug use is detected deserve additional research attention. Of course, these arrangements are only feasible with patients who have something significant to lose or are in a position to provide a sufficient deposit to function as an effective reinforcer. The most viable way of leveraging patient resources to provide incentives may come from using the patients' own fee payments. Many substance abuse treatment programs require out-of-pocket payments from patients. Results from the first randomized controlled trials of abstinence-contingent fee rebates provide support for the efficacy, practicality, and economic feasibility of this approach. Fee rebates contingent upon drug abstinence effectively reduced drug use and increased retention. Fee rebates were practical because existing, client-provided revenue was used, the procedure was simple to implement, and staff were already accustomed to handling and tracking client fees. Finally, in two different cities and three different clinics, making the fee rebates contingent upon being up to date on fee payments was economical, increasing fee compliance and net clinic revenue. This last aspect, which makes the fee rebate approach attractive to clinic managers and owners, may provide a great impetus toward the dissemination of CM procedures to community-based substance abuse treatment organizations.

Overall, some clearly exciting and promising new strategies for financing the incentives used in CM programs exist. Continued creative examination of existing resources may lead to other CM incentive sources that are similarly practical and feasible. Further research on these strategies in a wide range of substance abuse treatment settings will be essential for demonstrating their generality and assessing their attractiveness for adoption by community-based organizations.

ACKNOWLEDGMENTS

Preparation of this chapter was supported by National Institute on Drug Abuse Grant No. RO1 DA13638.

REFERENCES

Amass, L., Bickel, W. K., Crean, J., Higgins, S. T., & Badger, G. J. (1996). Preferences for clinic privileges, retail items and social activities in an outpatient buprenorphine treatment program. *Journal of Substance Abuse Treatment, 13,* 43–49.

Amass, L., Ennis, E., Mikulich, S. K., & Kamien, J. B. (1998). Using fee rebates to reinforce abstinence and counseling attendance in cocaine abusers. In L. S. Harris (Ed.), *Problems of drug dependence 1997* (NIDA Research Monograph 178, p. 99). Washington, DC: U.S. Government Printing Office.

Amass, L., & Kamien, J. B. (2004). A tale of two cities: Financing two voucher programs for substance abusers through community donations. *Experimental and Clinical Psychopharmacology, 12,* 147–155.

Amass, L., Kamien, J. B., & Samiy, T. (2003, June 14–19). *A randomized controlled trial of community financed, voucher-based reinforcement therapy for smoking cessation in women receiving community-based drug treatment.* Presented at the 65th annual meeting of the College on Problems of Drug Dependence. Bal Harbour, FL.

Amass, L., Kamien, J. B., Samiy, T., Reiber, C., Noe, C. B., Gelacio, S. A., et al. (2005, June 17–24). *Contingent fee rebates: A practical, affordable, revenue-generating and effective way to reduce drug use and drop-out during outpatient treatment of opioid dependence.* Presented at the 67th annual meeting of the College on Problems of Drug Dependence, Orlando, FL.

Bigelow, G., Stickler, D., Liebsen, I., & Griffiths, R. (1976). Maintaining disulfiram ingestion among outpatient alcoholics: A security-deposit contingency contracting procedure. *Behaviour Research and Therapy, 14,* 378–381.

Crowley, T. J. (1999). Research on contingency management treatment of drug dependence: Clinical implications and future directions. In S. T. Higgins & K. Silverman (Eds.), *Motivating behavior change among illicit-drug abusers: Research on contemporary contingency management interventions* (pp. 345–370). Washington, DC: American Psychological Association.

Donatelle, R. J., Prows, S. L., Champeau, D., & Hudson, D. (2000). Randomised controlled trial using social support, financial incentives for high risk pregnant smokers: Significant Other Supported (SOS) program. *Tobacco Control, 9*(Suppl. 3), iii67–iii69.

Elder, J. P., Campbell, N. R., Mielchen, S. D., Hovell, M. F., & Litrownick, A. J. (1991). Implementation and evaluation of a community sponsored smoking cessation contest. *American Journal of Health Promotion, 5,* 200–206.

Elliott, R., & Tighe, T. (1968). Breaking the cigarette habit: Effects of a technique involving threatened loss of money. *Psychological Record, 18,* 503–513.

Ferster, C. B., & Skinner, B. F. (1957). *Schedules of reinforcement.* Englewood Cliffs, NJ: Prentice-Hall.

Festinger, D. S., Marlowe, D. B., Croft, J. R., Dugosh, K. L., Mastro, N. K., Lee, P. A., et al. (2005). Do research payments precipitate drug use or coerce participation? *Drug and Alcohol Dependence, 78,* 275–281.

Hanson, G. R., Leshner, A. I., & Tai, B. (2002). Putting drug abuse treatment to use in real-life settings. *Journal of Substance Abuse Treatment, 23,* 69–70.

Henderson, L. (1984). *The ten lost commandments of fundraising: Davis and Henderson's bicentennial* [Booklet]. Toronto, Ontario: Council for Business and the Arts in Canada.

Iwata, B. A., & Becksfort, C. M. (1981). Behavioral research in preventative dentistry: Educational and contingency management approaches to the problem of patient compliance. *Journal of Applied Behavioral Analysis, 14,* 111–120.

Jones, H. E., Haug, N. A., Stitzer, M. L., & Svikis, D. S. (2000). Improving treatment outcomes for pregnant drug-dependent women using low-magnitude voucher incentives. *Addictive Behaviors, 25,* 263–267.

Kellogg, S. H., Burns, M., Coleman, P., Stitzer, M., Wale, J. B., & Kreek, M. J. (2005). Something of value: The introduction of contingency management interventions into the New York City Health and Hospital Addiction Treatment Service. *Journal of Substance Abuse Treatment, 28,* 57–65.

Kirby, K., Amass, L., & McLellan, A. T. (1999). Disseminating contingency-management research to drug abuse treatment practitioners. In S. T. Higgins & K. Silverman (Eds.), *Motivating behavior change among illicit-drug abusers: Research on contemporary contingency management interventions* (pp. 327–344). Washington, DC: American Psychological Association.

Lando, H. A. (1977). Successful treatment of smokers with a broad-spectrum behavioral approach. *Journal of Consulting and Clinical Psychology, 45,* 361–366.

Lando, H. A., Pirie, P. L., Dusich, K. H., Elsen, C., & Bernards, J. (1995). Community incorporation of quit and win contests in Bloomington, Minnesota. *American Journal of Public Health, 85,* 263–264.

Lussier, J. P., Heil, S. H., Mongeon, J. A., Badger, G. J., & Higgins, S. T. (2006). A meta-analysis of voucher-based reinforcement therapy for substance use disorders. *Addiction, 101,* 129–203.

Paxton, R. (1980). The effects of a deposit contract as a component in a behavioural programme for stopping smoking. *Behaviour Research and Therapy, 18,* 45–50.

Paxton, R. (1981). Deposit contracts with smokers: Varying frequency and amount of repayments. *Behaviour Research and Therapy, 19,* 117–123.

Paxton, R. (1983). Prolonging the effects of deposit contracts with smokers. *Behaviour Research and Therapy 21,* 425–433.

Peirce, J. M., Petry, N. M., Stitzer, M. L., Blaine, J., Kellogg, S., Satterfield, F., et al. (2006). Effects of lower-cost incentives on stimulant abstinence in methadone maintenance treatment: A national drug abuse treatment Clinical Trials Network study. *Archives of General Psychiatry, 63,* 201–208.

Petry, N. M. (2000). A comprehensive guide to the application of contingency management procedures in clinical settings. *Drug and Alcohol Dependence, 58,* 9–25.

Petry, N. M., Peirce, J. M., Stitzer, M. L., Baine, J., Roll, J. M., Cohen, A., et al. (2005). Effect of prize-based incentives on outcomes in stimulant abusers in outpatient psychosocial treatment programs. A national drug abuse treatment Clinical Trials Network study. *Archives of General Psychiatry, 62,* 1148–1156.

Petry, N. M., Tedford, J., Austin, M., Nich, C., Carroll, K. M., & Rounsaville, B. J. (2004). Prize reinforcement contingency management for treating cocaine users: How low can we go, and with whom? *Addiction, 99,* 349–360.

Rettig, R. A., & Yarmolinsky, A. (Eds.). (1995). *Federal regulation of methadone treatment.* Washington, DC: National Academy Press.

Roll, J. M., Chudzynski, J. E., & Richardson, G. (2005). Potential sources of reinforcement and punishment in a drug-free treatment clinic: Client and staff perceptions. *American Journal of Drug and Alcohol Abuse, 31,* 21–33.

Roll, J. M., Petry, N. M., Stitzer, M. L., Brecht, M. L., Peirce, J. M., McCann, M. J., et al. (2006). Contingency management for the treatment of methamphetamine use disorders. *American Journal of Psychiatry, 163,* 1993–1999.

Silverman, K., Chutaupe, M. A., Bigelow, G. E., & Stitzer, M. L. (1999). Voucher-based reinforcement of cocaine abstinence in treatment-resistant methadone patients: Effects of reinforcer magnitude. *Psychopharmacology, 146,* 128–138.

Silverman, K., Svikis, D., Wong, C. J., Hampton, J., Stitzer, M. L., & Bigelow, G. E. (2002). A reinforcement-based therapeutic workplace for the treatment of drug abuse: Three-year abstinence outcomes. *Experimental and Clinical Psychopharmacology, 10,* 228–240.

Spring, F. L., Sipich, J. F., Trimble, R. W., & Goeckner, D. J. (1978). Effects of contingency and noncontingency contracts in the context of a self-control-oriented smoking modification program. *Behavioral Therapeutics, 9,* 967–968.

Stitzer, M. L., Bickel, W. K., Bigelow, G. E., & Liebson, I. A. (1986). Effect of methadone dose contingencies on urinalysis test results of polydrug-abusing methadone-maintenance patients. *Drug and Alcohol Dependence, 18,* 341–348.

Stitzer, M. L., & Bigelow, G. E. (1978). Contingency management in a methadone maintenance program: Availability of reinforcers. *International Journal of the Addictions, 13*(5), 737–746.

Stitzer, M. L., & Bigelow, G. E. (1983). Contingent payment for carbon monoxide reduction: Effects of pay amount. *Behavioral Therapy, 14,* 647–656.

Stitzer, M. L., & Bigelow, G. E. (1984). Contingent payment for carbon monoxide reduction: Within-subject effects of pay amount. *Journal of Applied Behavioral Analysis, 17,* 477–483.

Stitzer, M. L., Bigelow, G. E., Lawrence, C., Cohen, J., D'Lugoff, B., & Hawthorne, J. (1977). Medication take-home as a reinforcer in a methadone maintenance program. *Addictive Behavior, 2,* 9–14.

Tighe, T. J., & Elliott, R. (1968). A technique for controlling behavior in natural life settings. *Journal of Applied Behavior Analysis, 1,* 263–266.

Winett, R. A. (1973). Parameters of deposit contracts in the modification of smoking. *Psychological Record, 23,* 49–60.

CHAPTER 16

CONTINGENCY MANAGEMENT IN AN ENTITLEMENT REHABILITATION SETTING

An Example from the Veterans Health Administration

Charles Drebing, Bruce J. Rounsaville,
and Robert Rosenheck

CONTINGENCY MANAGEMENT TARGETS FOR MENTALLY ILL SUBSTANCE ABUSERS

Extensive research over the past three decades has demonstrated that contingency management (CM) interventions are effective at reducing substance use, including the use of nicotine, alcohol, marijuana, cocaine, opiates, and benzodiazepines (Higgins et al., 2000; Peirce et al., 2006; Petry, Alessi, Marx, Austin, & Tardif, 2005; Roll, 2005). There have been a large number of clinical trials documenting the efficacy of these procedures for addressing substance abuse either through stand-alone interventions or in combination with other forms of clinical treatment. A growing body of evidence has supported the view that CM interventions can significantly reduce drug abuse among the severely mentally ill as well (Mueser, Drake, Sigmon, & Brunette, 2005).

While the majority of CM interventions with drug abusers have provided incentives aimed specifically at drug use, other recovery-oriented activities and treatment goals have been successfully targeted. Numerous studies have demonstrated the efficacy of CM interventions for enhancing attendance and retention in needed clinical services (Lewis & Petry, 2005; Petry & Simcic, 2002; Wong, Dillon, Sylvest, & Silverman, 2004b). In a study that points to a wide range of potential applications, Petry, Tedford, and Martin (2001) allowed participants in substance abuse treatment to select clinical goals for their CM program from a wide array of 90 possible goals.

From a behavioral perspective, the work setting and wages from employment can become an ongoing source of "natural reinforcers" that compete with disordered behaviors among adults with psychiatric and substance use disorders (Hebert, Drebing, Mueller, & Van Ormer, 2006). Unfortunately, most studies show that only 15–20% of adults with psychiatric disabilities are actively engaged in employment at any one time (Anthony & Blanch, 1987). This is likely due to the range of barriers faced by this group, including the disruptive nature of their clinical symptoms, reduced self-efficacy for obtaining and maintaining employment, cultural stigma associated with mental illness, and economic disincentives such as disability income programs.

In previous research, CM interventions have been successful in increasing targeted work-related activities in substance abuse settings. Several studies have used access to employment or work therapy as a reward for maintaining abstinence within substance abuse treatment settings (see Donlin, Knealing, & Silverman, Chapter 17, this volume). Silverman and colleagues (Silverman, Svikis, Robles, Stitzer, & Bigelow, 2001; Silverman et al., 2002; Wong, Dillon, Sylvest, & Silverman, 2004a; Wong et al., 2004b), in a program identified as the Therapeutic Workplace, made access to paid work contingent upon drug abstinence for drug abuse treatment participants. In one study (Silverman et al., 2001), participants in the contingent group were almost twice as likely as those in the control group to remain abstinent (33% vs. 59%). In another study, Milby, Schumacher, Raczynski, and Caldwell (1996) found that 48% of homeless substance abusers remained abstinent and participated in work activities when access to work and housing were used as incentives, compared to only 29% of a comparison group (see Milby & Schumacher, Chapter 9, this volume).

CM has also been used to reward work-related activities directly. Silverman and colleagues found that attendance at job training among a sample of unemployed methadone patients was significantly improved when attendance was reinforced with voucher-based incentives (Silverman, Chutuape, Bigelow, & Stitzer, 1996). As noted earlier, Petry et al. (2001) offered participants in substance abuse treatment a range of clinical goals for their CM program. Fifty-nine percent of the sample chose at least one work-related goal to be rewarded. Work-related goals on average were successfully completed 79% of the time, with rates of successful completion varying across the various types of target behaviors (e.g., working on a resume, 50%; identifying potential jobs, 66%; submitting job applications, 87%; attending work, 69%). In summary, several studies have documented the potential of applying CM interventions in order to influence work-related behavior.

APPLYING CM FOR ADULTS WITH SEVERE MENTAL ILLNESS AND SUBSTANCE USE DISORDERS IN VETERANS ADMINISTRATION VOCATIONAL REHABILITATION SETTINGS

The documented success of CM for reducing substance abuse and fostering employment in substance abusers suggested the promise of a behavioral incentive program to improve employment outcomes and reduce treatment failure for adults with severe mental illness (SMI) and substance use disorders participating in a Veterans Administration (VA) vocational rehabilitation (VR) setting.

In designing the CM intervention, we were interested in two major issues:

1. What are the optimal targets for CM interventions for drug abusers with SMI in a VR program?
2. What adaptations in the CM program are needed to manage the potential disincentives for obtaining employment for patients who are receiving disability payments?

This chapter describes our design, application, and efficacy testing of a CM intervention strategy in this specialized setting.

THE VA SETTING

The Veterans Health Administration (VHA) operates over 150 substance abuse programs, serving an average of 118,000 veterans per year, with about 15,000 veterans currently enrolled on any single day (Substance Abuse and Mental Health Services Administration [SAMHSA], 2005). VHA substance abuse programs tend to be relatively large in size, with a daily median census of about 105 compared to the median for non-VA programs of 36. They also tend to offer a wider range of services relative to non-VA programs, possibly reflecting the fact that 93% are located in hospital settings, compared to 47% of a comparable sample of non-VA programs (SAMHSA, 2005).

The VA is also responsible for administering veteran benefits programs that include a wide array of services such as disability compensation programs, education benefits, housing benefits, and others. In addition to social security disability compensation programs, the VA disability compensation programs provide income for veterans injured as part of their military service and more limited income for qualified veterans disabled by injuries acquired after their military service. Eligibility and restrictions on VA entitlements differ significantly between VA programs and with respect to non-VA programs ("Disability evaluation under social security," 1998; Red Book on Work Incentives, 1995; Survey of Disabled Veterans, 1989).

RATIONALE FOR ADDING CM TO VA VR

Employment is a crucial aspect of sustained recovery from mental illness. From a behavioral perspective, employment can serve as a powerful contingency whereby engaging in employment activities provides social and financial reinforcement that can compete with disordered behaviors (Hebert et al., 2006). Unfortunately, as was noted previously, most studies show that only 15–20% of adults with psychiatric disabilities are actively engaged in employment at any one time (Anthony & Blanch, 1987). While outcomes vary between VR models, even in the most successful models the percentage of participants with SMI who work steadily in competitive jobs tends to peak at around 40% (Bond, 2004). This is true for the VA's Compensated Work Therapy (CWT) program, one of the largest VR programs in the United States. Administrative outcome data collected by the Northeast Program Evaluation Center suggest that about 42% of the more than 13,000 veterans participating in CWT annually are competitively employed at discharge, while another 40% drop out (Resnick, Medak, Baldino, Corwel, & Rosenheck, 2004). Although these employment rates have been rising in recent years, consumers, administrators, and researchers have called for further efforts to improve employment outcomes (Blow, Gillon, & Dornfeld, 2001; Noble, Honberg, Hall, & Flynn, 1997; Xie, Dain, Becker, & Drake, 1997).

All of the 100 CWT programs share a basic model of services which, while being somewhat unique, shares many elements with the "diversified placement model" of VR (Koop et al., 2004). The programs are located at VA medical centers and participants must have a "vocational problem" and a clinical problem and must be referred by a health care provider to be eligible to participate. Administrative data indicate that participants in CWT primarily consist of veterans with psychiatric disorders (96.9%) and substance abuse disorders (86.9%) (Seibyl, Baldino, Corwel, Medak, & Rosenheck, 2002). Veterans are placed in structured work settings, usually in private companies or at the medical center, and compensated for their work. They are typically paid by the CWT program, which contracts with the company for their labor. The mean hourly wage varies by site, with a mean wage at the Bedford site of $7.28 per hour (Seibyl et al., 2002). While the veterans are working, CWT staff help them negotiate and resolve difficulties on the job and prepare for obtaining their own competitive job. The CWT program at Bedford is similar in structure and outcome rates to the other CWT programs around the country (Rosenheck, 2001). For dually diagnosed participants, the average length of stay is 17 weeks and the transition to competitive employment for those who do transition occurs after 22 weeks (Drebing, Penk, & Rosenheck, 2000). The only random assignment evaluation of CWT found that participation was associated with reduced drug and alcohol abuse, fewer episodes of homelessness and incarceration, and protection from a decline in physical health relative to a control group (Kashner et al., 2002).

We conducted two studies to evaluate the efficacy of adding CM initiatives to the VA VR program in order to improve program outcomes as measured by return to competitive employment. The studies examined whether enhancing traditional VR pay-for-work regimens by adding payments for meeting specific clinical goals improves the rate at which VR participants with comorbid psychiatric and substance use disorders transition to competitive employment. We chose to focus on dually diagnosed veterans because of the complexity of their clinical condition, their high risk for noncompliance and dropout, and the fact that more than half of VR participants in the VA are dually diagnosed (Drebing, Fleitas, et al., 2002).

STUDY 1

Methods

We first conducted a pilot study in which 19 dually diagnosed veterans entering VR were randomly assigned to VR only ($n = 8$) or to VR with CM ($n = 11$) (Drebing et al., 2005). Over the first 16 weeks of rehabilitation, those in the VR + CM condition could earn up to $1,006 in cash incentives for meeting two sets of clinical goals: (1) remaining abstinent from opiates, cocaine, and alcohol; and (2) taking steps to obtain and maintain competitive employment.

To be "dually diagnosed" participants in this study were required to have a current psychiatric diagnosis of schizophrenia, bipolar disorder, major depression, posttraumatic stress disorder (PTSD), or other anxiety disorder and current drug or alcohol dependence. We chose to limit the sample to those with substance dependence for alcohol, cocaine, or opiates, with active substance abuse in the prior 90 days. Participants also had to have a history of competitive employment during the prior 3 years and a stated goal of returning to competitive employment within 8 months and to have demonstrated "potential" for returning to competitive employment. Veterans over the age of 55, those who had a chronic medical problem which would make it unlikely that they would be able to obtain and sustain a competitive job within 8 months, and those who did not intend to stay in VR for at least 4 months or live in the local region for 12 months were excluded (Drebing, Losardo, et al., 2002).

Vocational Rehabilitation

When they enter CWT, veterans are almost immediately placed in structured work settings, typically in VA facilities or private companies, and compensated for their work. There is minimal if any formal assessment or other services prior to beginning work. While in these placements, participants are paid by the CWT program, which is paid by companies that have contracted for labor. While the veterans are working, CWT staff provides onsite and/or offsite job coaching. Placements are typically not time limited, but there is often a progression through placements in terms of difficulty, hours of work, or independence. Over time, staff assist the veterans to identify goals for competitive employment, and they provide some support during the job search process. Typically, once the veteran obtains a competitive job, he or she is discharged from the CWT program.

The CM Intervention

The VR + CM condition combined the incentives available to all who participate in the basic VR program, such as wages and social reinforcement, with additional cash awards or "bonuses" offered only to those assigned to this condition. Payment of the additional cash awards was contingent upon the completion of target steps related to obtaining and maintaining competitive employment, maintaining abstinence from substance abuse, and, indirectly, retention in VR. The "incentives" schedule was designed for dually diagnosed participants based on principles demonstrated in other empirical studies of CM (Petry, 2000) with close adherence to well-validated interventions (Higgins et al., 2000).

   We chose to target abstinence because of its direct tie to VR dropout (Drebing et al., 2000) and its responsiveness to CM interventions (Petry, 2000). The "incentive" regimen for encouraging abstinence was modeled closely after approaches developed and validated by Higgins and colleagues (Higgins et al., 2000). A series of increasing cash incentives was offered for drug and alcohol screens that were negative for alcohol, cocaine, or opiates. To ensure rapid and accurate onsite urine screening, the OnTrak Test Cup 5 Roche Diagnostics (Indianapolis, Indiana) and the OnSite Alcohol Assay were used. Screens were conducted twice weekly at unannounced times over the 16 weeks of the study. Screening results had to indicate no evidence of alcohol, cocaine, and opiate use to be considered "clean." The incentive for the initial clean screen was worth $2.50 and increased by $1 for each consecutive negative screen, such that the second consecutive negative screen was worth $3.50, the third was worth $4.50, and so on. Additional $10 incentives were awarded for weeks in which all screens were negative. No payments were given if the screen was positive or if the participant did not produce a urine screen for any reason. In addition, positive screens or failure to provide a scheduled specimen reset the value of the incentives back to their original low level from which they could increase again with consecutive negative screens. Four consecutive clean screens following a reset returned the incentive value to where it was prior to the reset. To encourage the acquisition and maintenance of a competitive job, we rewarded the following target behaviors: creating a usable resume, attending a job interview, obtaining a job, and working at a job for up to 4 consecutive weeks. The following guidelines were used.

1. VR staff were available to help participants with each step in getting a job and then provided support once they were working, for as long as they wished. If they lost their job for any reason, staff were available to help them find another job.

2. Payments were available for the following tasks related to obtaining and retaining a competitive job:

Producing a usable resume $20
Attending a job interview $30
Obtaining a job and working 1 week $40
Working a second consecutive week $50
Working a third consecutive week $60
Working a fourth consecutive week $70
Total employment payments $270

To earn the $20 for producing a usable resume, the resume had to meet three criteria: (a) provides appropriate information, including name, address, phone number, educational background, work history; (b) is organized in a manner that is typical of prototypes in resume workbooks; (c) is professional in appearance—neatly printed on clean paper.

3. The $30 incentive for attending a job interview required that participants produce written evidence of having done so.

4. Once participants obtained a job, they could receive a payment for each of the first 4 weeks they work at least 20 hours, as documented by a pay stub or other written documentation. The payment for the first week was worth $40. For each consecutive week they worked, the payment increased by $10 up to a maximum of $70 across 4 weeks. If they did not work at least 20 hours in a week, they did not receive the payment. If they

earned a payment for working but then failed to earn a subsequent payment for working, the value of the next payment they could earn for working returned to $40. Participants receiving payments for 4 weeks of employment could not earn payments for further employment but were still eligible for other incentives.

The participant was required to be enrolled and fully participating in VR services in order to earn payments for abstinence or work. Because they could not earn an incentive if they were discharged from VR for any reason, the payments indirectly rewarded compliance with VR and attendance at psychiatric appointments, which were required to continue in VR. If a participant in the VR + CM condition remained abstinent throughout the study, he or she could receive up to $736 in payments. Participants who completed all work-related activities and obtained and maintained a job for 4 consecutive weeks could receive up to $270 in payments. Over the 16 weeks of the study, participants had the potential to earn payments totaling $1,006 across the abstinence and vocational contingencies.

Outcome of VR Study 1

Relative to participants in the VR only group, those in the VR + CM condition engaged in more than twice as many job search activities and initiated those activities earlier in their rehabilitation. They were also more likely to remain abstinent, were more likely to obtain competitive employment, and earned an average of 68% more in wages (mean wages for the VR + CM condition, excluding incentives = $4,700 vs. $2,795 for the VR only condition).

When time-to-first-events (resume completion, first job interview, first job, first positive screen) was examined, participation in the CM condition was associated with a significantly shorter time to resume completion and first job interview and longer time to first positive screen, as is shown in Figure 16.1.

Whether someone was receiving disability income did not appear to influence outcomes. There were two participants in the VR only group receiving disability income and four participants in the VR + CM group. Of those in the VR + CM group, three were receiving VA disability income of 40% or less and one was receiving social security disability income (SSDI). In the VR + CM group, those receiving disability income all completed resumes compared to five of seven not receiving disability income. Similarly, all those receiving disability income completed job interviews compared to five of seven not receiving disability income. Two of four obtained competitive jobs compared to three of the seven who were not receiving pensions. One of the four participants receiving disability income relapsed compared

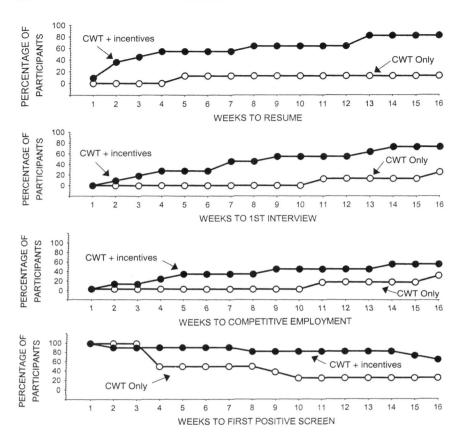

FIGURE 16.1. Percentage of participants in the CWT Only and Compensated Work Therapy + Incentives conditions in study 1 who were documented as having completed job search tasks and maintained abstinence during the 16-week treatment period.

to three of the seven not receiving pensions. With respect to earned income, there was little difference between the two groups ($5,014 for those receiving disability income vs. $5,148 for those not receiving disability income).

STUDY 2

Methods

We are nearing completion of a larger trial evaluating the efficacy of a revised version of this CM intervention. One hundred VR participants with comorbid psychiatric and substance use disorders have been enrolled and randomly assigned to one of the two conditions: VR only (n = 50) or to VR + CM (n = 50). The CM condition differs from that used in our first study in several ways:

1. To further increase employment outcomes, more money was designated for incentives for job search and acquisition such that the maximum possible amount of incentives was increased from $270 to $605. To avoid substantially raising the total cost of the intervention, the incentives for drug abstinence were decreased from $736 to $565. This was accomplished through the elimination of the $10 weekly bonuses, through minor reductions in incentive magnitude, and by increasing the total amount of incentives from $1,006 to $1,170.
2. The number and schedule of job search incentives was also modified so that an incentive could be earned every week for the first 16 weeks of the study, as opposed to eight total incentives that could be earned at any time over the course of the prior trial.
3. Procedures to ensure participant comprehension of the incentives and easy use of the CM schedule were added, including the addition of a screening test of comprehension and materials such as wallet-size summary cards.

Preliminary Outcomes

Preliminary results (n = 36) (Drebing, 2005) indicate that relative to participants in the VR only group, those in the VR + CM were more likely to obtain competitive employment (63% VR + CM vs. 31% VR only) and worked more days in competitive employment (51.3 days for the VR + CM group vs. 11.1 days for the VR only group). Examining only those who obtained competitive employment, participants in the VR + CM group worked more than twice the number of days (83.9 days vs. 36.0 days). Work outcomes over the 9 months of follow-up document that the benefits of the CM intervention grew over time with the greatest advantage in terms of days of employment per month, noted well after the incentives were no longer available, suggesting that the CM participants did successfully transition to natural incentives for employment (see Figure 16.2). Abstinence rates were better for the incentive group (69% vs. 50%), though the difference was not statistically significant.

Examining the impact of disability pension status, we again failed to find early evidence of a significant impact. Six of 37 participants were receiving either SSDI or VA disability income. Relative to participants receiving no disability income, those receiving disability income were somewhat less likely to obtain competitive employment (33% for the disability income group vs. 48% for those not receiving disability income) and did

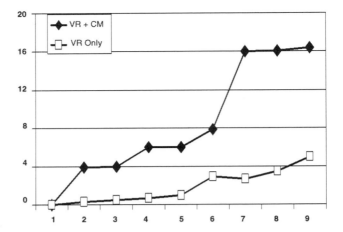

FIGURE 16.2. Mean days of competitive employment per month for the vocational rehabilitation (VR) only and the vocational rehabilitation + contingency management (CM) groups in study 2 during the 9-month period of follow-up.

work fewer days (23.8 days for the disability income group vs. 32.1 days for those not receiving disability income), though the differences were not statistically significant. If we examine only those in the CM intervention, those receiving disability income were no more likely to obtain competitive employment (50% for the disability income group vs. 50% for those not receiving disability income) and worked about the same number of days (49.5 days for the disability income group vs. 51.5 days for those not receiving disability income) as those without disability income. Similarly, those receiving disability income were slightly more likely to use substances at least once during the follow-up (33% for the disability income group vs. 22% for those not receiving disability income) and those in the CM group were also more likely to use substances at least once (50% for the disability income group vs. 36% for those not receiving disability income), though the differences were, again, not statistically significant.

DISCUSSION

These results are encouraging in several ways. First, the CM interventions were successful at increasing the rate of participants who met a long-term rehabilitation goal of obtaining employment. The array of competing incentives and disincentives for employment are complex and are implicated in the low employment rate for adults with mental illness (Hebert et al.,

2006). The evidence that a CM intervention can have an impact within such a complex field of incentives is encouraging and raises hope that other complex clinical targets can be met with similar interventions.

It is possible that these positive findings are reflective of a good match between CM interventions and VR treatment settings. Theoretically, there does appear to be a natural synergy between VR programs and CM techniques, as each addresses the other's limitations. VR is often undermined by misuse of drugs and alcohol and by participants' concerns about transitioning to competitive employment but has the advantage of providing long-term reinforcement in the form of both earnings and less tangible rewards such as social status and self-esteem. CM techniques can enhance the ability to meet treatment goals such as retention or abstinence but can result in dropoff in effects when the contrived reinforcers are removed. VR programs also appear to be a more natural setting for CM than other clinical programs. Petry (2000) has previously noted that "despite compelling evidence regarding their efficacy and the wide acceptability and applicability of these procedures, contingency management approaches are rarely implemented in (substance abuse) treatment programs" (p. 21). This appears to reflect concern about the impact of contingency payments on total program cost and discomfort by clinicians and administrators with what appears to be the artificiality of paying clients for meeting clinical goals and with working with money. These concerns are less relevant to VR settings, where there is adequate infrastructure for working with money and where clients are often paid. With respect to the concerns about cost, it is a relatively small step to restructure the existing financial payments in many VR settings to include explicit, contingent links to achieving clinical goals.

These results may also support the view that a wider range of clinical applications of CM techniques is possible. In this application we chose a combination of targets for CM: drug abstinence, which is crucial for employment in the real world, and achievement of milestones toward paid employment. Typically, CM interventions are used to achieve the repetition of targeted behaviors in order to either (1) unlearn undesirable habits and increase learning of desired behavior patterns (i.e., reducing repeated drug use and substituting other rewards) or (2) increase compliance with treatment so that participants can receive a sufficient dose to achieve a clinical goal, typically either medication or attendance. In this intervention we have identified key barriers to employment, identified behavioral targets that allow those barriers to be breached, and then rewarded these behavioral targets. This novel approach to designing CM incentives appears to be quite conducive to facilitating the chain of behaviors required to successfully acquire and maintain employment. A similar approach appears to be particularly well suited for improving outcomes for a range of other rehabilitation services and goals, such as services designed to enhance acquisition of successful housing, the resolution of legal issues, and the development of a social network.

Finally, these findings provide some limited information about the role of environmental disincentives and competing incentives. Although there are several studies that document that disability income represents a disincentive for employment, the present data suggest that in samples of VR participants screened for interest in returning to competitive employment, those receiving disability income are not clearly less responsive to a CM intervention. This is encouraging for clinicians working within a large entitlement system like the VHA health care system, suggesting that despite the complex array of benefits and rules, a CM intervention can have a significant impact on target behaviors, at least in select participants.

CONCLUDING COMMENTS

The rehabilitation of adults with psychiatric and substance abuse problems is a national priority both inside and outside the VA. Systematic efforts to enhance success rates of rehabilitation programs will require careful identification of barriers to success followed by the design of interventions to overcome those barriers. Some barriers have been identified and points in the rehabilitation process in which participants are particularly vulnerable to failing to progress have also been identified (Comander, Odell, Williams, Sashidharan, & Surtees, 1999; Drebing, Rosenheck, Schutt, Seibyl, & Penk, 2003; Johannessen et al., 2005). The studies summarized in this chapter suggest to us that new CM interventions need to be designed to assist participants to overcome those identified barriers and to successfully navigate key transitions as part of a fully complete transition to independent functioning. We are currently engaged in a pilot study of a new CM intervention designed to increase the probability that homeless, dually diagnosed veterans will successfully transition to independent housing. The transition to independent housing is often a key point in the rehabilitation process where the participant becomes integrated back into the community. Similar efforts could be developed for the range of mental health and rehabilitation services, including services designed to address legal issues, financial issues, education, socialization, case management and treatment compliance, and additional vocational issues.

REFERENCES

Anthony, W. A., & Blanch, A. (1987). Supported employment for persons who are psychiatrically disabled: An historical and conceptual perspective. *Psychosocial Rehabilitation Journal, 11*, 5–23.

Blow, F. C., Gillon, L., & Dornfeld, M. (2001). *Comprehensive national evaluation of VHA Compensated Work Therapy.* Ann Arbor, MI: Serious Mental Illness Treatment Research and Evaluation Center (SMITREC).

Bond, G. R. (2004). Supported employment: Evidence for an evidence-based practice. *Psychiatric Rehabilitation Journal, 27*(4), 345–359.

Comander, M. J., Odell, S. O., Williams, K. J., Sashidharan, S. P., & Surtees, P. G. (1999). Pathways to care for alcohol use disorders. *Journal of Public Health Medicine, 21*(1), 65–69.

"Disability evaluation under Social Security." (1998). Washington, DC: Social Security Administration.

Drebing, C. E. (2005). *Paying people to get better: Incentive enhancement and vocational rehabilitation.* Paper presented at the annual convention of the American Psychological Association, Washington, DC.

Drebing, C. E., Fleitas, R., Moore, A., Krebs, C., Van Ormer, E. A., Penk, W., et al. (2002). Patterns in work functioning and vocational rehabilitation associated with co-morbid psychiatric and substance use disorders. *Rehabilitation Counseling Bulletin, 46*(1), 5–13.

Drebing, C. E., Losardo, M., Van Ormer, E. A., Krebs, C., Penk, W., Nasser, E., et al. (2002). Vocational rehabilitation and older adults: Patterns in participation and outcome. *Journal of Rehabilitation, 68*(3), 28–32.

Drebing, C. E., Penk, W., & Rosenheck, R. (2000). *Readiness for competitive employment: Predicting "success" of CWT graduates.* Paper presented at the annual convention of the American Psychological Association, Washington, DC.

Drebing, C. E., Rosenheck, R., Schutt, R., Seibyl, C., & Penk, W. (2003). Patterns in referral and admission to vocational rehabilitation associated with co-existing psychiatric and substance use disorders. *Rehabilitation Counseling Bulletin, 47*(1), 15–23.

Drebing, C. E., Van Ormer, E. A., Krebs, C., Rosenheck, R., Rounsaville, B., Herz, L., et al. (2005). The impact of enhanced incentives on vocational rehabilitation outcomes for dually diagnosed veterans. *Journal of Applied Behavior Analysis, 38*, 359–372.

Hebert, M., Drebing, C., Mueller, L., & Van Ormer, E. A. (2006). Job search decision making among vocational rehabilitation participants: A behavioral economics perspective. *American Journal of Psychiatric Rehabilitation, 9*, 191–218.

Higgins, S. T., Budney, A. J., Bickel, W. K., Foerg, F., Donham, R., & Badger, M. S. (1994). Incentives improve outcome in outpatient behavioral treatment of cocaine dependence. *Archives of General Psychiatry, 51*, 568–576.

Higgins, S. T., Wong, C. J., Badger, G. J., Ogden, D. E., Haug, D., & Dantona, R. L. (2000). Contingent reinforcement increases cocaine abstinence during outpatient treatment and one year of follow-up. *Journal of Consulting and Clinical Psychology, 68*, 64–72.

Johannessen, J. O., Larsen, T. K., Joa, I., Melle, I., Friis, S., Opjordsmoen, S., et al. (2005). Pathways to care for the first-episode psychosis in an early detection healthcare sector: Part of the Scandinavian TIPS Study. *British Journal of Psychiatry, 187*(Suppl. 48), S24–S28.

Kashner, T. M., Rosenheck, R., Campinell, A. B., Suris, A., Crandall, R., Garfield, N. J., et al. (2002). Impact of work on health status among homeless, substance dependent veterans: A randomized controlled trial. *Archives of General Psychiatry, 59*(10), 938–945.

Koop, J. I., Rollins, A. L., Bond, G. R., Salyers, M. P., Dincin, J., Kinley, T., et al. (2004). Development of the DPA Fidelity Scale: Using fidelity to define an existing vocational model. *Psychiatric Rehabilitation Journal, 28*(1), 16–24.

Lewis, M. W., & Petry, N. M. (2005). Contingency management treatments that reinforce completion of goal-related activities: Participation in family activities and its association with outcomes. *Drug and Alcohol Dependence, 79*(2), 267–271.

Milby, J. B., Schumacher, J. E., Raczynski, J. M., & Caldwell, E. (1996). Sufficient conditions for effective treatment of substance abusing homeless persons. *Drug and Alcohol Dependence, 43*, 39–47.

Mueser, K. T., Drake, R. E., Sigmon, S. C., & Brunette, M. F. (2005). Psychosocial interventions for adults with severe mental illness and co-occurring substance use disorders: A review of specific interventions. *Journal of Dual Diagnosis, 1*(2), 57–82.

Noble, J. H., Honberg, R. S., Hall, L. L., & Flynn, L. M. (1997). *A legacy of failure: The inability of the federal-state vocational rehabilitation system to serve people with severe mental illnesses*. Arlington, VA: National Alliance for the Mentally Ill.

Peirce, J. M., Petry, N. M., Stitzer, M. L., Blaine, J., Kellogg, S., Satterfield, F., et al. (2006). Effects of lower-cost incentives on stimulant abstinence in methadone maintenance treatment: A national drug abuse treatment Clinical Trials Network study. *Archives of General Psychiatry, 63*(2), 201–208.

Petry, N. M. (2000). A comprehensive guide to the application of contingency management procedures in clinical settings. *Drug and Alcohol Dependence, 58*, 9–25.

Petry, N. M., Alessi, S. M., Marx, J., Austin, M., & Tardif, M. (2005). Vouchers versus prizes: Contingency management treatment of substance abusers in community settings. *Journal of Consulting and Clinical Psychology, 73*(6), 1005–1014.

Petry, N. M., & Simcic, F. (2002). Recent advances in the dissemination of contingency management techniques: Clinical and research perspectives. *Journal of Substance Abuse Treatment, 23*(2), 81–86.

Petry, N. M., Tedford, J., & Martin, B. (2001). Reinforcing compliance with non-drug-related activities. *Journal of Substance Abuse Treatment, 20*(33–44).

Red Book on Work Incentives. (1995). Washington, DC: Social Security Administration.

Resnick, S. G., Medak, S., Baldino, R., Corwel, L., & Rosenheck, R. (2004). *Eight progress report on the Compensated Work Therapy (CWT)/Veterans Industries (VI) program*. West Haven, CT: Department of Veterans Affairs Northeast Program Evaluation Center.

Roll, J. M. (2005). Assessing the feasibility of using contingency management to modify cigarette smoking by adolescents. *Journal of Applied Behavior Analysis, 38*(4), 463–467.

Rosenheck, R. (2001). *Fiscal Year 2000 draft tables CWT progress report*. West Haven, CT: Northeast Program Evaluation Center.

Seibyl, C. L., Baldino, R., Corwel, L., Medak, S., & Rosenheck, R. (2002). *Final progress report on the Compensated Work Therapy (CWT)/Veterans Industries (VI) programs: Fiscal year 2001*. West Haven, CT: Veterans Administration Northeast Program Evaluation Center.

Silverman, K., Chutuape, M. D., Bigelow, G. E., & Stitzer, M. L. (1996). Voucher-based reinforcement of attendance by unemployed methadone patients in a job skills training program. *Drug and Alcohol Dependence, 41*, 197–207.

Silverman, K., Svikis, D., Robles, E., Stitzer, M. L., & Bigelow, G. E. (2001). A reinforcement-based Therapeutic Workplace for the treatment of drug abuse: Six-month abstinence outcomes. *Experimental and Clinical Psychopharmacology, 9*(1), 14–23.

Silverman, K., Svikis, D., Wong, C. J., Hampton, J., Stitzer, M. L., & Bigelow, G. E. (2002). A reinforcement-based Therapeutic Workplace for the treatment of drug abuse: Three-year abstinence outcomes. *Experimental and Clinical Psychopharmacology, 10*(3), 228–240.

Substance Abuse and Mental Health Services Administration. (2005). *National Survey on Drug Use and Health*. Washington, DC: Office of Applied Studies.

Survey of Disabled Veterans. (1989). Washington, DC: Department of Veterans Affairs.

Wong, C. J., Dillon, E. M., Sylvest, C. E., & Silverman, K. (2004a). Contingency management of reliable attendance of chronically unemployed substance abusers in a Therapeutic Workplace. *Experimental and Clinical Psychopharmacology, 12*(1), 39–46.

Wong, C. J., Dillon, E. M., Sylvest, C. E., & Silverman, K. (2004b). Evaluation of a modified contingency management intervention for consistent attendance in therapeutic workplace participants. *Drug and Alcohol Dependence, 74*(3), 319–323.

Xie, H., Dain, B. J., Becker, D. R., & Drake, R. E. (1997). Job tenure among persons with severe mental illness. *Rehabilitation Counseling Bulletin, 40*(4), 230–239.

CHAPTER 17

EMPLOYMENT-BASED REINFORCEMENT IN THE TREATMENT OF DRUG ADDICTION

Wendy D. Donlin, Todd W. Knealing,
and Kenneth Silverman

Contingency management interventions have been extraordinarily effective in promoting drug abstinence (see Chapters 1–7, this volume) and medication adherence in addiction treatment (see Chapter 8, this volume) for diverse populations, including individuals who have failed to respond to conventional approaches (see Chapters 1–12, this volume). Despite this effectiveness, contingency management interventions have not been used widely in routine clinical practice (e.g., McGovern, Fox, Xie, & Drake, 2004).

Dissemination-oriented research has focused on integrating contingency management into traditional drug abuse treatment clinics. Due to limited resources in these settings (McLellan, Carise, & Kleber, 2003), researchers have focused on using readily available or low-cost reinforcers, devising creative ways to pay for the interventions, and arranging short-duration reinforcement contingencies. These approaches have shown great promise and are described in other chapters in this book (see Chapters 13–15, this volume).

Although low-cost and short-duration interventions have clearly been effective and are useful for many individuals, they have not been effective in initiating targeted behavior change in all individuals, and they have not reliably produced successful long-term outcomes in those who do initiate the desired behavior change. To augment the effectiveness of these interventions, a small number of researchers have investigated interventions that utilize reinforcers that are available outside the drug abuse treatment clinic that might be harnessed for therapeutic purposes. Researchers pursuing this approach have used housing for homeless drug-addicted adults (Chapter 9, this volume), social security disability benefits for drug users with co-occurring mental illness (Chapter 11, this volume), and consequences in the criminal justice system for convicted offenders (Chapter 18, this volume). A few researchers have investigated the potential of using contingent access to employment to reinforce therapeutically important behaviors. This chapter discusses the scientific foundation underlying the use of employment-based reinforcement; reviews research illustrating and evaluating employment-based reinforcement interventions; and reviews policies and practices that exist in community workplaces and supported employment environments, which may accommodate the therapeutic use of employment-based reinforcement.

SCIENTIFIC FOUNDATION FOR THE USE OF EMPLOYMENT-BASED REINFORCEMENT

Abstinence reinforcement, in which reinforcement is delivered contingent upon objective evidence of drug abstinence, is arguably the most important and useful type of contingency management intervention for the treatment of drug addictions. Abstinence reinforcement has been effective in promoting abstinence from most commonly abused drugs and in diverse populations. However, not all those exposed to these interventions initiate abstinence, and some who do initiate abstinence relapse to drug use when the intervention is discontinued.

Increasing the Proportion of Patients That Respond to Interventions

In virtually all studies of abstinence reinforcement, some participants continue to use the targeted drug despite exposure to the abstinence-reinforcement intervention. A recent randomized controlled multisite study illustrates this point (Peirce et al., 2006). That study evaluated an abstinence-reinforcement intervention in six community methadone programs. The cost of the reinforcement system was kept relatively low to enhance its potential for real-world application. Under the abstinence-reinforcement system, participants could earn up to $420 in prizes for providing stimulant-negative urine samples over 12 weeks. Participants exposed to the prize reinforcement system achieved almost a twofold increase in the rates of stimulant-negative urine samples compared to a usual-care control group. Although the abstinence-reinforcement intervention was clearly effective, 46% of the urine samples provided by participants exposed to the abstinence-reinforcement intervention were positive for stimulants and over half of the participants provided predominantly stimulant-positive urine samples.

We do not fully understand why only some participants respond in a particular abstinence-reinforcement application. Several studies have shown that participants with the highest baseline rates of drug use are less likely to respond to abstinence-reinforcement interventions than those with lower rates. A few studies have shown that methadone patients with the highest baseline rates of cocaine use were least likely to achieve sustained abstinence when exposed to an intervention in which they could earn monetary vouchers for providing cocaine-negative urine samples (e.g., Silverman et al., 1998). Similarly, Stitzer, Iguchi, and Felch (1992) found that methadone patients with the highest baseline rates of polydrug use were least likely to respond to an intervention in which they could earn take-home methadone doses for providing drug-free urine samples. Stitzer, Rand, Bigelow, and Mead (1986) also found that cigarette smokers with the highest base rates of smoking were least likely to achieve abstinence when exposed to monetary-based abstinence reinforcement.

Reviews and meta-analyses suggest the effectiveness of abstinence-reinforcement increases, for example, as reinforcement magnitude increases (Lussier, Heil, Mongeon, Badger, & Higgins, 2006), as delay to reinforcement decreases and when abstinence from single versus multiple drugs is required (Griffith, Rowan-Szal, Roark, & Simpson, 2000; Lussier et al., 2006). Of the explored parameters, the effects of reinforcement magnitude have been the most clearly established both within (Dallery, Silverman, Chutuape, Bigelow, & Stitzer, 2001; Petry et al., 2004; Silverman, Chutuape, Bigelow, & Stitzer, 1999; Stitzer & Bigelow, 1984) and across studies (Lussier et al., 2006). In one study (Silverman et al., 1999), methadone patients were exposed to varying voucher magnitudes after failing to achieve sustained cocaine abstinence when exposed to a cocaine-abstinence-reinforcement intervention in which they could earn up to $1,155 in vouchers over 12 weeks. These participants only initiated sustained cocaine abstinence when exposed to a 9-week voucher condition in which they could earn up to about $3,400 in vouchers for providing cocaine-free urine samples; lower-magnitude conditions had no effect. Dallery et al. (2001) showed similar results in a study in which abstinence from both opiates and cocaine was reinforced. While these studies did not identify the minimum reinforcement magnitudes that would have been required to initiate abstinence in these individuals, they do suggest that some patients require high-magnitude reinforcement.

Producing Long-Term Abstinence Outcomes

The common description of drug addiction as a "chronic relapsing disorder" (McLellan, Lewis, O'Brien, & Kleber, 2000) derives in part from the fact that patients exposed to all types of treatment frequently relapse to drug use at some point after treatment ends. Some abstinence-reinforcement interventions have produced long-term increases in abstinence that are evident after the intervention is discontinued (Higgins, Badger, & Budney, 2000), apparently by increasing the duration of abstinence that individuals achieve during treatment (Higgins et al., 2000). However, as with other treatments, many individuals who initiate abstinence under abstinence reinforcement resume their drug use at some point after the discontinuation of the reinforcement. Relapse following abstinence reinforcement has been seen in cigarette smokers (e.g., Winett, 1973), benzodiazepine users (e.g., Stitzer, Bigelow, Liebson, & Hawthorne, 1982), opiate users (e.g., Silverman, Wong, et al., 1996), and cocaine users (e.g., Silverman et al., 1999).

To address the problem of postintervention relapse, McLellan et al. (2000) suggested the adoption of long-term care strategies similar to those used in the treatments of other chronic disorders such as diabetes and hypertension. Indeed, many treatments must be maintained over extended periods to sustain effectiveness. Recent research shows that abstinence reinforcement can be used effectively as a maintenance intervention (e.g., Preston, Umbricht, Wong, & Epstein, 2001; Silverman, Robles, Mudric, Bigelow, & Stitzer, 2004). Silverman et al. (2004) maintained increased cocaine abstinence for an entire year in methadone patients by sustaining a year-long abstinence-reinforcement contingency.

EMPLOYMENT-BASED REINFORCEMENT IN THE TREATMENT OF DRUG ADDICTION

This preceding research suggests that for some treatment-refractory individuals, high-magnitude abstinence reinforcement may be required to initiate abstinence, and that long-duration abstinence reinforcement may be useful to promote long-term abstinence outcomes. The need for high-magnitude and long-duration abstinence reinforcement raises an obvious practical problem: How can such contingencies be financed? To address this problem, several investigators have integrated abstinence-reinforcement contingencies into workplaces and have used contingent access to paid employment to reinforce abstinence (e.g., Cohen, Bigelow, Hargett, Allen, & Halsted, 1973; Crowley, 1986; Milby et al., 1996; Miller, 1975; Silverman, Svikis, Robles, Stitzer, & Bigelow, 2001; Silverman et al., 2002). In many ways, workplaces are ideal contexts to arrange abstinence reinforcement (Silverman, 2004, p. 219):

1. Workplaces control powerful reinforcers, most notably salary, which could be used to reinforce drug abstinence.
2. Individuals maintain regular contact with their places of employment, which could allow for the routine collection of urine samples and reinforcement of abstinence based on urinalysis results.
3. Employment is typically maintained over extended periods of time, which could allow for the long-term maintenance of abstinence-reinforcement contingencies.
4. Through the growth of employee assistance programs (EAP), workplaces are becoming common and accepted providers of substance abuse services (Hartwell, Steele, French, & Rodman, 1996; Substance Abuse and Mental Health Services Administration, 2002).
5. Workplaces are everywhere, which could facilitate the dissemination of employment-based abstinence-reinforcement contingencies.

To arrange employment-based abstinence reinforcement, a contingency can be arranged in which employees must remain abstinent to work and earn wages. Drug use can be monitored through routine collection of biological samples (e.g., urine samples) that are tested for the targeted drugs of abuse. The opportunity to work and earn wages can then be made contingent upon verified abstinence. Such contingencies can be maintained over time to sustain abstinence over time. Similar contingencies can be arranged to promote the use of addiction treatment medications such as disulfiram or naltrexone.

TREATMENT OF ALCOHOL ADDICTION

In the 1970s, researchers developed employment-based reinforcement contingencies to treat persistent alcohol problems. In an early study, Cohen et al. (1973) treated four male Baltimore City Hospital employees who were on the verge of employment dismissal if they could not control their drinking. The treatment program was designed to increase abstinence and the use of an alcohol treatment medication, disulfiram. The treatment was individualized but included the following general procedures. Each participant signed a contract agreeing to the terms of the treatment. Three of the participants were required to take a daily dose of disulfiram under the observation of a nurse and to provide breath alcohol samples on one-quarter of the workdays (randomly selected). For one participant, disulfiram was contraindicated; he was required to provide daily breath alcohol samples before work. On days that a participant took the scheduled dose of disulfiram (if required) and provided a breath sample that was negative for alcohol (if required), he was allowed to work. If a participant failed to take a dose of disulfiram or provided a sample that was positive for alcohol, he was suspended from work for 1 day without pay. Termination from employment for repeated failures to comply was mentioned, but the conditions under which that might occur were not specified.

Positive outcomes were reported for two of the participants in this study, but effectiveness of these procedures is not known because of the lack of any experimental design. One supervisor refused to impose the programmed consequences for failing to take disulfiram, a result that might suggest a potential obstacle to implementing such contingencies in the workplace. This study suggests that employment-based reinforcement contingencies may promote medication compliance and abstinence in employees with drug abuse problems.

In an experimental evaluation of an employment-based reinforcement intervention (Robichaud, Strickler, Bigelow, & Liebson, 1979), 21 industrial employees were referred by their employers to treatment due to drinking-related problems on the job. Under the intervention, participants had to ingest disulfiram under a nurse's observation daily for 14 days and every other day thereafter. At the start of treatment, the participant, the employer, and the clinic agreed on the duration of treatment. Every 2 weeks throughout treatment a letter was sent to employers indicating that the participant had attended treatment. The report did not specify the precise consequences for failing to take disulfiram. Treatments lasted an average of 10.6 months, and ranged from 3 to 30.3 months. During the 24 months prior to enrollment in treatment, participants were absent on 10% of the workdays. During treatment, absenteeism dropped to less than 2%. After the treatment ended, absenteeism increased to 7%. The rates of absenteeism during the treatment period were significantly lower than the rates before or after treatment. The study illustrated how a drug abuse treatment clinic could coordinate with employers to integrate employment-based contingencies into treatment.

Miller (1975) devised a novel application of employment-based reinforcement for a group of unemployed, homeless, "skid row alcoholics" with a history of repeated arrests for public drunkenness. Because these men were generally unemployed and lacked many essentials of living, the local social services agencies offered them employment opportunities and other necessities such as housing, food, and clothing. To promote abstinence in these individuals, Miller arranged a contingency management intervention in which they could receive the employment opportunities and other benefits only as long as they remained abstinent from alcohol. If they were ever observed using alcohol (as assessed on random breath alcohol tests or by direct observation of gross intoxication), they lost access to the employment opportunities and other privileges for 5 days. A small, randomized controlled study showed that this contingency management intervention decreased arrests for public drunkenness and increased the days of employment, relative to a control group. Although the role of the employment-based reinforcement contingency in producing the positive results cannot be determined, the report provides an early illustration of a potential employment-based reinforcement intervention for chronically unemployed individuals.

Contingency Contracting for Licensed Health Professionals

Crowley developed a classic contingency management intervention to treat licensed health care professionals addicted to various drugs (Crowley, 1984, 1986). Under this intervention, Crowley created a written contract with patients that specified the terms of a novel employment-based abstinence-reinforcement contingency. The contract specified that (1) the health care professional would submit to random, observed urine testing throughout the term of the contract; and (2) if the health care professional ever provided a drug-positive urine sample or failed to provide a scheduled sample while the contract was in effect, the therapist would send a letter to the appropriate licensing board, indicating a drug relapse during treatment and the surrender of the health care professional's medical license.

In one of the reports, Crowley (1984) described the application of contingency contracting with 17 physicians, nurses, and dentists. Twelve of those individuals had professional privileges restricted or suspended, and three others had been threatened with similar restrictions if they did not receive effective treatment. Contract lengths varied from 1 month to 38 months, and half were at least 12 months in duration. About half of the patients (53%) remained abstinent from drugs for 12 months after signing the contract, 29% used drugs while the contract was in effect, 12% lost their license through the contract, and 29% used drugs after the contract ended. The published reports (Crowley, 1984, 1986) described the application of this intervention but did not demonstrate the effectiveness of this intervention through a controlled study. The reports did provide promising descriptive data and an important illustration of a novel and potentially useful contingency management application.

Work Therapy for Homeless Adults

In an innovative approach to treating homeless drug abusers, Milby and colleagues developed a comprehensive intervention that included intensive behavioral counseling and abstinence-contingent access to housing and employment (e.g., Milby et al., 1996). Under this intervention, urine samples were collected routinely and analyzed for drug use. Individuals were given access to a furnished apartment and to paid employment contingent upon drug abstinence. Contingent employment was typically minimum-wage construction jobs refurbishing houses. Participants could maintain housing and work as long as they continued to provide drug-negative urine samples. If a participant ever provided a drug-positive urine sample, the individual was immediately moved from the apartment to a local shelter and denied access to employment and could not return until providing 2 consecutive weeks of drug-free urine samples. The overall intervention was shown effective in retaining participants in treatment and increasing abstinence; however, the effects of the employment-based abstinence reinforcement were never isolated (see Chapter 9, this volume, for a review of this research).

A Therapeutic Workplace for Chronically Unemployed and Treatment-Resistant Adults

Silverman et al. (2001) developed an employment-based reinforcement intervention to treat chronically unemployed adults with long histories of drug addiction who have failed to respond to conventional treatment approaches. The intervention has a few key features: Participants are hired and paid to work in a model Therapeutic Workplace. To promote abstinence participants are required to provide drug-negative urine samples to gain access to the workplace and to maintain maximum rate of pay. If a participant ever provides a drug-positive urine sample or fails to provide a scheduled sample the participant is not allowed to work that day or any day thereafter until the participant provides a new drug-negative urine sample. Importantly, employment is never terminated for providing drug-positive urine samples; the participant is always encouraged to return on subsequent days to try again. To promote sustained abstinence and attendance, a schedule of escalating reinforcement modeled after the schedule developed by Higgins et al. (1991) is arranged in which the pay rate increases as the participant's duration of sustained abstinence and workplace attendance increases.

Targeting chronically poor and unemployed individuals with few job skills, the intervention includes two sequential phases. In the initial phase, each participant works on intensive and individualized training programs designed to teach prerequisites and job skills needed for employment. During this phase, participants receive vouchers exchangeable for goods and services to reduce the chance that earnings could be used to purchase drugs, similar to the system developed by Higgins et al. (1991). Participants who initiate sustained abstinence and acquire needed skills progress to the second phase of treatment, in which they are hired to perform real jobs and earn wages in the Therapeutic Workplace income-producing business. Participants are guaranteed a base pay equal to minimum wage as well as an opportunity to earn additional pay based on the amount and quality of their work performance. However, if a participant ever provides a drug-positive urine sample or fails to provide a scheduled sample, the participant is not allowed to work that day and receives a temporary decrease in the rate of productivity pay available for work performance.

Initially, the intervention was implemented manually (Silverman et al., 2001; Silverman et al., 2002). An instructor taught the basic academic and job skills; attendance, work hours, and performance were monitored through manual recording; and a complex set of reinforcement contingencies for abstinence, attendance, and professional demeanor were arranged through primarily manual procedures. To simplify implementation, Silverman et al. (2005) developed a web-based application that computerized most aspects of the intervention.

A Therapeutic Workplace Prototype

The original Therapeutic Workplace intervention targeted methadone patients from the Center for Addiction and Pregnancy, a comprehensive treatment program for pregnant and recently postpartum women located in Baltimore, Maryland (Silverman et al., 2001). Forty patients from the Center for Addiction and Pregnancy who continued to use opiates and cocaine during that treatment were randomized to the Therapeutic Workplace or usual-care control group. Both groups continued to receive treatment at the Center for Addiction and Pregnancy as long as it was available and were monitored over time. Participants were initially enrolled for 6 months, and then re-enrolled repeatedly in 6-month blocks for over 4 years.

Therapeutic Workplace participants could attend the workplace 3 hours every weekday dependent on providing an observed urine sample that tested negative for opiates and cocaine. The program provided training in basic academic skills and computer data entry. Participants who provided a drug-negative urine sample, arrived on time, and worked a complete work shift earned a base-pay voucher. Initially, the base-pay voucher was worth $7, but it increased in value by $0.50 for every consecutive day that the participant provided a drug-free urine sample and worked a complete work shift (to a maximum of $27). The value of the base-pay voucher was reset to $7 if a participant ever provided a drug-positive sample, failed to provide a mandatory urine sample (i.e., a Monday, Wednesday, or Friday sample), or had an unexcused late arrival or incomplete work shift. Participants earned additional vouchers for professional demeanor, reaching daily learning aims, and entering batches of data into a computer. Over the course of a 24-week period, participants could earn up to about $4,000.

About 45% of the participants attended the Therapeutic Workplace consistently for over 3 years (Silverman et al., 2001; Silverman et al., 2002). Compared to the usual-care control group, Therapeutic Workplace participants provided significantly more urine samples negative for opiates and cocaine during the first 6 months of treatment (33% vs. 59% negative, respectively) (Silverman et al., 2001) and significant differences were maintained for 3 years after intake. In monthly assessments conducted 18 to 36 months after study intake, compared to usual-care controls, Therapeutic

Workplace participants provided almost twice the rate of urine samples negative for cocaine (28% vs. 54% negative, respectively) and opiates (37% vs. 60% negative, respectively). Six women in the Therapeutic Workplace group (30%) provided cocaine- and opiate-negative urine samples on 100% of the monthly assessment opportunities during that period, whereas only one woman (5%) achieved that outcome in the usual-care control group.

Eight of the 20 Therapeutic Workplace participants (40%) were hired as data entry operators in a Phase 2 Therapeutic Workplace business, Hopkins Data Services, and functioned effectively in that business (Silverman et al., 2005). Hopkins Data Services provided double-entry data entry (typically research surveys) into computer files. The operators earned $5.25 per hour in base pay plus productivity bonuses of about $5 per batch of data entered minus $0.08 per error. Approximately one batch could be entered per hour. Data entry operators were required to provide drug-negative urine samples to continue to work and earn wages. If a participant provided a drug-positive urine sample, he or she was not allowed to work that day and received a temporary reduction in the productivity bonus. The eight data entry operators entered about 15 million characters in the first year of operation of Hopkins Data Services and maintained an overall data entry accuracy of 99.6% correct. Although the data entry business was not financially self-sustaining, it was successful in attracting customers and in maintaining repeat business from 40% of the customers in the first year of operation (Silverman et al., 2005).

Silverman et al. (2002) also illustrated a potential means of arranging abstinence-reinforcement contingencies for individuals employed in community workplaces. Three participants in the Therapeutic Workplace group obtained employment in community workplaces during the study. To maintain abstinence in those participants, the investigators allowed them to provide urine samples each Monday, Wednesday, and Friday and paid them the Phase 1 base-pay vouchers for providing drug-free urine samples and evidence (e.g., paychecks) that they had maintained their offsite employment.

The Therapeutic Workplace for Cocaine Users in Methadone Treatment: A Partial Failure to Engage

Knealing, Wong, Diemer, Hampton, and Silverman (2006) attempted to replicate the effects of the manual Therapeutic Workplace intervention with the web-based Therapeutic Workplace application program in crack cocaine users enrolled in community-based methadone programs in Baltimore City. All participants were unemployed, met criteria for cocaine dependence, and provided a cocaine-positive urine sample at intake. Participants were randomly assigned to a Therapeutic Workplace ($n = 22$) or usual-care control ($n = 25$) group. Therapeutic Workplace participants were invited to earn vouchers in the workplace every workday for 9 months. About one-third (7 of the 22 participants) initiated sustained periods of abstinence and workplace attendance. Another third of the participants (8 of 22) never provided a drug-free urine sample and thus never had the opportunity to work and earn salary. Analyses of the monthly urine samples collected from both groups throughout the study showed that the Therapeutic Workplace and control participants provided similar rates of urine samples that were negative for cocaine (22.3% vs. 21.8%, respectively), opiates (56.1% vs. 47.1%, respectively), and both cocaine and opiates (25.8% vs. 17.3%, respectively). In this study, the Therapeutic Workplace intervention was not effective in initiating abstinence.

Initiating Cocaine Abstinence in Injection Drug Users in Methadone Treatment

Silverman et al. (in press) reported preliminary results from a trial that attempted to replicate the original effects of the Therapeutic Workplace and to experimentally isolate the effects of the employment-based abstinence-reinforcement contingency embedded in the Therapeutic Workplace intervention. Unemployed adults enrolled in community methadone programs in Baltimore who provided a cocaine-positive urine sample and had visible injection marks were invited to attend the workplace for 4 weeks. Initially, participants could work and earn vouchers independent of their urinalysis results. Participants who attended the workplace consistently and continued to provide cocaine-positive samples were randomly assigned to a work only or abstinence + work group. Participants in both groups could attend the workplace four hours per day for 26 weeks and could earn up to $8 per hour in base pay and $2 per hour for work performance. Work only participants could work and earn wages independent of Monday, Wednesday, and Friday urinalysis results. However, abstinent work participants could work only when urinary benzoylecgonine concentrations decreased by 20% per day from the last sample provided; if a participant failed to provide a scheduled sample or provided a sample that did not meet the abstinence requirement, the participant was not allowed to work that day and the participant's base pay was reduced to $1 per hour. Preliminary results showed that the percentage of urine samples negative for cocaine was significantly higher in the abstinence + work (29%) compared to the work only (10%) group. These preliminary results showed that the Therapeutic Workplace could increase cocaine abstinence and that the abstinence contingency is critical to increasing cocaine abstinence.

Although we cannot know why the Therapeutic Workplace was successful in initiating abstinence in this study and not in an earlier replication attempt (Knealing et al., 2004), at least two key procedures differed, possibly accounting for different outcomes. First, all participants in the second study could work and earn wages independent of their urinalysis results for the initial 4 weeks of treatment. During this period, participants sampled the reinforcers available in the workplace and established the daily behaviors required to succeed in the workplace (e.g., establishing a personal daily schedule, traveling to and from the workplace, and establishing initial typing and keypad skills). In contrast, participants in the first study were required to provide drug-free urine samples beginning on the first day of treatment, before sampling voucher reinforcers or establishing a work routine. Second, the cocaine-abstinence contingency in the second study only required a decrease in the urinary benzoylecgonine concentration across days, modeled after the procedures developed by Preston, Silverman, Schuster, and Cone (1997). Using this procedure, a participant could meet cocaine-abstinence requirements by abstaining from cocaine use for a 24-hour period. In contrast, in the earlier study, qualitative urinalysis testing required a benzoylecgonine concentration at or below a standard cutoff of 300 ng/mL to work and earn wages. Using this qualitative testing approach, participants with high initial urinary benzoylecgonine concentrations might have to remain abstinent for several days before meeting requirements to enter the workplace. Indeed, in the study by Knealing et al. (2006) it appeared that some participants arrived at the workplace expecting to gain entrance but were turned away for failing to meet the stringent qualitative abstinence requirement. The insensitivity of qualitative urinalysis testing to detect and reinforce recent abstinence may have contributed to the failure to engage some of the participants in that study.

The Therapeutic Workplace in Homeless Alcohol-Dependent Adults

Wong, Kolodner, Fingerhood, Bigelow, and Silverman (2005) reported preliminary results of a randomized controlled study of the Therapeutic Workplace for unemployed homeless alcohol-dependent adults. Participants were randomly assigned to one of three groups: work only, abstinence + work, or no vouchers. All 88 participants could work in the Therapeutic Workplace 4 hours per day for 26 weeks. Breath samples were tested for alcohol prior to start of each workday and at random times throughout each week. Participants in the work only and abstinence + work groups could earn up to $5 per hour in base pay and additional earnings for performance on training programs. Work only participants could work and earn wages independent of their breath results. Abstinent and work participants could work and earn wages only when their daily and random breath samples tested negative for alcohol. In addition, if a participant provided a positive sample, the participant's base pay rate was temporarily reduced to a low amount. No Voucher participants could work in the workplace independent of daily and random breath sample results and did not receive vouchers.

Work only and abstinence + work participants attended the workplace at similar rates, averaging 40% and 43% of workdays; significantly more than the no voucher participants, who attended on 18% of the workdays. Breath-sample collection rates for no voucher participants were significantly lower than for work only and abstinence + work participants, complicating comparisons to the no voucher group. Work only participants were significantly more likely (odds ratio [OR] = 2.36) to provide an alcohol-positive breath sample and to report heavy drinking (OR = 2.43) than abstinence + work participants. Consistent with results obtained in an early study in unemployed methadone patients (Silverman, Chutuape, Bigelow, & Stitzer, 1996), this reduced attendance of No Voucher participants showed that payment for participation in training appears critical for this population. The comparison of the work only and abstinence + work groups suggests that employment-based abstinence reinforcement can increase alcohol abstinence in homeless alcohol-dependent individuals.

APPLICATIONS OF EMPLOYMENT-BASED REINFORCEMENT

The research reviewed in this chapter has illustrated a variety of applications of employment-based reinforcement. Experimental evidence is accumulating that shows that employment-based abstinence reinforcement can be an effective means of promoting therapeutic behavior change. In general, there are two broad contexts in which employment-based reinforcement could be applied: in employment programs for chronically unemployed and drug-addicted individuals and in community workplaces. Importantly, common policies and procedures in these two contexts are conducive to the application of employment-based abstinence-reinforcement contingencies.

Integration in Intensive Employment Programs for the Chronically Unemployed

A number of employment programs for chronically unemployed adults provide intensive education, jobs-skills training, and supported work; some provide stipends for participation in training and supported work (Dickinson, 1981); and some have policies intended to require that participants maintain abstinence from drugs to continue to train and earn training or supported work stipends (e.g., Kashner et al., 2002). Kashner et al. (2002) reported on an evaluation of one of the largest and most recognized of those programs, the U.S. Department of Veterans Affairs' Compensated Work Therapy (CWT) program, which offers supported employment opportunities "(continued employment, higher wages, hours, promotion, and responsibility) based on client work performance (productivity, reliability, presentation, an punctuality) and health behaviors (sobriety and use of recommended addiction services)" (p. 939). Although the CWT program arranges contingencies for abstinence, the nature of the contingencies and the consequences for drug use do not appear systematic or well defined. The contingencies are guided by clinical judgment through "client observation, random drug screenings, and chart reviews"; and "consequences for inappropriate behaviors (positive drug screenings) vary from a reprimand to program dismissal and loss of CWT employment" (p. 939). This study showed that the CWT program can decrease drug-related problems, homelessness, and incarcerations. This study also showed that, in principle, employment-based abstinence reinforcement is accepted and used routinely in this large Veterans Affairs program. Integrating well-defined employment-based reinforcement techniques that have been proven effective (e.g., Silverman, Wong, et al., in press) might well enhance the effectiveness of programs such as CWT (see Chapter 16, this volume, for a description of related research).

Integration in Community Workplaces

Although illicit drug and heavy alcohol use is generally higher in unemployed than in employed individuals, the majority of illicit drug and heavy alcohol users are employed. The National Survey on Drug Use and Health (Substance Abuse and Mental Health Services Administration, 2005) estimated that in 2004 there were about 16.4 million illicit-drug-using adults in the United States and that 12.3 million (75%) were employed part or full time. Similarly, the survey estimated there were about 16 million heavy alcohol users and that 12.7 million (80%) were employed part or full time.

The Drug-Free Workplace Act of 1988

The Drug-Free Workplace Act (1988) was enacted to prohibit the unlawful "manufacturing, distribution, dispensation, possession or use" of a controlled substance on a worksite that receives federal funding. Under the Act, federally funded worksites must develop a written policy prohibiting activities involving illicit drugs and establish an employee education and awareness program. Employment can be terminated or rehabilitation required if the drug policy is violated. The U.S. Department of Labor (1990) has published guidelines to facilitate compliance with this Act.

Employee Assistance Programs

Through the growth of EAPs in the United States, workplaces have increasingly become recognized as an important entry point to substance abuse treatment (Hartwell et al., 1996). EAPs systematically identify and address personal problems affecting employee work performance, including, but not limited to substance abuse (Blum, Roman, & Harwood, 1995). Employees referred to the company's EAP are directed toward appropriate assistance. The primary goal of EAPs is to prevent loss of employment by helping the employee return to an adequate level of work performance. Based on the 2000 National Household Survey of Drug Abuse (Substance Abuse and Mental Health Services Administration, 2002), 53% of workers were aware of EAP programs for substance abuse at their workplace. Approximately 4.5% of employees utilize their EAP in any given 12-month period; approximately 33% of that caseload related to substance abuse (Blum, 1989).

Drug Testing in the Workplace

Drug testing is common in community workplaces. In 1997, 49% of U.S. workers indicated that their workplace had some type of drug testing; testing was most frequently reported in larger workplaces (Substance Abuse and Mental Health Services Administration, 2002). Respondents reported testing procedures at hiring (39% of workplaces), randomly (25% of workplaces), upon suspicion (30% of workplaces), and after accidents (29% of workplaces).

The U.S. Department of Transportation (DOT) policy for safety-sensitive employees provides a detailed illustration of accepted use of workplace drug testing (DOT, 2005). In the DOT, safety-sensitive employees are subject to pre-employment testing, postaccident testing, reasonable suspicion testing, and random testing (from every 2 weeks to not less than once a year). A drug-positive urine submission on any of these tests necessitates two final types of drug testing: return to duty and follow-up testing. Employment consequences following the first drug-positive submission are at the discretion of direct supervisors, but upon the second positive drug test, the employee must be permanently removed from performing any safety-sensitive duty within the DOT.

Controlled evaluations of the effects of workplace drug testing in community workplaces have not been done; however, some descriptive data suggest that workplace testing is associated with lower rates of drug use (French, Roebuck, & Kebreau Alexandre, 2004). The drug-testing infrastructures in workplaces could be used to facilitate integration of employment-based abstinence-reinforcement contingencies, although their application may be limited in some states by local attitudes or laws. In some states, drug testing is highly restricted (National Conference of State Legislators, 2005). Attitudes toward drug testing in the workplace vary based on the type of job and testing schedule. Surveys have shown that Americans are more accepting of drug testing in safety-sensitive jobs (95% approval) than in office work (69% approval). In 2002, 19% of employees did not approve of drug testing, although 57% indicated that they would comply with drug testing if refusal meant losing their job (Fendrich & Yun Soo Kim, 2002).

Impaired Physician Programs

In 1972, the American Medical Association started a program to rehabili-
tate physicians with substance abuse problems (American Medical Association, 1973). Under the programs, contracts require the physician to enter
treatment and to provide random urine samples for urinalysis testing. Noncompliance can result in the physician being reported to his or her state
medical board and losing his or her license. Many states have organized
and reported on their programs (e.g., Bohigan, Bondurant, & Croughan,
2005). Although the effectiveness of these programs has not been established, between 66% and 90% of physicians successfully complete the
treatment and continue to work.

ETHICAL ISSUES

The use of employment-based reinforcement contingencies can have serious
consequences for the drug user: Individuals can temporarily lose access to a
training program or workplace and lose the opportunity to work and earn
wages or salary. Given the severity of the consequences, these programs
seem most appropriate for individuals who have failed to respond to less
intrusive intervention approaches. Ideally, individuals should enroll in
employment-based reinforcement programs voluntarily. For training programs, contingencies should be explained prior to enrollment, allowing
choice on whether or not to participate. In community workplaces,
employment-based reinforcement might be particularly attractive as an alternative to firing.

CONCLUDING COMMENTS

A limited number of reports have described the use of employment-based
reinforcement contingencies to promote abstinence and medication compliance.
Recently, carefully controlled evaluations have shown that employment-
based reinforcement can increase drug abstinence in individuals who continue to use drugs despite exposure to conventional treatments. Controlled
research in this area is new, and much remains to be learned about ways to
increase the effectiveness of these contingencies and to extend their use to
new populations and work settings. The widespread use of drug testing,
EAPs, and drug-free workplace policies suggests that workplaces could be
viable and appropriate places for the implementation of employment-based
reinforcement contingencies in the treatment of drug addiction. Employment-
based reinforcement contingencies could be used to augment efforts made
by drug abuse treatment programs to initiate and sustain abstinence using
counseling, clinic-based contingency management interventions, and pharma-

cotherapies (e.g., methadone, naltrexone, or disulfiram). Given the persistent nature of drug use in some individuals, coordinating and combining influences from home (e.g., significant others), work (e.g., employment-based reinforcement), formal drug abuse treatment, and other areas of a person's life (e.g., the criminal justice system) may be a highly productive approach to producing substantial and lasting change for many persistent drug users.

ACKNOWLEDGMENTS

Preparation of the chapter was supported by Grant Nos. R01 DA13107, R01 DA19386, R01 DA019497, and T32-DA07209 from the National Institute on Drug Abuse.

REFERENCES

American Medical Association. (1973). The sick physician: Impairment by psychiatric disorders, including alcoholism and drug dependence. *Journal of the American Medical Association, 223*, 684–687.

Blum, T. C. (1989). The presence and integration of drug abuse intervention in human resource management. *NIDA Research Monograph, 91*, 245–269.

Blum, T. C., Roman, P. M., & Harwood, E. M. (1995). Employed women with alcohol problems seek help from employee assistance programs. In M. Galanter (Ed.), *Recent developments in alcoholism: Vol. 12. Women and alcoholism* (pp. 125–156). New York: Kluwer.

Bohigan, G. M., Bondurant, R., & Croughan, J. (2005). The impaired and disruptive physician: The Missouri Physicians' Health Program—An update (1995–2002). *Journal of Addictive Diseases, 24*, 13–23.

Cohen, M., Bigelow, G., Hargett, A., Allen, R., & Halsted, C. (1973). The use of contingency management procedures for the treatment of alcoholism in a work setting. *Alcoholism, 9*, 97–104.

Crowley, T. J. (1984). Contingency contracting treatment of drug-abusing physicians, nurses, and dentists. *NIDA Research Monograph, 46*, 68–83.

Crowley, T. J. (1986). Doctors' drug abuse reduced during contingency-contracting treatment. *Alcohol and Drug Research, 6*(4), 299–307.

Dallery, J., Silverman, K., Chutuape, M. A., Bigelow, G. E., & Stitzer, M. L. (2001). Voucher-based reinforcement of opiate plus cocaine abstinence in treatment-resistant methadone patients: Effects of reinforcer magnitude. *Experimental and Clinical Psychopharmacology, 9*(3), 317–325.

Dickinson, K. P. (1981). Supported work for ex-addicts: An exploration of endogenous tastes. *Journal of Human Resources, 16*(4), 551–599.

Drug Free Workplace Act, 42 U.S. Code Section 701 (1988).

Fendrich, M., & Yun Soo Kim, J. (2002). The experience and acceptability of drug testing: Poll trends. *Journal of Drug Issues, 32*(1), 81.

French, M. T., Roebuck, M. C., & Kebreau Alexandre, P. (2004). To test or not to test: Do workplace drug testing programs discourage employee drug use? *Social Science Research, 33*(1), 45–63.

Griffith, J. D., Rowan-Szal, G. A., Roark, R. R., & Simpson, D. D. (2000). Contingency management in outpatient methadone treatment: A meta-analysis. *Drug and Alcohol Dependence, 58*(1–2), 55–66.

Hartwell, T., Steele, P., French, M., & Rodman, N. (1996). Prevalence of drug testing in the workplace. *Monthly Labor Review, 119*(11), 35–49.

Higgins, S. T., Badger, G. J., & Budney, A. J. (2000). Initial abstinence and success in achieving longer term cocaine abstinence. *Experimental and Clinical Psychopharmacology, 8*(3), 377–386.

Higgins, S. T., Delaney, D. D., Budney, A. J., Bickel, W. K., Hughes, J. R., Foerg, F., et al. (1991). A behavioral approach to achieving initial cocaine abstinence. *American Journal of Psychiatry, 148*(9), 1218–1224.

Kashner, T. M., Rosenheck, R., Campinell, A. B., Suris, A., Crandall, R., Garfield, N. J., et al. (2002). Impact of work therapy on health status among homeless, substance-dependent veterans: A randomized controlled trial. *Archives of General Psychiatry, 59*(10), 938–944.

Knealing, T. W., Wong, C. J., Diemer, K. N., Hampton, J., & Silverman, K. (2006). A randomized controlled trial of the therapeutic workplace for community methadone patients: A partial failure to engage. *Experimental and Clinical Psychopharmacology, 14*(3), 350–360.

Lussier, J. P., Heil, S. H., Mongeon, J. A., Badger, G. J., & Higgins, S. T. (2006). A meta-analysis of voucher-based reinforcement therapy for substance use disorders. *Addiction, 101*(2), 192–203.

McGovern, M. P., Fox, T. S., Xie, H., & Drake, R. E. (2004). A survey of clinical practices and readiness to adopt evidence-based practices: Dissemination research in an addiction treatment system. *Journal of Substance Abuse Treatment, 26*(4), 305–312.

McLellan, A. T., Carise, D., & Kleber, H. D. (2003). Can the national addiction treatment infrastructure support the public's demand for quality care? *Journal of Substance Abuse Treatment, 25*(2), 117–121.

McLellan, A. T., Lewis, D. C., O'Brien, C. P., & Kleber, H. D. (2000). Drug dependence, a chronic medical illness: Implications for treatment, insurance, and outcomes evaluation. *Journal of the American Medical Association, 284*(13), 1689–1695.

Milby, J. B., Schumacher, J. E., Raczynski, J. M., Caldwell, E., Engle, M., Michael, M., et al. (1996). Sufficient conditions for effective treatment of substance abusing homeless persons. *Drug and Alcohol Dependence, 43*(1–2), 39–47.

Miller, P. M. (1975). A behavioral intervention program for chronic public drunkenness offenders. *Archives of General Psychiatry, 32*(7), 915–918.

National Conference of State Legislators. (2005). *State statute chart on drug testing in the workplace.* Retrieved January 4, 2006, from *www.ncsl.org/programs/employ/drugtest.htm.*

Peirce, J. M., Petry, N. M., Stitzer, M. L., Blaine, J., Kellogg, S., Satterfield, F., et al. (2006). Effects of lower-cost incentives on stimulant abstinence in methadone maintenance treatment: A national drug abuse treatment Clinical Trials Network study. *Archives of General Psychiatry, 63*(2), 201–208.

Petry, N. M., Tedford, J., Austin, M., Nich, C., Carroll, K. M., & Rounsaville, B. J. (2004). Prize reinforcement contingency management for treating cocaine users: How low can we go, and with whom? *Addiction, 99*(3), 349–360.

Preston, K. L., Silverman, K., Schuster, C. R., & Cone, E. J. (1997). Assessment of cocaine use with quantitative urinalysis and estimation of new uses. *Addiction, 92*(6), 717–727.

Preston, K. L., Umbricht, A., Wong, C. J., & Epstein, D. H. (2001). Shaping cocaine absti-nence by successive approximation. *Journal of Consulting and Clinical Psychology,* 69(4), 643–654.

Robichaud, C., Strickler, D., Bigelow, G., & Liebson, I. (1979). Disulfiram maintenance employee alcoholism treatment: A three-phase evaluation. *Behaviour Research and Therapy,* 17(6), 618–621.

Silverman, K. (2004). Exploring the limits and utility of operant conditioning in the treat-ment of drug addiction. *The Behavior Analyst,* 27, 209–230.

Silverman, K., Chutuape, M. A., Bigelow, G. E., & Stitzer, M. L. (1996). Voucher-based re-inforcement of attendance by unemployed methadone patients in a job skills training program. *Drug and Alcohol Dependence,* 41(3), 197–207.

Silverman, K., Chutuape, M. A., Bigelow, G. E., & Stitzer, M. L. (1999). Voucher-based re-inforcement of cocaine abstinence in treatment-resistant methadone patients: Effects of reinforcement magnitude. *Psychopharmacology,* 146(2), 128–138.

Silverman, K., Robles, E., Mudric, T., Bigelow, G. E., & Stitzer, M. L. (2004). A random-ized trial of long-term reinforcement of cocaine abstinence in methadone-maintained patients who inject drugs. *Journal of Consulting and Clinical Psychology,* 72(5), 839–854.

Silverman, K., Svikis, D., Robles, E., Stitzer, M. L., & Bigelow, G. E. (2001). A reinforce-ment-based therapeutic workplace for the treatment of drug abuse: Six-month absti-nence outcomes. *Experimental and Clinical Psychopharmacology,* 9(1), 14–23.

Silverman, K., Svikis, D., Wong, C. J., Hampton, J., Stitzer, M., & Bigelow, G. (2002). A re-inforcement-based therapeutic workplace for the treatment of drug abuse: Three-year abstinence outcomes. *Experimental and Clinical Psychopharmacology,* 10(3), 228–240.

Silverman, K., Wong, C. J., Grabinski, M. J., Hampton, J., Sylvest, C. E., Dillon, E. M., et al. (2005). A web-based Therapeutic Workplace for the treatment of drug addiction and chronic unemployment. *Behavior Modification,* 29(2), 417–463.

Silverman, K., Wong, C. J., Higgins, S. T., Brooner, R. K., Montoya, I. D., Contoreggi, C., et al. (1996). Increasing opiate abstinence through voucher-based reinforcement ther-apy. *Drug and Alcohol Dependence,* 41(2), 157–165.

Silverman, K., Wong, C. J., Needham, M., Diemer, K. N., Knealing, T. W., Crone-Todd, D., et al. (in press). A randomized trial of employment-based reinforcement of cocaine-abstinence in injection users. *Journal of Applied Behavior Analysis.*

Silverman, K., Wong, C. J., Umbricht-Schneiter, A., Montoya, I. D., Schuster, C. R., & Preston, K. L. (1998). Broad beneficial effects of cocaine abstinence reinforcement among methadone patients. *Journal of Consulting and Clinical Psychology,* 66(5), 811–824.

Stitzer, M. L., & Bigelow, G. E. (1984). Contingent methadone take-home privileges: Ef-fects on compliance with fee payment schedules. *Drug and Alcohol Dependence,* 13(4), 395–399.

Stitzer, M. L., Bigelow, G. E., Liebson, I. A., & Hawthorne, J. W. (1982). Contingent rein-forcement for benzodiazepine-free urines: Evaluation of a drug abuse treatment inter-vention. *Journal of Applied Behavior Analysis,* 15(4), 493–503.

Stitzer, M. L., Iguchi, M. Y., & Felch, L. J. (1992). Contingent take-home incentive: Effects on drug use of methadone maintenance patients. *Journal of Consulting and Clinical Psychology,* 60(6), 927–934.

Stitzer, M. L., Rand, C. S., Bigelow, G. E., & Mead, A. M. (1986). Contingent payment pro-cedures for smoking reduction and cessation. *Journal of Applied Behavior Analysis,* 19(2), 197–202.

Substance Abuse and Mental Health Services Administration. (2002). *National Household Survey on Drug Abuse: Main findings, 2000. NHSDA Series H-13 (DHHS Publication No. [SMA] 01-3549).* Rockville, MD: Office of Applied Studies.

Substance Abuse and Mental Health Services Administration. (2005). *Results from the 2004 National Survey on Drug Use and Health: National Findings* (NSDUH Series H-28, DHHS Publication No. SMA 05-4062). Rockville, MD: Office of Applied Studies.

U.S. Department of Labor. (1990). *An employer's guide to dealing with substance abuse.* Washington, DC: Author.

U.S. Department of Transportation. (2005). 49 CFR Part 40. *Federal Register.*

Winett, R. (1973). Parameters of deposit contracts in the modification of smoking. *Psychological Record, 23*(1), 49–60.

Wong, C. J., Kolodner, K., Fingerhood, M., Bigelow, G. E., & Silverman, K. (2005). *A therapeutic workplace for homeless alcohol-dependent individuals.* Paper presented at the College on Problems of Drug Dependence, Orlando, FL.

CHAPTER 18

CONTINGENCY MANAGEMENT IN ADULT CRIMINAL DRUG COURTS

Douglas B. Marlowe *and* Conrad J. Wong

SUBSTANCE ABUSE AMONG CRIMINAL OFFENDERS

Substance abusers are disproportionately represented in criminal justice settings. Nationally, it is estimated that 80% of prison and jail inmates (Belenko & Peugh, 1998), 67% of probationers (Bureau of Justice Statistics [BJS], 1998), and 80% of parolees (BJS, 2001) are substance involved, meaning they (1) were convicted of a drug- or alcohol-related offense, (2) were intoxicated at the time of their offense, (3) reported committing their offense to support a drug habit, or (4) have a substantial history of substance abuse or substance abuse treatment. Approximately 50% of inmates meet diagnostic criteria for current substance abuse or dependence, and approximately 60–70% meet criteria for lifetime substance abuse or dependence (Peters, Greenbaum, Edens, Carter, & Ortiz, 1998; Teplin, 1994; Teplin, Abrams, & McClelland, 1996).

Conversely, a substantial proportion of clients in community-based drug abuse treatment are involved with the criminal justice system. Approximately two-thirds of clients in long-term residential drug abuse treatment, one-half in outpatient drug abuse treatment, and one-quarter in methadone maintenance treatment are awaiting a criminal trial or sentencing, were sentenced to community supervision on probation, or were conditionally released from prison on parole (Craddock, Rounds-Bryant, Flynn, & Hubbard, 1993).

THE LESSONS OF HISTORY

History is littered with failed efforts to intervene with drug-abusing offenders. Traditional correctional approaches have been consistently unsuccessful. The average effect size of prison sentences on crime and drug use is close to zero (Gendreau, Goggins, Cullen, & Andrews, 2000). Within 3 years of release from prison, approximately two-thirds of all inmates, including drug offenders, are rearrested for a new crime, one-half are convicted beyond a reasonable doubt of a new crime, and one-half are reincarcerated for a new crime or parole violation (Langan & Levin, 2002). Equally discouraging, approximately 70–85% of drug-abusing offenders return to regular drug use within 1 year of release from prison and 95% return to drug use within 3 years (e.g., Hanlon, Nurco, Bateman, & O'Grady, 1998; Martin, Butzin, Saum, & Inciardi, 1999; Nurco, Hanlon, & Kinlock, 1991; Satel, 1999).

"Intermediate sanctions" are community-based correctional programs that provide enhanced surveillance of offenders outside prison walls. For example, intensive supervised probation or parole (ISP) programs employ specially trained officers to closely monitor offenders' conduct, make home visits, demand spot-check urine samples, and phone-monitor compliance with home curfews or house arrest. Unfortunately, studies have revealed that intermediate sanctions had little impact on drug use or crime (e.g., Gendreau, Cullen, & Bonta, 1994). In fact, the enhanced monitoring of offenders in ISP programs has been paradoxically associated with seemingly worse outcomes because of the greater opportunities to detect infractions (Petersilia & Turner, 1993).

Treatment-oriented strategies have been equally discouraging. Approximately 70% of probationers and parolees drop out of drug abuse treatment or attend irregularly within 2–6 months (Langan & Cunniff, 1992; Nurco et al., 1991; Taxman, 1999; Young, Usdane, & Torres, 1991) and over 90% drop out in 12 months (Satel, 1999). Evidence from the Drug Abuse Treatment Outcome Study (DATOS) suggests that 3 months of treatment may be a minimum threshold for detecting dose–response effects; that is, prior to 3 months there may not be a significant relationship between tenure in treatment and outcomes (Simpson, Joe, & Brown, 1997). It also appears that 6–12 months may be a further threshold for observing enduring reductions in drug use. Approximately 50% of clients who complete 12 months or more of treatment remain abstinent for a year following completion of treatment (McLellan, Lewis, O'Brien, & Kleber, 2000). Given offenders' precipitous attrition from treatment prior to reaching these thresholds, one should expect as few as 5–15% of the intent-to-treat population to contact a minimal therapeutic dose of service. As far as the public and policymakers are concerned, this is unacceptable.

DRUG COURTS

Drug courts were created largely in response to the disappointing results obtained from other programs for drug-abusing offenders. Drug courts are special criminal court dockets that provide a judicially supervised regimen of drug abuse treatment and case management services in lieu of prosecution or incarceration. According to the National Association of Drug Court Professionals (NADCP, 1997), the "key components" of a drug court include (1) ongoing status hearings before the judge in court, (2) mandatory completion of drug abuse treatment and relevant adjunctive services, (3) random urine drug screens, and (4) negative sanctions for program infractions and positive rewards for achievements. The sanctions and rewards are typically arranged on an escalating gradient, in which the magnitude increases in response to each successive infraction or accomplishment. Common examples of sanctions include verbal reprimands, writing assignments, increased counseling, fines, community service, and brief intervals of jail detention. Common examples of rewards include praise, token gifts, certificates of recognition, and reductions in treatment or supervisory obligations.

In preadjudication drug courts, offenders who satisfactorily complete the program have their criminal charges dropped and may be eligible for record expungement after remaining arrest free for an additional waiting period. Record expungement permits the individual to respond, truthfully, on an employment application or similar document that he or she was not arrested for a drug offense. In postadjudication drug courts, graduates can avoid incarceration, reduce their probationary obligations, or receive a sentence of time served in the drug court program.

Reviews of dozens of evaluations concluded that an average of 60% of drug court clients completed 1 year or more of drug treatment and roughly one-half graduated from the program (Belenko, 1998, 1999). This compares quite favorably to typical retention rates in community-based drug treatment programs where, as noted, over 70% of probationers and parolees drop out within a few months. Drug court clients also exhibited significant reductions of approximately 20–30 percentage points in drug use and crime compared to probationers while enrolled in the program, and reductions of 15 percentage points in rearrest rates at 2 to 3 years postadmission (Belenko, 1998, 1999, 2001; Marlowe, DeMatteo, & Festinger, 2003; U.S. Government Accountability Office, 2005). Data are largely lacking on other postprogram outcomes, such as substance use, employment, or family functioning.

CONTINGENCY MANAGEMENT IN DRUG COURTS

The correctional system is, in essence, a contingency management program designed to reduce antisocial conduct and enhance adaptive functioning of offenders. Unfortunately, the contingencies are rarely managed in a systematic manner to maximize effects. Consequences are often applied in the absence of certainty or predictability and after unacceptably long time delays (e.g., Marlowe, 2002). Drug courts represent an explicit effort to manage contingencies for offenders more systematically and in accordance with effective principles of behavior modification (e.g., Burdon, Roll, Prendergast, & Rawson, 2001; Harrell & Roman, 2001; Marlowe & Kirby, 1999). Few drug court practitioners are behavioral scientists by background or training, and few may have a sophisticated grasp of the principles of operant conditioning. Regardless, the founders of drug courts had an intuitive sense of how to influence behavior and were successful in translating that anecdotal knowledge into workable best-practice standards for the courts. In so doing, they borrowed concepts not only from operant conditioning, but also from sociological and criminological theories that view perceptions of contingencies as exerting an important influence on offenders' conduct. Some of the constructs may be unfamiliar to behavioral scientists; however, they frequently describe processes that are reasonably analogous to contingency management (CM) principles, and many of the terms can be crosswalked to operant conditioning concepts.

Drug courts were designed to apply a full range of operant conditioning techniques. At the risk of oversimplification, the basic techniques of operant conditioning may be depicted as follows:

	REWARD	SANCTION
GIVE	Positive Reinforcement	Punishment
TAKE	Response Cost	Negative Reinforcement

Logically, there are four ways to influence the behavior of offenders through the administration of sanctions or rewards contingent upon desirable or undesirable behavior. It is possible to:

• *Give a reward contingent upon desirable behavior (positive reinforcement).* Providing a drug offender with praise, token gifts, or certificates of accomplishment for attending counseling sessions is an example of positive reinforcement.

• *Give a sanction contingent upon undesirable behavior (punishment).* Giving a writing assignment or jail sanction for using drugs is an example of punishment.

• *Take away a reward or something valued contingent upon undesirable behavior (response cost).* Imposing a monetary fine or revoking an offender's driver's license for criminal activity is an example of response cost. Response cost is similar to punishment in that they both cause distress and are designed to reduce unwanted behaviors. With response cost, the sanction involves losing something of value (in this example, money or driving privileges) that was previously in the offender's possession (e.g., Martin & Pear, 1999).

• *Take away a sanction contingent upon desirable behavior (negative reinforcement).* Drug courts often structure reinforcement in the negative. That is, participants are commonly rewarded with reductions in treatment or supervisory obligations, or with the avoidance of a criminal record or incarceration. Negative reinforcement is similar to positive reinforcement in that they are both desirable to the individual and designed to increase wanted behaviors. Negative reinforcement involves relief from previously unpleasant circumstances, whereas positive reinforcement is characterized by the giving of a new, prospective reward (e.g., Hineline, 1976; Sidman, 1966).

Drug courts utilize all four of these techniques and this combination of strategies is believed to elicit synergistic effects by simultaneously squelching undesired behaviors and reinforcing desired behaviors (e.g., Marlowe & Kirby, 1999; NADCP, 1997). More important, drug courts can apply these procedures in a highly effective manner. There are several critical parameters that influence the effectiveness of any CM intervention. If these parameters are applied incorrectly, the effectiveness of the intervention will be diminished (e.g., Martin & Pear, 1999).

Certainty

One critically important parameter is certainty (e.g., Harrell & Roman, 2001; Stitzer & McCaul, 1987; Taxman, 1999). This may be expressed as a ratio of sanctions to infractions or a ratio of rewards to achievements. For example, if drug court clients were sanctioned every time they failed to attend a treatment session, the ratio of sanctions to infractions would be 1:1. From an operant conditioning perspective, this would be analogous to a "fixed ratio-1" or "FR 1" schedule. If they were sanctioned for every two missed sessions, this would be an FR-2 schedule, and so forth. Generally speaking, the smaller this ratio, the greater the effects for suppressing unde-sirable behaviors or initiating desired behaviors (Azrin & Holz, 1966; Mar-tin & Pear, 1999; Van Houten, 1983).

Unfortunately, certainty is often conspicuously absent in the criminal justice system. Offenders typically engage in repetitive instances of drug use or crime before being detected by law enforcement (e.g., Nurco et al., 1991). Once they have been arrested, the prosecutor might not file charges because of insufficient evidence, insufficient resources, or insufficient inter-est. If the case does go to trial, the state bears the heavy burden of proving guilt "beyond a reasonable doubt" (sometimes expressed as > 95% likeli-hood). This makes the odds of imposing a criminal sanction decidedly small. Finally, convicted drug-possession offenders are typically sentenced to probation for their first few offenses. Because probation officers often have high caseloads and insufficient resources, it may be exceedingly diffi-cult to monitor probationers effectively or impose consequences for viola-tions (Goldkamp, 2000; Taxman, 1999). Taking these factors into consid-eration, one should assume that the ratio of sanctions to infractions would ordinarily be too small to exert a meaningful influence on behavior.

Drug courts were designed to increase the certainty of contingent con-sequences in several ways. First, drug courts ordinarily require clients to de-liver urine specimens in direct observation of clinical staff on at least a ran-dom weekly basis during the first several months of the program (NADCP, 1997). In addition, clients are usually required to attend weekly appoint-ments with a clinical case manager and appear at regular status hearings in court (NADCP, 1997). The judge receives progress reports from the case managers concerning drug-screen results and counseling attendance, and treatment providers or case managers may appear in court to give testi-mony about clients' progress. This reduces the likelihood that accomplish-ments or infractions will go undetected or that clients will "slip through the cracks" and elude deserved sanctions or be denied deserved rewards.

In addition, drug courts can maneuver around many of the "proce-dural due process" obstacles that typically complicate or delay the imposi-tion of judicial sanctions (Marlowe, Elwork, Festinger, & McLellan, 2003). For example, in a traditional criminal trial or violation of probation (VOP) hearing, defendants are usually entitled to a panoply of procedural protections, such as the right to advance notice of the hearing, to have de-fense counsel present, to admit evidence, to cross-examine witnesses, and to refuse to testify. By contrast, status hearings in drug courts are considerably less formalistic. In exchange for the opportunity to avoid a criminal record or incarceration, defendants in drug courts are ordinarily required to waive many of these procedural formalities. For instance, judges in drug courts may speak directly to offenders rather than through their attorneys, and there may be no formal opportunity for defense attorneys to challenge evidence or cross-examine witnesses. As a result, greater information can be made readily available to the court, which makes it substantially more likely for a client to be found in violation and to receive a sanction for non-compliance in the program.

Celerity

Another critical parameter of operant conditioning is what drug courts term *celerity,* which also means rapidity or immediacy. The effects of sanctions and rewards may begin to degrade within only hours or days after an offender engages in a target behavior (Azrin & Holz, 1966; Taxman, 1999). Worse still, this decline is not necessarily linear but may be exponential (Sidman, 1966). One partial explanation for this precipitous decline in efficacy is that there is interference from new behaviors. Assume, for example, that an offender uses drugs on Monday and then is abstinent and compliant with treatment for the remainder of the week. If that same individual is sanctioned on Friday for the drug use that occurred on Monday, it should be evident that the desirable behaviors transpiring on Tuesday through Thursday are closer in time to the sanction than the drug use. This may explain why the effects of sanctions decline exponentially. New behaviors occur more recently in time and operant conditioning works, in part, by proximity in time. In this example, the effects of the sanction could be, paradoxically, to "punish" the desirable behaviors that occurred most recently. This, of course, would be ineffective or counterproductive.

Celerity, too, is conspicuously absent in the criminal justice system. The constitutional requirements of procedural due process make it virtually impossible for a finding of guilt or a criminal sentence to be imposed in less than 6 months, usually considerably longer. Discovery proceedings, pretrial motions, motions for reconsideration, and appeals typically take months or years to resolve. Once an offender has been convicted and sentenced to probation, there are further time delays associated with bringing VOP petitions for subsequent violations. In Philadelphia, for example, it takes roughly 30 to 45 days from the filing of a VOP petition to the date of a court hearing and up to roughly 4 to 6 months for a final disposition. Given such inordinate delays, the effects of sanctions should be expected to be minimal. In contrast, status hearings in drug courts are typically held in front of the judge on a weekly or biweekly basis, possibly tapering to monthly after several months. This enables the court to impose sanctions and rewards in a more time-efficient, and thus more effective, manner.

Magnitude

The issue of magnitude is more complicated than many criminal justice professionals recognize. There is a common misconception that sanctions and rewards are most effective at high magnitudes, which could explain the penchant of some authorities to impose long and arduous prison sentences. In fact, evidence suggests that sanctions tend to be least effective at the lowest and highest magnitudes and most effective at moderate magnitudes.

Sanctions that are too weak in magnitude can precipitate "habituation," in which the individual becomes inured to being sanctioned (e.g., Marlowe & Kirby, 1999). The problem with habituation is not only that low-magnitude sanctions may fall below an effective threshold—of greater concern, they can make it less likely for higher-magnitude sanctions to work in the future, because they can raise the client's tolerance for sanctioning. This may partially account for the "been-there, done-that" attitude that many drug offenders exhibit in response to threats of punishment. Over time, they become hardened to the threats; therefore, they may be apt to push the limits to the point of no return (e.g., to the point of imprisonment or drug-related death).

At the other extreme, sanctions that are too high in magnitude can lead to "ceiling effects," in which further escalation of punishment is impracticable (e.g., Marlowe & Kirby, 1999). Once an offender has been imprisoned, for example, the authorities have used up their armamentarium of sanctions—and the offender *knows* they have exhausted their options. At this point, future efforts to improve behavior could be futile. More important, high-magnitude sanctions are apt to precipitate a host of iatrogenic reactions, such as avoidance and escape responses, learned helplessness, and antitherapeutic feelings of anger and despondency (e.g., Newsom, Favell, & Rincover, 1983; Sidman, 1988).

The criminal justice system tends to operate at the lowest and highest magnitudes of sanctions. Offenders often receive a mere "slap on the wrist," such as a reprimand or brief probation sentence, for their first few crimes (e.g., Nurco et al., 1991). This may stem from a well-intentioned desire to be lenient with youthful offenders or a lack of resources for first- or second-time offenders. Regardless, it presents a formidable risk of habituation. Subsequently, after multiple crimes, the only remaining sanction at the authorities' disposal may be imprisonment, which is the paradigm of a ceiling effect.

For this reason, drug courts crafted a wide and creative range of intermediate sanctions and rewards that can be ratcheted upward or downward in response to clients' behaviors. For example, clients may receive writing assignments, increased treatment requirements, fines, community service, or brief intervals of jail detention for failing to comply with treatment. Conversely, they may receive verbal praise, token gifts, or reductions in treatment or supervisory obligations for complying with treatment. This enables drug courts to navigate between habituation and ceiling effects by altering the magnitude of punishment in response to successive infractions. It also permits the criminal justice system to offer a substantially richer and more effective range of contingent rewards than is ordinarily available to individuals on probation, parole, or in prison.

Procedural Justice

The drug court model assumes that perceptions of contingencies are also very important. Particular attention is given to "procedural justice." Evidence from cognitive psychology suggests that individuals are more likely to perceive a decision as being correct and appropriate if they believe fair procedures were employed in reaching that decision (Thibaut & Walker, 1975). In fact, the perceived fairness of the procedures exerts a greater influence over participants' reactions than the outcome of the decision itself. Specifically, defendants are most likely to accept an adverse judgment if they feel they (1) had a fair opportunity to voice their position, (2) were treated in an equivalent manner to similar people in like circumstances, and (3) were accorded respect and dignity (Tyler, 1994). Importantly, evidence suggests that when these factors are absent, behavior not only fails to improve but may get worse and offenders may sabotage their own treatment goals (e.g., Sherman, 1993).

Offenders may be more likely to feel heard and to believe they are being treated in the same manner as other individuals if a judge handles their case, as opposed to a probation officer or clinician (e.g., Satel, 1998). Offenders frequently complain that probation officers act capriciously in applying sanctions. Because they rarely witness the officers interacting with other clients, they may become convinced that others are being treated more leniently than they. In contrast, drug court clients have the opportunity to see the judge interacting in a public forum with other clients. Moreover, given the "trappings" of the courtroom environment, the procedural requirements of due process, and the presence of defense attorneys, drug court clients may be more likely to feel they have had a say in their case and that their position has at least been considered.

Drug courts also place considerable emphasis on delineating clients' rights and responsibilities upfront at the point of admission into the program. At an "entry hearing," defendants are informed of the program rules, the specific behaviors that may trigger sanctions or rewards, the types of sanctions and rewards that can be legally imposed, criteria for graduation or termination, and the consequences of graduation or failure. This information is typically memorialized in a written manual, which is signed off by each of the relevant agencies, including the court, attorney general, public defender, treatment programs, and probation department. In addition, the information is the subject of an oral "colloquy" between the judge and client that is often memorialized in a stenographic record, and that ensures that each client understands the rights he or she is giving up and the risks being assumed by entering the program. These procedures are conducted in the presence of defense counsel, who can offer advice, dispel myths, guard against undue coercion, and advocate for clients' legal interests. As a result, it is believed clients in drug courts will be more readily accepting of negative sanctions should they need to be imposed.

Learned Helplessness: Predictability, Controllability, and Ratio Burden

Drug courts can be vulnerable to criticism when it comes to eliciting reactions of "learned helplessness" (Seligman, 1975). This refers to a process by which many individuals become angry, aggressive, or despondent if they are sanctioned for failing to comply with excessive or unrealistic demands. Under such circumstances, behavior may fail to improve and clients may sabotage their own treatment goals (e.g., Sherman, 1993).

The major factors that precipitate this iatrogenic reaction are an absence of predictability or controllability. Predictability refers to a client's ability to anticipate the precise behaviors that will elicit a sanction or reward. For example, if a client is told that he or she will be sanctioned for failing to be "mature," this might seem unfair if the client is unable to predict the specific behaviors the judge would interpret as reflecting immaturity, and thus deserving of a sanction. This could cause the client to become resentful or despondent or to give up. Controllability refers to a client's ability to engage in a desired target behavior or refrain from an undesired behavior. If, for example, a client was sanctioned for failing to obtain a GED (general equivalency diploma), the sanction could precipitate despondence if the individual suffered from an undiagnosed learning disability that prevented him or her from understanding study materials or completing educational exercises. Under such circumstances, incarceration would be unlikely to further educational aims and could interfere with other treatment goals.

Related to the factor of controllability is the issue of "ratio burden." Drug courts often place multiple, concurrent demands on clients that may be difficult to comply with simultaneously. For example, clients may be required to attend counseling sessions, appear at court hearings, deliver urine specimens, remain abstinent, and complete vocational training—and they may be sanctioned for failure to comply with any one of those directives. Under such circumstances, the sheer burden of response requirements could be so daunting as to trigger a learned-helplessness response.

In theory, drug courts are designed to address learned helplessness in several ways. First, as discussed previously, substantial efforts are made to clearly specify the concrete behaviors that can trigger a sanction or reward. This is intended to enhance perceptions of procedural justice and increase a sense of predictability in the program. In addition, most drug courts employ a phase structure that is intended to shape behavior by separating proximal from distal behavioral goals (NADCP, 1997). Proximal behaviors are those that (1) clients are readily capable of engaging in, and (2) are believed to be necessary for longer-term objectives to be attained. Examples include attendance at scheduled counseling sessions, attendance at court hearings, and delivery of urine specimens. Distal behaviors are those that are ultimately desired but may take clients some time to accomplish. Examples include drug abstinence, gainful employment, and improved parenting. Of course, behaviors that present an immediate threat to public safety, such as criminality or DWI (driving while intoxicated), are necessarily conceptualized as proximal because they cannot be permitted to continue. Offenders who fail to refrain from these behaviors are ordinarily considered poor candidates for drug court and are likely to be confined and treated in a prison or jail setting, correctional halfway house, or residential program.

During the early phases of drug court, the intent is to place greater emphasis on proximal behaviors such as counseling attendance, and gradually shift the emphasis to distal behaviors. This is usually accomplished by altering the magnitude (but not the certainty or celerity) of contingent responses over time (Meyer, 2002). During the first few weeks or months, relatively higher-magnitude sanctions and rewards would be imposed for proximal behaviors and lower-magnitude sanctions and rewards would be imposed for distal behaviors. For example, clients might receive verbal reprimands or writing assignments for providing drug-positive urine samples but might receive brief periods of jail detention for failing to show for a counseling session or provide a urine specimen. Gradually, the emphasis would shift to distal goals and higher-magnitude sanctions would be applied for positive urine drug screens as well. The goal is to navigate between habituation and ceiling effects by immediately and substantially reinforcing proximal pro-treatment behaviors, while reserving a larger range of responses for distal behaviors that could take some time for clients to accomplish.

Unfortunately, practice does not necessarily jibe with intentions. Some drug court judges may administer substantial sanctions such as jail detention for drug use occurring early in treatment (e.g., Hoffman, 2002). For clients who are truly addicted to drugs or alcohol, this can lead to learned helplessness or ceiling effects within only a few weeks or months of entry into the program. Conversely, other judges may tolerate repetitive instances of tardiness or absenteeism, which can lead to habituation and a pronounced failure to achieve distal objectives. Educating judges and other drug court professionals about the most effective techniques for shaping clients' behaviors remains a critical task for the drug court field. Efforts are under way to develop training curricula, workshops, and instructional materials to address these and related topics (e.g., Huddleston, Meyer, & Marlowe, 2006).

The Carrot versus the Stick

There is also a concern that some drug courts may place an inordinate emphasis on squelching undesired behaviors to the detriment of reinforcing desired behaviors (e.g., Burdon, Roll, Prendergast, & Rawson, 2001; Marlowe & Kirby, 1999). Although drug courts can be effective at reducing crime and drug use while clients are under the supervision of the judge, these effects would not be expected to endure unless the clients contacted alternative reinforcers in their natural environments that maintained the effects over time (e.g., Higgins et al., 1994). For instance, clients who find a job, develop hobbies, or improve their family relationships will be more likely to be continuously reinforced (e.g., with praise, social prestige, or wages) for prosocial behaviors and punished (e.g., by being ostracized from peers or fired from a job) for drug-related behaviors. In contrast, those who return to their previous habitats may find themselves back in an environment that reinforces drug use at the expense of prosocial attainments. The community reinforcement approach (CRA; Sisson & Azrin, 1989) is a counseling strategy that capitalizes on such natural systems of reinforcement to compete with the drug-abusing lifestyle.

To maintain treatment effects over time, it is essential that drug courts not merely punish crime and drug use but also reward productive activities that are themselves incompatible with crime and drug use. This represents one of the greatest challenges facing drug courts, because law professionals have not traditionally defined their role in this manner. Judges and prosecutors are trained to adjudicate controversies and reduce recidivism, and they have traditionally measured their success by these metrics. Only recently have the courts recognized "therapeutic jurisprudence" as a legitimate legal philosophy, in which improving the psychological health of citizens is viewed as an appropriate function of the judiciary (e.g., Hora et al., 1999). A critical task facing the drug court field is to educate law practitioners about the importance of using more positive reinforcement in their work and selecting behavioral goals for their clients that are consistent with the principles of the CRA.

THE RISK PRINCIPLE

The "risk principle" is a central construct in criminal justice research (e.g., Taxman & Marlowe, 2006). A substantial body of evidence reveals that intensive interventions such as drug courts are best suited for "high-risk" offenders who have more severe antisocial propensities or drug use histories but may be ineffective or contraindicated for "low-risk" offenders (e.g., Andrews & Bonta, 1998). Low-risk offenders are less likely to be on a fixed antisocial trajectory and are more likely to "adjust course" following a run-in with the law; therefore, intensive treatment and supervision may offer little incremental benefit at a substantial cost (e.g., DeMatteo, Marlowe, & Festinger, 2006). High-risk offenders, on the other hand, are likely to require intensive interventions to dislodge their entrenched behavioral patterns. The greatest risk factors for failure in correctional programs include (1) being younger, (2) having an early onset of crime or drug use, (3) multiple prior arrests, (4) a comorbid diagnosis of antisocial personality disorder (ASPD) or psychopathy, or (5) having previously failed in drug abuse treatment or a diversion program (Marlowe, Patapis, & DeMatteo, 2003; Peters, Haas, & Martin, 1999).

Research suggests that certain high-risk offenders may respond differently to sanctions and rewards than other individuals. For example, psychopathic offenders, those with ASPD, and youthful offenders are apt to discount the probability of receiving a serious sanction in the long-term in favor of earning an immediate reward (e.g., Patterson & Newman, 1993). They are also more likely to opt for smaller short-term rewards on delay-discounting tasks than to forestall gratification in favor of larger rewards to be earned in the future (e.g., Petry, 2002). This apparent hypersensitivity to rewards, imperviousness to sanctions, and impulsivity could reflect executive-control deficits stemming from damage or immaturity to the prefrontal cortex (e.g., Fishbein, 2000). Alternatively, it could reflect the vagaries of their learning histories. By virtue of their recidivist proclivities, antisocial offenders may be more likely to have habituated to or reached a ceiling effect on sanctions. This could make them seem neurologically unresponsive to sanctions, when they simply had maladaptive experiences with punishment in the past.

Etiology aside, evidence is convincing that structured behavioral interventions are ideally suited for high-risk offenders. Studies have reported that drug abuse clients with comorbid diagnoses of ASPD performed as well or better than non-ASPD clients in voucher-based CM interventions (e.g., Messina, Farabee, & Rawson, 2003; Silverman et al., 1998) and similarly structured behavioral programs (e.g., Brooner, Kidorf, King, & Stoller, 1998; Messina, Wish, Hoffman, & Nemes, 2002). It would appear that the higher the risk-level in a given population, the less margin of error there might be for applying CM interventions effectively (e.g., Higgins, 1996). Greater exactitude may be required in certainty, celerity, and procedural justice to achieve comparable gains for high-risk offenders as for other clients.

RESEARCH ON CONTINGENCY
MANAGEMENT IN DRUG COURTS

Drug courts have been surprisingly amenable to descriptive and experimental studies of their core components, including controlled studies of the contingent application of sanctions and rewards.

Graduated Sanctions

One experimental study in the District of Columbia (Harrell, Cavanagh, & Roman, 1999) randomly assigned drug-abusing arrestees in a pretrial supervision program to one of three conditions:

1. Participants assigned to the *standard condition* received the typical regimen of pretrial services, which included infrequent court appearances, infrequent urine testing, and nonmandatory referrals to treatment services.
2. Participants assigned to the *sanctions condition* provided urine specimens on a random weekly basis, and received sanctions for drug-positive urines that escalated in magnitude in response to successive positive results. The sanctions included jail stays of up to 3–7 days.
3. Finally, participants assigned to the *treatment condition* attended an intensive day-treatment program that provided clinical services, meals, and recreational activities several hours per week.

Contrary to expectations, participants preferred the sanctions condition to day treatment (Harrell et al., 1999). Only 40% of participants assigned to day treatment agreed to participate in treatment, whereas 66% of those assigned to the sanctions condition agreed to comply with the sanction requirements. Focus-group inquiries revealed that the participants objected to the time burden and intrusiveness of day treatment, which substantially outweighed the minimally intrusive procedures employed in weekly urine collection (Harrell & Smith, 1997). Importantly, participants in both the treatment condition and sanctions condition had lower rates of drug use than those receiving standard services; however, participants in the sanctions condition had the best outcomes because they also had lower rearrest rates extending out to 1 year postentry (Harrell et al., 1999). This represents one controlled study that must be replicated; however, the results suggest that graduated sanctions, including the threat of brief jail detention, can be acceptable and effective for some drug-abusing offenders.

Several researchers have conducted confidential focus groups with drug court participants to learn whether *they* perceived graduated sanctions to be a motivator to perform well in treatment. The results confirmed that participants generally viewed the threat of sanctions to be a powerful inducement to succeed in the program—but only when the sanctions were perceived as being imposed in accordance with the principles of procedural justice outlined earlier (Goldkamp, White, & Robinson, 2002; Satel, 1998; Cooper, 1997). Sanctions were viewed as detrimental to treatment goals when they were meted out in an arbitrary, inconsistent, or noncontingent manner. In contrast, they were viewed as helpful when participants felt they had a chance to articulate their side of the story, believed they were treated equivalently to other clients, and felt they were accorded respect and dignity throughout the process.

Graduated Rewards

No published controlled study has investigated the effects of judicially administered rewards in a drug court. Preliminary data from two ongoing studies suggest there might be a "ceiling effect" in some drug courts that can mask the influence of enhancing tangible positive rewards (Marlowe, Festinger, Lee, et al., 2005; Prendergast, Hall, & Roll, 2005). These studies provided additional payment vouchers or gift certificates for compliance with program requirements. Contrary to expectations, this procedure did not improve during-treatment outcomes. The powerful contingencies that are naturally in place in drug courts could have produced such high rates of counseling attendance and drug abstinence (at least while participants were enrolled in the program) that augmenting tangible rewards did not yield measurable incremental gains.

Importantly, however, planned interaction analyses in one of the studies conducted in the Philadelphia Treatment Court indicated that positive effects of enhanced rewards were elicited for high-risk participants who were younger or had a more serious criminal history (Marlowe, Festinger, Lee, et al., 2005). If these preliminary results are confirmed on a larger cohort, this would suggest that increasing the density of tangible rewards can improve outcomes for high-risk participants in drug court programs. It would also provide further validation of the risk principle and yield practical guidance about how to arrange reinforcement contingencies for drug offenders.

Perceived Deterrence

As noted previously, drug courts place substantial emphasis on perceptions of contingencies. Several commentators have suggested that the positive effects of drug courts might be accounted for, in part, by the theory of "perceived deterrence" (e.g., Harrell & Roman, 2001; Hora, Schma, & Rosenthal, 1999; Marlowe & Kirby, 1999). This theory posits that most individuals perform a type of "cost/benefit analysis" when deciding whether or not to engage in illegal or inappropriate conduct. The calculus of the cost–benefit ratio is believed to involve a consideration of (1) the perceived certainty of being detected for infractions, (2) the perceived certainty of receiving a sanction for infractions, and (3) the anticipated magnitude of the sanctions (e.g., Harrell & Roman, 2001; Gibbs, 1975; Zimrig & Hawkins, 1973). Although classical deterrence theory focused on the avoidance of negative behaviors, in its broadest formulation it also involves a rational consideration of the costs and benefits of engaging in prosocial behaviors in lieu of illegal behaviors (e.g., obtaining a job in lieu of committing a robbery). In this sense, the cost–benefit ratio is further influenced by (4) the perceived certainty of being recognized for achievements, (5) the perceived certainty of receiving a reward for those achievements, and (6) the perceived magnitude or desirability of the rewards (e.g., Akers, 1990).

A recent study in three drug courts assessed clients' perceptions of deterrence on a monthly basis and related those data to program outcomes (Marlowe, Festinger, Foltz, Lee, & Patapis, 2005). As expected, participants who perceived a more certain and immediate connection between their conduct and the imposition of sanctions and rewards had better outcomes. The best outcomes were associated with consistently elevated perceived-deterrence scores, whereas the worst outcomes were associated with scores that declined over time as the participants became acclimated or habituated to the program. Of course, these correlational findings leave open the question whether it is simply the schedule of contingencies as opposed to perceptions of contingencies that influenced outcomes, and how schedules of contingencies might influence client perceptions. Regardless, the results do suggest that perceptions of deterrence could serve as a useful marker of progress within drug court programs.

CONCLUDING COMMENTS

Substance abuse is ubiquitous in criminal justice populations and drug offenders have been largely unresponsive to traditional correctional and treatment-oriented strategies. Dissatisfied with this state of affairs, a group of judges set aside special court dockets to provide closer supervision and greater accountability for these individuals. Wittingly or unwittingly, these judges devised programs highly consonant with established scientific principles of operant conditioning. Specifically, they:

- Introduced greater certainty, celerity, and fairness into the process of imposing criminal justice sanctions.
- Combined various CM techniques to simultaneously squelch undesired conduct and increase desired conduct.
- Crafted a range of intermediate-magnitude sanctions and rewards that could be ratcheted upward or downward in response to offender conduct.
- Developed a phased-in structure to shape offender behavior and reduce learned helplessness and ratio burden.
- Introduced more positive reinforcement and therapeutic goals into the business of the courts.

Drug courts are far from perfect and may be assumed to be ineffective or contraindicated for some segments of the offender population under certain circumstances. More work is needed to pinpoint the appropriate target populations for drug courts and to fine-tune the behavioral components of these programs. This will necessitate the development of collaborative partnerships between drug court practitioners and behavioral scientists, and the forging of a planned research agenda that not only permits rigorous scientific hypothesis testing but also has meaningful relevance for criminal justice practice and drug policy.

ACKNOWLEDGMENTS

This chapter was supported by Grant Nos. R01-DA-14566, R01-DA-13096, and R21-DA-17885 from the National Institute on Drug Abuse (NIDA). The views expressed are those of the authors and do not reflect the views of NIDA. The Philadelphia Treatment Court is gratefully acknowledged for hosting experimental studies of rewards and sanctions in its felony drug court program.

REFERENCES

Akers, R. (1990). Rational choice, deterrence, and social learning theory in criminology: The path not taken. *Journal of Criminal Law and Criminology, 81*, 653–676.

Andrews, D. A., & Bonta, J. (1998). *The psychology of criminal conduct* (2nd ed.). Cincinnati: Anderson.

Azrin, N. H., & Holz, W. C. (1966). Punishment. In W. K. Honig (Ed.), *Operant behavior: Areas of research and application* (pp. 380–447). New York: Appleton-Century-Crofts.

Belenko, S. (1998). Research on drug courts: A critical review. *National Drug Court Institute Review, 1*, 1–42.

Belenko, S. (1999). Research on drug courts: A critical review: 1999 update. *National Drug Court Institute Review, 2*(2), 1–58.

Belenko, S. (2001). *Research on drug courts: A critical review: 2001 update.* New York: National Center on Addiction and Substance Abuse at Columbia University.

Belenko, S., & Peugh, J. (1998). *Behind bars: Substance abuse and America's prison population.* New York: National Center on Addiction & Substance Abuse at Columbia University.

Brooner, R., Kidorf, M., King, V., & Stoller, K. (1998). Preliminary evidence of good treatment response in antisocial drug abusers. *Drug and Alcohol Dependence, 49*, 249–260.

Burdon, W. M., Roll, J. M., Prendergast, M. L., & Rawson, R. A. (2001). Drug courts and contingency management. *Journal of Drug Issues, 31*, 73–90.

Bureau of Justice Statistics. (1998). *Substance abuse and treatment of adults on probation, 1995.* Washington, DC: U.S. Department of Justice.

Bureau of Justice Statistics. (2001). *Trends in state parole, 1990–2000.* Washington, DC: U.S. Department of Justice.

Cooper, C. S. (1997). *1997 Drug Court Survey Report: Executive summary.* Drug Court Clearinghouse and Technical Assistance Project, Office of Justice Programs, U.S. Department of Justice. Available at *www.gurukul.ucc.american.edu/justice/exec1.htm.*

Craddock, S. G., Rounds-Bryant, J. L., Flynn, P. M., & Hubbard, R. L. (1993). Characteristics and pretreatment behaviors of clients entering drug abuse treatment: 1969 to 1993. *American Journal of Drug and Alcohol Abuse, 23,* 43–59.

DeMatteo, D. S., Marlowe, D. B., & Festinger, D. S. (2006). Secondary prevention services for clients who are low risk in drug court: A conceptual model. *Crime and Delinquency, 52,* 114–134.

Fishbein, D. (2000). Neuropsychological function, drug abuse, and violence: A conceptual framework. *Criminal Justice and Behavior, 27,* 139–159.

Gendreau, P., Cullen, F. T., & Bonta, J. (1994). Intensive rehabilitation supervision: The next generation in community corrections? *Federal Probation, 58,* 72–78.

Gendreau, P., Goggins, C., Cullen, F. T., & Andrews, D. A. (2000). The effects of community sanctions and incarceration on recidivism. *Forum on Corrections Research, 12,* 10–13.

Gibbs, J. (1975). *Crime, punishment and deterrence.* New York: Elsevier.

Goldkamp, J. S. (2000). The drug court response: Issues and implications for justice change. *Albany Law Review, 63,* 923–961.

Goldkamp, J. S., White, M. D., & Robinson, J. B. (2002). An honest chance: Perspectives on drug courts. *Federal Sentencing Reporter, 6,* 369–372.

Hanlon, T. E., Nurco, D. N., Bateman, R. W., & O'Grady, K. E. (1998). The response of drug abuser parolees to a combination of treatment and intensive supervision. *Prison Journal, 78,* 31–44.

Harrell, A., Cavanagh, S., & Roman, J. (1999). *Final report: Findings from the evaluation of the District of Columbia Superior Court Drug Intervention Program.* Washington, DC: Urban Institute.

Harrell, A., & Roman, J. (2001). Reducing drug use and crime among offenders: The impact of graduated sanctions. *Journal of Drug Issues, 31,* 207–232.

Harrell, A., & Smith, B. (1997). *Evaluation of the District of Columbia Superior Court Drug Intervention Program: Focus group interviews.* Washington, DC: Urban Institute.

Higgins, S. T. (1996). Some potential contributions of reinforcement and consumer-demand theory to reducing cocaine use. *Addictive Behaviors, 21,* 803–816.

Higgins, S. T., Budney, A. J., Bickel, W. K., Foerg, F. E., Donham, R., & Badger, G. (1994). Incentives improve outcome in outpatient behavioral treatment of cocaine dependence. *Archives of General Psychiatry, 51,* 568–576.

Hineline, P. N. (1976). Negative reinforcement and avoidance. In W. K. Honig & J. E. R. Straddon (Eds.), *Handbook of operant behavior* (pp. 364–414). Englewood Cliffs, NJ: Prentice-Hall.

Hoffman, M. B. (2002). The rehabilitative ideal and the drug court reality. *Federal Sentencing Reporter, 14,* 172–178.

Hora, P. F., Schma, W. G., & Rosenthal, J. T. A. (1999). Therapeutic jurisprudence and the drug treatment court movement: Revolutionizing the criminal justice system's response to drug abuse and crime in America. *Notre Dame Law Review, 74,* 439–538.

Huddleston, C. W., Meyer, W., & Marlowe, D. B. (2006, January). *Rethinking court responses to client behavior: Incentives and sanctions—New tools to build a better drug court.* Alexandria, VA: National Drug Court Institute and Bureau of Justice Assistance.

Langan, P., & Cunniff, M. A. (1992). *Recidivism of felons on probation, 1986–1989.* Washington, DC: Bureau of Justice Statistics.

Langan, P. A., & Levin, D. J. (2002). *Recidivism of prisoners released in 1994.* Washington, DC: Bureau of Justice Statistics, U.S. Department of Justice.

Marlowe, D. B. (2002). Effective strategies for intervening with drug abusing offenders. *Villanova Law Review, 47,* 989–1025.

Marlowe, D. B., DeMatteo, D. S., & Festinger, D. S. (2003). A sober assessment of drug courts. *Federal Sentencing Reporter, 16,* 153–157.

Marlowe, D. B., Elwork, A., Festinger, D. S., & McLellan, A. T. (2003). Drug policy by popular referendum: This, too, shall pass. *Journal of Substance Abuse Treatment, 25,* 213–221.

Marlowe, D. B., Festinger, D. S., Foltz, C., Lee, P. A., & Patapis, N. S. (2005). Perceived deterrence and outcomes in drug court. *Behavioral Sciences and the Law, 23,* 183–198.

Marlowe, D. B., Festinger, D. S., Lee, P. A., Fox, G., Alexander, R., Mastro, N. K., et al. (2005, June). *Contingency management in drug court.* Paper presented at the 67th annual scientific meeting of the College on Problems of Drug Dependence, Orlando, FL.

Marlowe, D. B., & Kirby, K. C. (1999). Effective use of sanctions in drug courts: Lessons from behavioral research. *National Drug Court Institute Review, 2,* 1–31.

Marlowe, D. B., Patapis, N. S., & DeMatteo, D. S. (2003). Amenability to treatment of drug offenders. *Federal Probation, 67,* 40–46.

Martin, G., & Pear, J. (1999). *Behavior modification: What it is and how to do it* (6th ed.). Upper Saddle River, NJ: Prentice-Hall.

Martin, S. S., Butzin, C. A., Saum, S. A., & Inciardi, J. A. (1999). Three-year outcomes of therapeutic community treatment for drug-involved offenders in Delaware. *Prison Journal, 79,* 294–320.

McLellan, A. T., Lewis, D. C., O'Brien, C. P., & Kleber, H. D. (2000). Drug dependence, a chronic medical illness: Implications for treatment, insurance, and outcomes evaluation. *Journal of the American Medical Association, 284,* 1689–1695.

Messina, N., Farabee, D., & Rawson, R. (2003). Treatment responsivity of cocaine-dependent patients with antisocial personality disorder to cognitive-behavioral and contingency management interventions. *Journal of Consulting and Clinical Psychology, 71,* 320–329.

Messina, N., Wish, E. D., Hoffman, J. A., & Nemes, S. (2002). Antisocial personality disorder and TC treatment outcomes. *American Journal of Drug and Alcohol Abuse, 28,* 197–212.

Meyer, W. G. (2002). *Developing consensus on sanction and incentive guidelines in the drug court.* Alexandria, VA: National Drug Court Institute.

National Association of Drug Court Professionals. (1997). *Defining drug courts: The key components.* Washington, DC: Office of Justice Programs, U.S. Department of Justice.

Newsom, C., Favell, J. E., & Rincover, A. (1983). The side effects of punishment. In S. Axelrod & J. Apsche (Eds.), *The effects of punishment on human behavior* (pp. 285–316). New York: Academic Press.

Nurco, D. N., Hanlon, T. E., & Kinlock, T. W. (1991). Recent research on the relationship between illicit drug use and crime. *Behavioral Sciences and the Law, 9,* 221–249.

Patterson, C. M., & Newman, J. P. (1993). Reflectivity and learning from aversive events: Toward a psychological mechanism for the syndromes of disinhibition. *Psychological Review, 100,* 716–736.

Peters, R. H., Greenbaum, P. E., Edens, J. F., Carter, C. R., & Ortiz, M. M. (1998). Prevalence of DSM-IV substance abuse and dependence disorders among prison inmates. *American Journal of Drug and Alcohol Abuse, 24,* 573–587.

Peters, R. H., Haas, A. L., & Murrin, M. R. (1999). Predictors of retention and arrest in drug court. *National Drug Court Institute Review, 2,* 33–60.

Petersilia, J., & Turner, S. (1993). Intensive probation and parole. In M. Tonry (Ed.), *Crime and justice: An annual review of research* (Vol. 17, pp. 281–335). Chicago: University of Chicago Press.

Petry, N. M. (2002). Discounting of delayed rewards in substance abusers: Relationship to antisocial personality disorder. *Psychopharmacology, 162,* 425–432.

Prendergast, M. L., Hall, E. A., & Roll, J. M. (2005, June). *Judicial supervision and contingency management in treating drug-abusing offenders: Preliminary outcomes.* Poster presentation at the 67th annual scientific meeting of the College on Problems of Drug Dependence, Orlando, FL.

Satel, S. L. (1998). Observational study of courtroom dynamics in selected drug courts. *National Drug Court Institute Review, 1,* 43–72.

Satel, S. L. (1999). *Drug treatment: The case for coercion.* Washington, DC: American Enterprise Institute.

Seligman, M. E. P. (1975). *Helplessness.* San Francisco: Freeman.

Sherman, L. W. (1993). Defiance, deterrence, and irrelevance: A theory of the criminal justice sanction. *Journal of Research in Crime and Delinquency, 30,* 445–473.

Sidman, M. (1966). Avoidance behavior. In W. K. Honig (Ed.), *Operant behavior: Areas of research and application* (pp. 448–497). New York: Appleton-Century-Crofts.

Sidman, M. (1988). *Coercion and its fallout.* Boston: Authors Cooperative.

Silverman, K., Wong, C., Umbricht-Schneiter, A., Montoya, I., Schuster, C., & Preston, K. (1998). Broad beneficial effects of cocaine abstinence reinforcement among methadone patients. *Journal of Consulting and Clinical Psychology, 66,* 811–824.

Simpson, D. D., Joe, G. W., & Brown, B. S. (1997). Treatment retention and follow-up outcomes in the Drug Abuse Treatment Outcome Study (DATOS). *Psychology of Addictive Behaviors, 11,* 294–307.

Sisson, R. W., & Azrin, N. H. (1989). The community reinforcement approach. In R. K. Hester, & W. R. Miller (Eds.), *Handbook of alcoholism treatment approaches: Effective alternatives* (pp. 242–258). Elmsford, NY: Pergamon Press.

Stitzer, M. L., & McCaul, M. E. (1987). Criminal justice interventions with drug and alcohol abusers: The role of compulsory treatment. In E. K. Edwards & C. J. Braukmann (Eds.), *Behavioral approaches to crime and delinquency* (pp. 331–361). New York: Plenum Press.

Taxman, F. S. (1999). Graduated sanctions: Stepping into accountable systems and offenders. *The Prison Journal, 79,* 182–204.

Taxman, F. S., & Marlowe, D. B. (Eds.). (2006). Risk, needs, responsivity: In action or inaction? [introduction to Special Issue]. *Crime and Delinquency, 52,* 3–6.

Teplin, L. A. (1994). Psychiatric and substance abuse disorders among male urban jail detainees. *American Journal of Public Health, 84,* 290–293.

Teplin, L. A., Abram, K. M., & McClelland, G. M. (1996). Prevalence of psychiatric disorders among incarcerated women. *Archives of General Psychiatry, 53,* 505–512.

Thibaut, J. W., & Walker, L. (1975). *Procedural justice: A psychological analysis.* Hillsdale, NJ: Erlbaum.

Tyler, T. R. (1994). Psychological models of the justice motive: Antecedents of distributive and procedural justice. *Journal of Personality and Social Psychology, 67,* 850–863.

U.S. Government Accountability Office. (2005). *Adult drug courts: Evidence indicates re-cidivism reductions and mixed results for other outcomes* (No. GAO-05-219). Washington, DC: Author.

Van Houten, R. (1983). Punishment: From the animal laboratory to the applied setting. In S. Axelrod & J. Apsche (Eds.), *The effects of punishment on human behavior* (pp. 13–44). New York: Academic Press.

Young, D., Usdane, M., & Torres, L. (1991). *Alcohol, drugs and crime: Vera's final report on New York State's interagency initiative.* New York: Vera Institute of Justice.

Zimring, F., & Hawkins, G. (1973). *Deterrence: The legal threat in crime control.* Chicago: University of Chicago Press.

AUTHOR INDEX

355

SUBJECT INDEX